Congenital Cataract

Ian Christopher Lloyd • Scott R. Lambert
Editors

Congenital Cataract

A Concise Guide to Diagnosis and Management

Springer

Editors
Ian Christopher Lloyd
Department of Clinical and Academic Ophthalmology
Great Ormond Street Hospital for Children
London
UK

Scott R. Lambert
Opthalmology
Stanford University School of Medicine
Stanford, CA
USA

ISBN 978-3-319-27846-9 ISBN 978-3-319-27848-3 (eBook)
DOI 10.1007/978-3-319-27848-3

Library of Congress Control Number: 2016954327

Printed on acid-free paper

This Springer imprint is published by Springer Nature
The registered company is Springer International Publishing AG Switzerland

Foreword

Management of the young child with cataracts, as opposed to the adult with acquired cataracts, involves its own unique set of challenges. This often requires a team approach, with ophthalmologists working closely with pediatricians, geneticists, anesthesiologists, contact lens fitters, and, most importantly, the parents. The benefits, and risks, of early surgery for congenital cataracts are well established, but early surgery requires early identification, usually by a pediatrician. Surgical techniques for removal of a cataract in a young child address several uniquely different problems than those utilized in adult cataract surgery. Postoperative contact lens fitting may be necessary in some cases, a distinctly time-consuming and costly endeavor. Whether and how to implant an intraocular lens is a critical decision in most of these cases. The importance of appropriate amblyopia therapy that addresses the need to improve vision, with as little disruptive effect on binocular function as possible, is a keystone of successful treatment. Regrettably, the high incidence of postoperative complications, especially glaucoma, adds an additional burden to an already highly demanding process.

Christopher Lloyd and Scott Lambert now have edited this comprehensive and detailed text to address all these issues. It does not sacrifice clarity for comprehensiveness. It will serve as the definitive reference text for all who provide care for children with cataracts for years to come. All of the contributing authors are world-famous experts in dealing with the problems associated with cataracts in young children. They bring years of experience from five continents. As a result, the discussion of each topic is not based solely on review of the scientific literature, but also on the extensive clinical experience of the authors. Where controversies or vagaries about certain aspects of care exist, the authors have clearly and fairly documented the reasons for these uncertainties. This book is well referenced and illustrated.

Christopher Lloyd and Scott Lambert bring unique qualities to the task of editing this book. Both have dedicated a significant portion of their time to improving the outcomes in children with cataracts. Their research has been fundamental for many of the critical advances in managing the myriad of problems associated with cataracts in children. They are leaders in the field and this book testifies to their commitment to leading the way forward to provide better care for children with visually disabling cataracts. All of us who read this book and return to it, again and again, will remain indebted to them.

San Francisco, CA, USA — Creig Hoyt

Preface

Congenital cataract remains a major worldwide cause of both childhood and lifelong visual impairment. The physical, social and socio-economic impact of this condition upon affected children and their families is profound. Prompt and effective management of such children has the potential to substantially improve their vision and, in so doing, transform their lives.

There has been much exciting work in this area, and in putting together this book we have attempted to provide a comprehensive yet relatively concise update of current knowledge. We have been very fortunate in being able to draw upon excellent contributions from clinicians and scientists who are real leaders in the field. Chapters addressing historical perspective, epidemiology, genetics, pre-operative assessment, surgical techniques, complications, refractive management and outcomes are included, while two chapters provide insight and perspective on the factors unique to paediatric cataract management in the developing world. The ground-breaking IATS study is discussed together with an overview of the early results from the large British cohort study IOLu2.

We hope that paediatric ophthalmologists and all clinicians and scientists involved in the often challenging care of children with cataracts find this book readable and useful.

We are very grateful to Sowmya Ramalingam, Liz Pope and everyone in the team at Springer who have assisted us along the way. Thanks also to Dr. Caroline Kilduff who provided fantastic graphic artwork – unfortunately, we could not use all of it!

Lastly we send our love and thanks to our wives Fiona and Elizabeth for their unwavering support and in particular their tolerance of our use of family time spent glued to laptop keyboards. We could not have managed this without them!

London, UK — Ian Christopher Lloyd
Stanford, CA, USA — Scott R. Lambert

Contents

Contributors

Jane L. Ashworth, PhD, FRCOphth Department of Paediatric Ophthalmology, Manchester Royal Eye Hospital, University of Manchester, Manchester, UK

Eileen E. Birch, PhD Crystal Charity Ball Pediatric Vision Laboratory, Retina Foundation of the Southwest, Dallas, TX, USA

Department of Ophthalmology, University of Texas Southwestern Medical Center, Dallas, TX, USA

Susmito Biswas, FRCOphth Department of Paediatric Ophthalmology, Manchester Royal Eye Hospital, University of Manchester, Manchester, UK

Graeme C.M. Black, DPhil, FRCOphth Manchester Centre for Genomic Medicine, Genomic Medicine, The University of Manchester, Manchester, UK

Erick D. Bothun, MD Department of Ophthalmology, Mayo Clinic, Rochester, MN, USA

Richard Bowman, MA, MD, FRCOphth Department of Clinical and Academic Ophthalmology, Great Ormond Street Hospital for Children, London, UK

Jan Tjeerd de Faber, MD The Rotterdam Eye Hospital, Rotterdam, The Netherlands

Carolyn Drews-Botsch, PhD, MPH Department of Epidemiology, Rollins School of Public Health, Emory University, Atlanta, GA, USA

Cecilia Fenerty, MD, FRCOphth Manchester Royal Eye Hospital, Manchester, UK

Manchester University, Manchester, UK

Godfrey Furahini, BSc (ed), MD, MMed, FCOphth.ECSA Ophthalmologist, Kilimanjaro Christian Medical Centre, Moshi, Kilimanjaro, Tanzania

Department of Ophthalmology, Kilimanjaro Christian Medical University College, Moshi, Kilimanjaro, Tanzania

Department of Clinical Research, Faculty of Infectious and Tropical Diseases, London School of Hygiene and Tropical Medicine, London, UK

Rachel L. Gillespie, PhD Manchester Centre for Genomic Medicine, Genomic Medicine, The University of Manchester, Manchester, UK

John Grigg, MBBS, MD, FRANZCO, FRACS Ophthalmology Save Sight Institute, Sydney Eye Hospital Campus, Sydney Medical School, The University of Sydney, Sydney, NSW, Australia

Sydney Eye Hospital, The Children's Hospital Westmead, Sydney, NSW, Australia

E. Eugenie Hartmann, PhD Department of Vision Sciences, University of Alabama at Birmingham, Birmingham, AL, USA

Ramesh Kekunnaya, MD, FRCS (Ophthal) Paediatric Ophthalmology and Strabismus Services, Child Sight Institute, Jasti V Ramanamma Children's Eye Care Center, Hyderabad, India

Scott R. Lambert, MD Department of Ophthalmology, Stanford University School of Medicine, Stanford, CA, USA

Ian Christopher Lloyd, MB, FRCS, FRCOphth Department of Clinical and Academic Ophthalmology, Great Ormond Street Hospital for Children, London, UK

Paediatric Ophthalmology, Manchester Royal Eye Hospital, University of Manchester, Manchester, UK

David G. Morrison, MD Department of Ophthalmology and Visual Sciences, Vanderbilt University, Nashville, TN, USA

Ken K. Nischal, MD, FRCOphth Pediatric Ophthalmology and Strabismus, Children's Hospital of Pittsburgh of UPMC, School of Medicine, University of Pittsburgh, Pittsburg, PA, USA

Anna O'Connor, PhD Orthoptics and Vision Science, School of Health Science, University of Liverpool, Liverpool, UK

David A. Plager, MD Eugene and Marilyn Glick Eye Institute, Indiana University Medical Center, Indianapolis, IN, USA

Section of Pediatric Ophthalmology and Adult Strabismus, Riley Hospital for Children, Indianapolis, IN, USA

Jugnoo Sangeeta Rahi, PhD, FRCOphth Lifecourse Epidemiology and Biostatistics Section, Population, Policy and Practice Programme, UCL Institute of Child Health/Great Ormond Street Hospital and Institute of Ophthalmology UCL/Moorfields Eye Hospital, London, UK

Great Ormond Street Hospital Biomedical Research Centre, London, UK

Moorfields Eye Hospital Biomedical Research Centre, London, UK

Ulverscroft Vision Research Group, London, UK

Virender Sachdeva, MS Paediatric Ophthalmology and Strabismus Services, Child Sight Institute, Jasti V Ramanamma Children's Eye Care Center, Hyderabad, India

Jay Self, BM, FRCOphth, PhD University of Southampton, Southampton, UK

Ameenat Lola Solebo, PhD, FRCOphth Lifecourse Epidemiology and Biostatistics Section, Population, Policy and Practice Programme, UCL Institute of Child Health/Great Ormond Street Hospital and Institute of Ophthalmology UCL/Moorfields Eye Hospital, London, UK

Great Ormond Street Hospital Biomedical Research Centre, London, UK

Moorfields Eye Hospital Biomedical Research Centre, London, UK

Ulverscroft Vision Research Group, London, UK

David Taylor, FRCS, FRCP, FRCOphth, DSc(Med) Paediatric Ophthalmology, Institute of Child Health, University College London, London, UK

Rupal H. Trivedi, MD Department of Ophthalmology, Storm Eye Institute, Medical University of South Carolina, Charleston, SC, USA

Cindy Tromans, PhD, BSc(Hons), MCOptom, FEAOO Manchester Royal Eye Hospital, Manchester, UK

Deborah K. VanderVeen, MD Department of Ophthalmology, Boston Children's Hospital, Harvard Medical School, Boston, MA, USA

Helen Wilson, BSc(Hons), MCOptom, Dip Tp(IP) Manchester Royal Eye Hospital, Manchester, UK

M. Edward Wilson, MD Department of Ophthalmology, Storm Eye Institute, Medical University of South Carolina, Charleston, SC, USA

Katherine S. Wood, MS-II Department of Ophthalmology, Storm Eye Institute, Medical University of South Carolina, Charleston, SC, USA

Part I
Overview

The History of the Management of Congenital Cataract

1

David Taylor

1.1 The Pre-anaesthetic and Antisepsis Era

Arguably, the most important advance in the management of congenital cataract was the invention of various forms of anaesthesia. Prior to that era, immobility was achieved by dint of extreme self-control by adults aided by strong assistants or by brutal restraint (Fig. 1.1a, b). Surgery had to be brief with, effectively, only one chance of success. The instruments used, whilst finer, were conceived on the battlefield. Pain relief and some immobility relied on the torpor induced by alcohol, opiates and other drugs, aided by cocaine after the Austrian, Carl Koller [1] performed eye surgery under cocaine in 1884. Even in the mid-twentieth century, delicious sweet Port wine was still used as a sedative for relatively low pain 'minor' procedures and suture removal in children. What were the great advances in surgery based on?

D. Taylor, FRCS, FRCP, FRCOphth, DSc(Med)
Paediatric Ophthalmology, Institute of Child Health, University College London, London, UK
e-mail: dsit@btinternet.com

1.2 The Post-anaesthetic and Antisepsis Era

1.2.1 Anaesthesia

Joseph Priestley and Thomas Beddoes, members of the philosophical-scientific eighteenth century Lunar Society, and Humphrey Davy, discovered the anaesthetic properties of Nitrous Oxide but were not involved in its later use in surgery. Chloroform and Ether were used for years but the former was cardio- and hepato-toxic and the latter a volatile explosive. Modern anaesthetics for children have totally revolutionised the management of surgical ophthalmology in children of all ages.

1.2.2 Anti-sepsis

Alexander Gordon (Scotland), Louis Pasteur (France), Oliver Wendell Holmes (USA), Ignaz Semmelweiss (Hungary) and Charles White (England) all pointed towards the germ theory of infection: Joseph Lister proved it with the effects of Carbolic Acid and layered dressings for surgery, opening the door to a previously unbelievably low infection rate for all surgery.

1.2.3 Antibiotics

The discovery of sulphonamides by Gerhardt Domagk and of Penicillin by Alexander

I.C. Lloyd, S.R. Lambert (eds.), *Congenital Cataract*, DOI 10.1007/978-3-319-27848-3_1

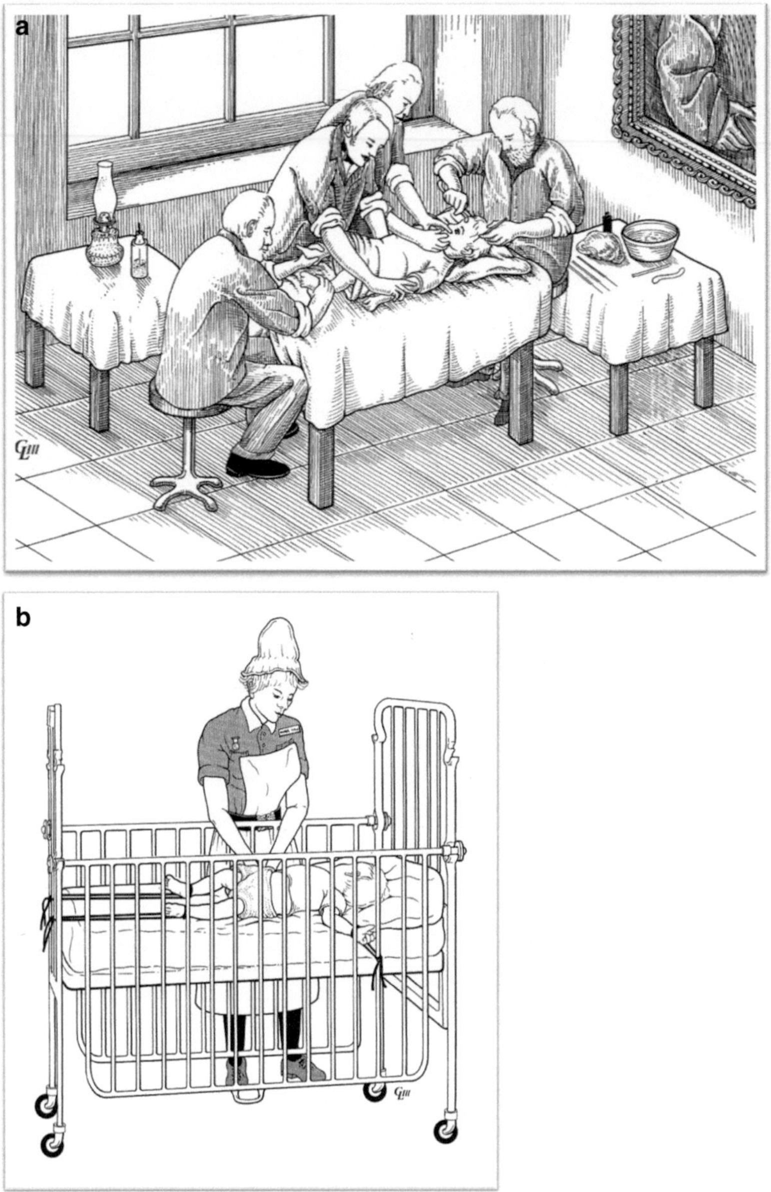

Fig. 1.1 (**a**) John Cunningham Saunders' restraint for surgery [3] in 1811. "The child must now be placed on a table parallel with a window, from which the eye, that is to be submitted to the operation, is farthest. Four assistants and in stouter children five, are required to confine the patient…. The surgeon seated on a high chair behind the patient proceeds in the following manner……" (Figure courtesy of Gillian Lee FMAA). (**b**) Restraint was still practised in the mid-1970s. This figure shows how an infant was restrained after cataract surgery by having each limb tied to the four corners of the cot. Such restraint became less frequent for normal cases once it was realised how well infants responded to comfort, were allowed early breast or bottle feeding, cuddling and being held by their parent (Figure courtesy of Gillian Lee FMAA)

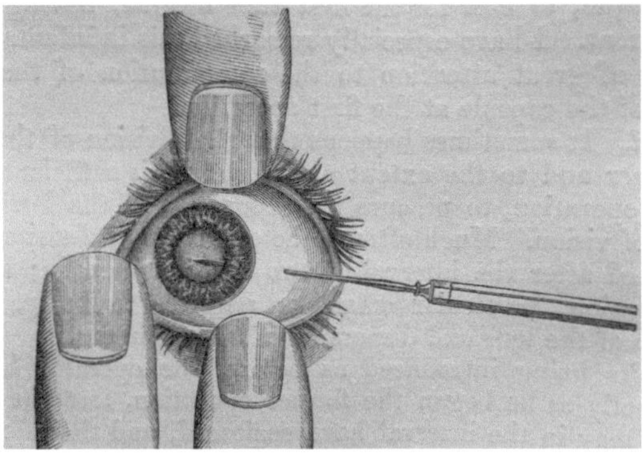

Fig. 1.2 Innumerable fine instruments were made by skilled instrument makers [2]. Instruments such as this needle for "dissolution" of soft cataract was one half the size of a displacement (couching) needle and introduced through the sclera into the anterior chamber, the lens capsule is lacerated, the cortex cut into pieces (discission). Mackenzie practised this on infants

Fleming, Ernst Chain and Howard Florey, revolutionised management of eye diseases in children: care is needed to ensure we do not return to before that era!

1.3 Surgical Techniques

Early couching would likely have been helped by the skills of the Arab metalworkers but the instruments were necessarily simple. In Europe, the nineteenth century saw the manufacture of instruments to previously unreachable fineness and quality (Figs. 1.2, 1.3, 1.4, and 1.5), driven by the industrial skills of the instrument makers, metallurgical advances and the obsessive-compulsive drive of the surgeons.

1.4 Couching

Antyllus, a contemporary of the Greek, Galen, in the Aesculapium in Pergamum removed cataracts by couching [5]. This was attributed to him by Rhazes (854 CE–925 CE), the Persian polymath and physician. Couching probably started long before then in South Asia and, possibly, earlier in Egypt and it was many centuries before Jaques Daviel developed the art of surgical removal of cataracts in the eighteenth century.

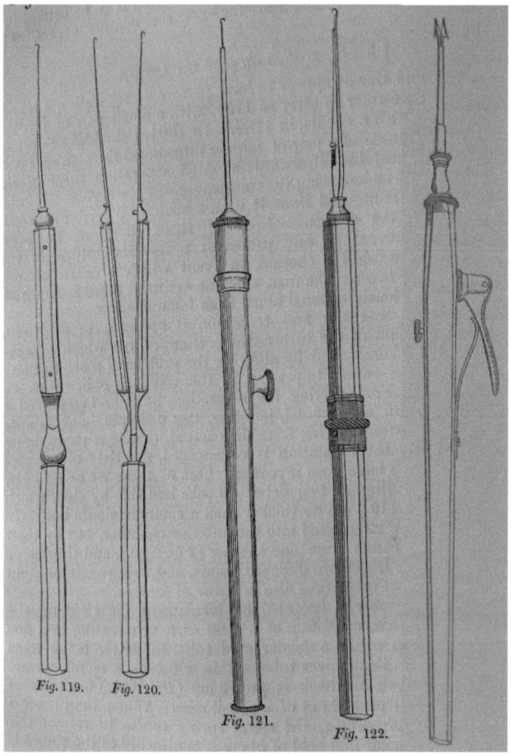

Fig. 1.3 By the mid eighteenth century, under the influence of watch-and clock-makers many of whom were highly skilled Huguenots fleeing France in the late seventeenth century, very fine quality instruments were made. Mackenzie [2] attributed the intra-ocular scissors on the right to Wilde of Dublin: they were interchangeable with a forceps. On the left there are various hooks for forming an artificial pupil by iridectomy

Couching was performed by inserting a sharp and often fairly broad needle through the limbus anterior to the iris or through the sclera posterior to the iris, across the anterior surface of the lens and it is then directed backwards, rupturing the superior zonules and thrusting it down below the inferior pupil margin where, hopefully, it remained. If the lens floated up on partial withdrawal, the procedure was repeated before the needle was withdrawn. Alternatively, later, a knife incision was made and a blunt, flattish needle used to dislocate the lens downward. It is likely that couching was performed on children with cataracts but the likely high complication

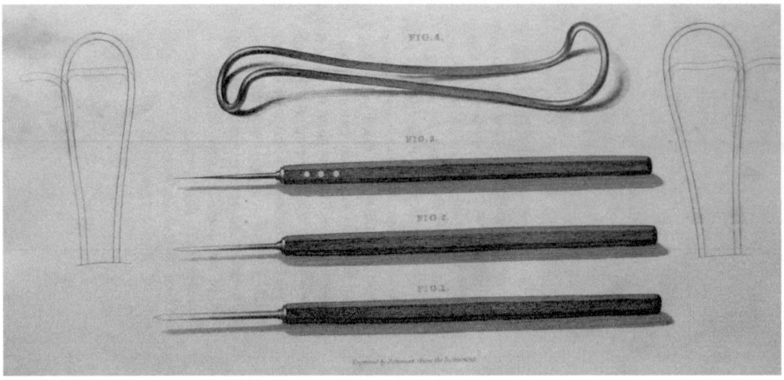

Fig. 1.4 A speculum and needles used for cataract surgery by discission [3], the lower being larger and the upper two being the smaller; The Fig. 1.3 in this illustration shows the lateral view. The needles tapered, the tips sharp on both edges and were used to "cut up the texture of the lens and its capsule"- discission

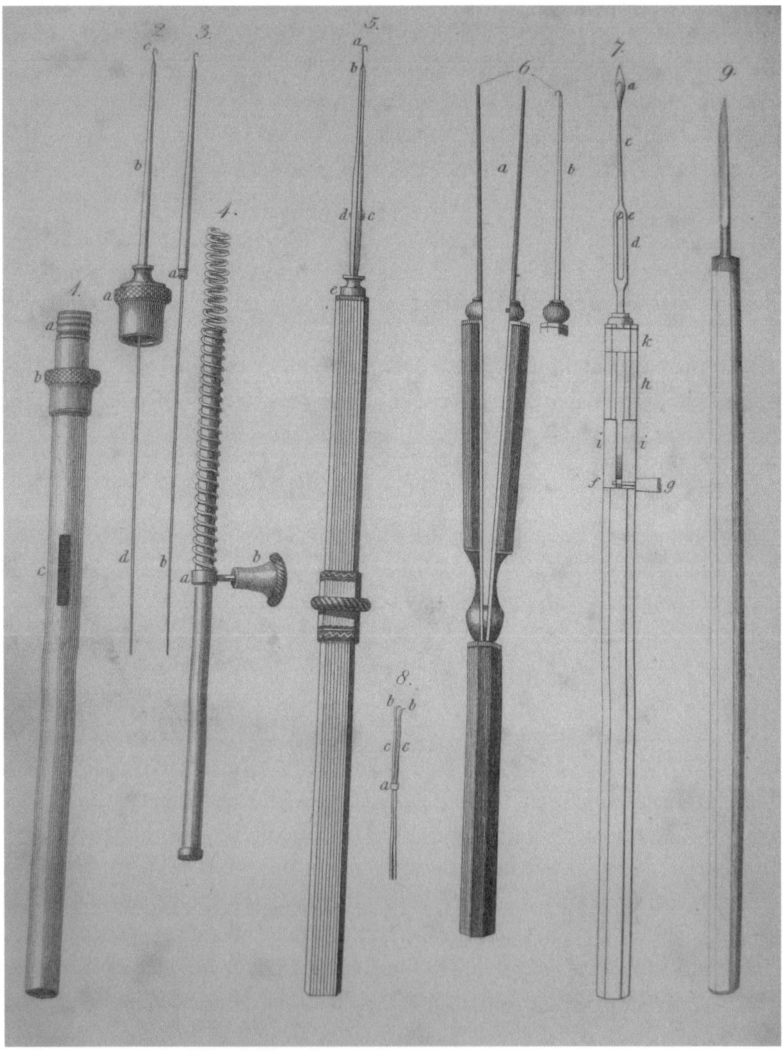

Fig. 1.5 Instruments from Guthrie's 1819 book [4]. *1–4* on the left, Langenbeck's "Coreonceon" in 'exploded' view. *5*. The Iriankistron of Dr Schlagintweit. *6*. Dr Reisinger's double-hooked forceps. *7*. Dr Embden's Raphiankistron. *8*. Gräefe's Coreoncion. *9*. Iris scalpel, sharp on one side only

rate from the strength of the juvenile zonule was not recorded.

Percival Pott [6] (1714–1788) the surgeon to St Bartholomew's hospital in London in 1775 (a year before the United States was founded), however, had strong opinions on couching.

(the practice of the day was to use an f instead of a non-pluralizing s.)

P712: "*The objections, which are made againft the operation of couching, at leaft thofe which have any femblance of truth, or force, are reducible to four:*

The firft is, that if the cataract be perfectly soft, the operation will not be fuccefsful, from the impoffibility of accomplifhing the propofed end of it.

The fecond is, that if it be the mixed kind, partly soft, and partly hard, it will alfo most probably fail of fuccefs, not only from the impossibility of depreffing the fofter parts, but alfo becaufe the more firm ones will either elude the point of the needle, and remaining in the posterior chamber, still form a cataract; or getting through the pupil into the anterior chamber, will there bring on pain and inflammation, and induce a neceffity of dividing the cornea for their difcharge.

The third is, that if the cataract is of the firm, solid kind…….it will remain undiffolved, folid and opake……yet prove fome hindrance to perfect vision.

The fourth objection………the operation will neceffarily occasion fuch violation, and derangement of the internal parts of the eye, as muft cause confiderable mischief".

Benjamin Gibson [7], the Manchester ophthalmologist, attributed Cheselden as, in about 1728, having used a couching needle (sharp on one side only) mostly on cases which were couched and then the pupil had closed. In infants he just used a couching needle, or an instrument resembling it….."*it is more certain to remove the disease in these young subjects.*"

1.5 Discission

Pott [2] invented the operation, discission, which was to remain popular for decades. His description was clear: *P 718*: "……*I have fometimes, when I have found the cataract to be of the mixed kind, not attempted depreffion: but have contented myfelf with a free laceration of the capfula; and having turned the needle round and round between my finger and thumb, within the body of the cryftalline, have left all the parts within their natural fituation: in which cafes I have hardly ever known them fail of diffolving fo entirely, as not to leave the fmalleft veftige of a cataract.*"

Benjamin Travers (1783–1858), the ophthalmologist to St Thomas' Hospital in London, in a hand written book of lectures felt that Pott's invention was poorly recognised: "*Mr Potts' operation of breaking up the substance of the cataract of the cataract by introducing a needle and turning it about in the lens did not excite the attention, which is merited, perhaps it would not have been prosecuted further, had it not been for Mr Saunders who first watched the progress of the operation on a shoemaker who had accidentally wounded his lens by an awl. It was he who first devised and applied this operation to Congenital Cataract as also the flocculent. He performed on infants of all ages with the most complete success, the result was the restoration of very good vision……… I cannot help considering it, as one of the greatest discoveries in modern surgery. Mr Saunders intended to ascertain its result in adults but was prevented by death. I have followed up his intentions but must own it has proved inadequate to my expectations*".

Discission was still practised in the twentieth century. Zeigler [8], an ophthalmologist in Philadelphia, invented a sickle- shaped knife-needle (Fig. 1.6). "*Discission is a cutting through of lens in toto rather than an incision of the anterior capsule or cutting up the lens into fragments.*" "*Boldness in incision is a virtue and conversely, timidity a vice!*" "*Do not stir up the cortex or vitreous but saw in a straight line. Incision of the vitre-*

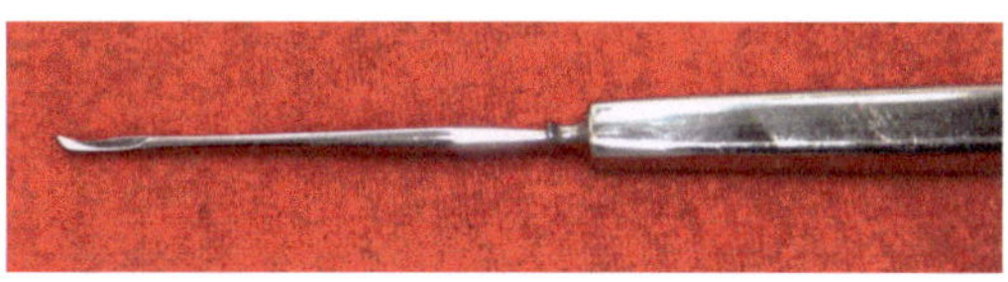

Fig. 1.6 A version of Zeigler's knife-needle [8]

ous is, in itself, not dangerous if you make a clean cut.....". The operation had few other advocates but the knife found many uses elsewhere, particularly in the cutting of fibrous membranes and anomalies in congenital cataracts, PHPV etc.

Nutt, in 1957 [9] was still practising discission. "....first to make an adequate incision in the (*anterior*) lens capsule and second to disintegrate the lens substance as much as possible without damaging the posterior lens capsule or vitreous".

Henry Smith, an Indian Army Medical Service Colonel in the early twentieth century, regarded it safe to operate on infants from 6 months to a year [10]. He practised needling, a form of discission, for infant cataracts except he preferred a fine Graefe's knife, sharp only for 3/16ths of an inch (4.8 mm) at the tip, blunted elsewhere. He found Daviel's procedure [11] the most satisfactory in older children. He performed a capsulectomy with iris forceps at the same sitting. "If a bead of vitreous does escape, it should be snipped off with the scissors- it is of no consequence".

In about 1980, I was one of an international panel of about six ophthalmologists asked to examine a young Royal Prince of a Middle Eastern country who was a combat aircraft pilot. He had been injured in one eye resulting in a cataract and at least 180° angle recession. All except one of the panel agreed that a simple lens aspiration accompanied or followed by an intra-ocular lens was the safest way forward. The panellist from the Soviet Union disagreed: discission and when the lens material had absorbed, an IOL: clearly the young man was going to end up with angle obstruction, glaucoma et sequitur. By chance, I was passing through 6 months later and was asked to see him. He was aphakic, waiting for his IOL, with 6/6 corrected acuity, normal intraocular pressure and a clear, intact, posterior capsule!

1.6 Daviel's Operation

Jaques Daviel (1696–1762) [11], a physician trained in Rouen and Paris, invented an operation in 1747, it is said, after an unsuccessful first couching on a man blind in both eyes from cataract. Before operating the second eye, he developed the technique on human cadaver and animal eyes in which the eye was opened with a broad keratome and enlarged with knife and scissors [3]. The cataract material was removed usually by a spoon-spatula: it was the first extracapsular extraction but it employed a large incision, unsutured and must have had a high complication rate, especially if applied to children.

1.7 Linear Extraction

Gibson [7] couched infant cataracts "......*and I have been in the habit of operating, for ten years, upon subjects of all ages; although I prefer an infant, from half a year, to a year or two old*". But he found that with soft cataract, which was difficult to couch, he would convert to an anterior capsulotomy and discission "*to break down the substance of the cataract by passing the couching needle cautiously through it, in different directions, that the aqueous humour may more readily act upon it, and reduce it to a pulpy state*". Two or three weeks later he went back, opened the eye through a corneal incision using a large cornea knife. Aqueous and some lens material would spontaneously evacuate: that left behind was removed with a curette.

Gibson's instruments (Fig. 1.7) "*were pointed out to me some time ago, by Dr Flajani, physician to his Holiness the Pope, upon shewing him those (in Brambilla's plates of instruments), which had been constructed for me by Mr Savigny*".

By the twentieth century, the operation had reached a degree of sophistication. Alexander [12] described a six stage procedure (1) Dilate the pupil and a full but unenlarged keratome incision. (2) Iridectomy. (3) Forceps capsulectomy-often with Fuch's forceps. (4) Stir up the lens with an iris repositor having a hockey-stick bend. (5) Express the lens. (6) Free irrigation.

"....*I would not hesitate to operate as early as 9 months*". "*It is only since doing the last case that I find I have been unwittingly following the lead given by Colonel H. Smith.......*"

In discussion Colonel Lister said "......*In one case he (Colonel Smith) did it on a girl aged 8, who had been blind from birth, and it was very interesting to watch the girl learning to see, as at first she had to feel an object to identify it, and then she learnt to recognize it by seeing it*".

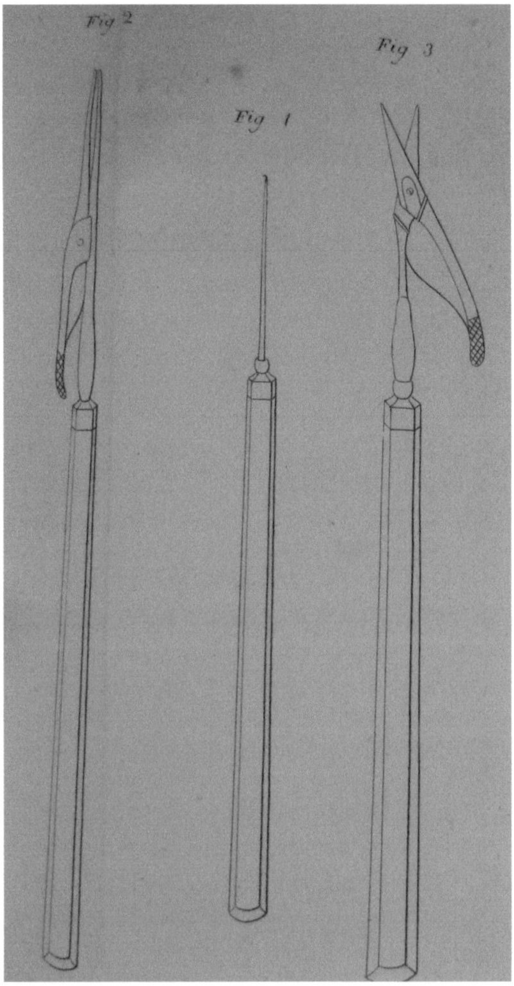

Fig. 1.7 Some of Benjamin Gibson's instruments [7] from 1811

Nutt [9] considered Linear Extraction (which he attributed to Gibson in 1811) was "....*still the most satisfactory, viz. discission followed a few days later by an evacuation of the soft lens matter with a spoon through a 3 mm 'puncture' incision of the cornea*".

1.8 Intracapsular Lens Extraction

Intracapsular extraction started slowly. Daviel converted an extracapsular procedure to an intracapsular one when he found the lens capsule thickened. Georg Joseph Beer (1763–1821), the founder of the Vienna 'School' was an advocate at the end of the eighteenth century but it was rarely used until the twentieth century when Henry Smith wrote a treatise on the treatment of cataract, liberally illustrated by Derrick Vail, from Cincinnati, USA (Fig. 1.8). Smith practised Daviel's method until he had a few occasions when that procedure was complicated by the patient straining and expressing the whole lens with some vitreous with 'good visual results'.

As regards the vitreous loss he wrote "*I then began to doubt the existence of the facts on which was based the holy horror of the escape of vitreous.......was never seriously questioned and carefully examined by the light of facts*". He did, himself then try to avoid vitreous loss. "*For this operation there is nerve required in the operator........extraction of cataract in the capsule is the most highly technical operation in the whole range of surgery*". Smith did not use this operation for childhood cataract, preferring needling or Daviel's method.

In discussing intracapsular extraction, Nutt [9] wrote "*I have no experience of intracapsular extraction for congenital cataract but it does not appeal as a very rational procedure*". He cited Guyton in 1947 who overcame the strength of the young zonule by "*.....grasping the lens at the equator at 6 o'clock and pulling hard enough to stretch the ciliary processes and bring the zonule into view: he then stripped the zonule from the lens with an iris spatula, after which the lens was tumbled. He reported no undue reaction........but one cannot help speculation on the possible influence of this procedure on detachment of the retina in later life*".

1.9 Suction Methods

Teale [14], of Leeds: "*During the autumn of last year I was led to inquire whether the principle of suction might not be made use of in withdrawing from the eye through a small wound all such cataracts...... as have neither a hard nucleus from old age nor have undergone calcareous degeneration*". He dilated the pupil, ruptured anterior capsule with two needles, opened the cornea with a broad needle the size of the suction curette and sucked out the cataract. Teale noted that the

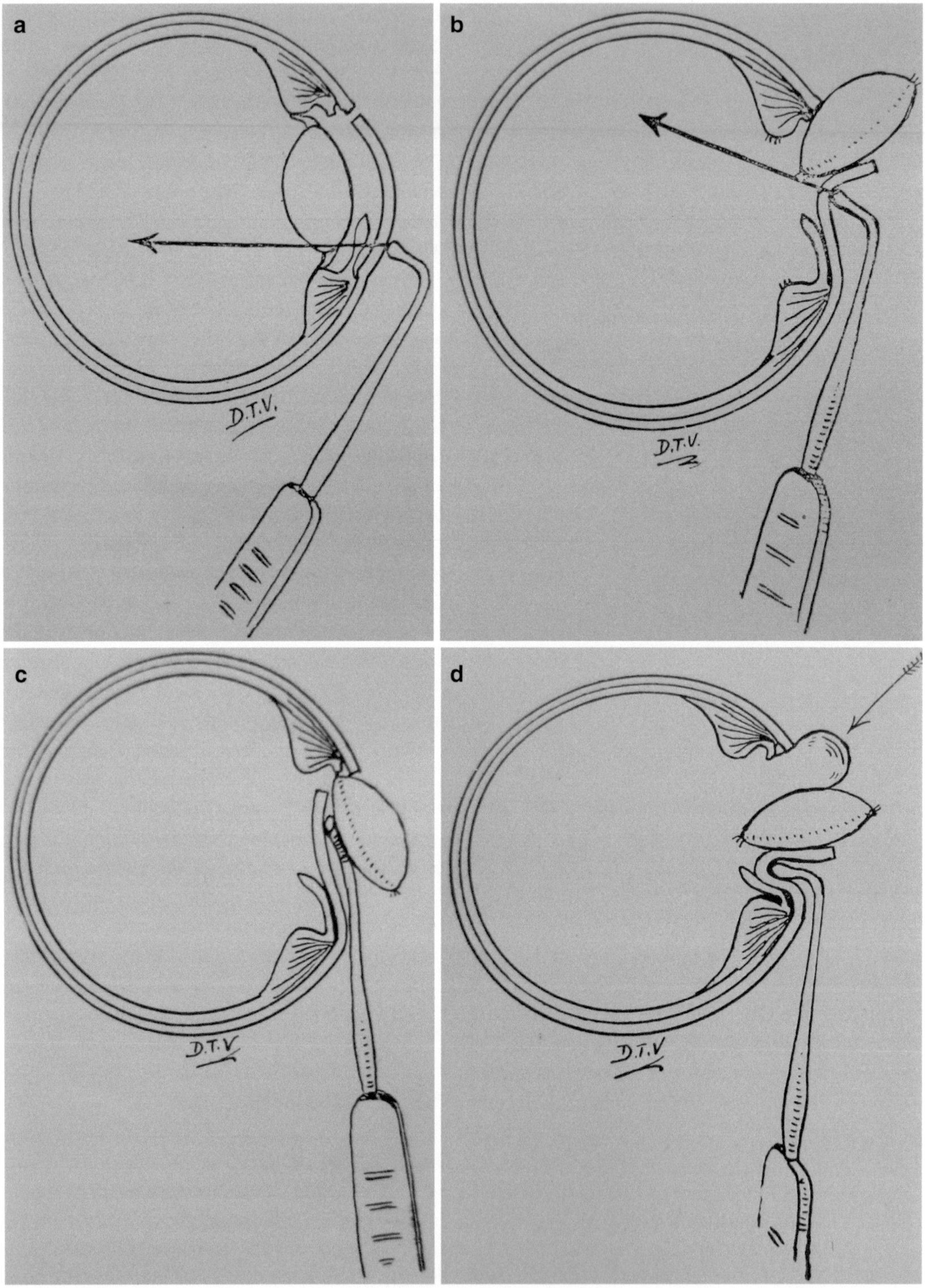

Fig. 1.8 (**a**) Pressure being applied with the lens hook in a direction to tilt the lens so that the upper pole opens the superior wound in the cornea to let it gape (From Smith [13]. Drawing by Derrick Vail). (**b**) The lens is coming out fairly upright with the cornea in near apposition. The direction of the pressure is changed to tuck the cornea in behind the lens (From Smith [13]. Drawing by Derrick Vail). (**c**) The upper edge of the lens is delivered first and flops over and the cornea tucked in behind the lens from where the latter can be easily be removed (From Smith [13]. Drawing by Derrick Vail) (**d**) "Tumbling" the lens inappropriately has resulted in the zonules rupturing above and vitreous has escaped (From Smith [13]. Drawing by Derrick Vail)

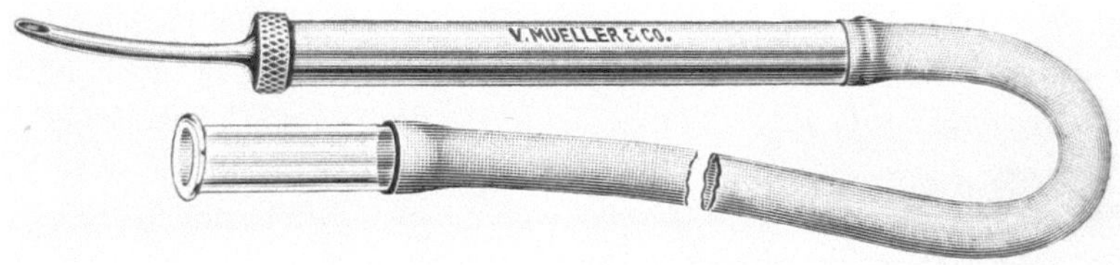

Fig. 1.9 The suction tube used by Teale [14] found by Dean [15] in London in 1893. Mouth suction was applied through the glass tube

Persians were said by Avicenna to have sucked out cataracts.

The American, FW Dean [15] travelled far to improve his technique "*While in London, in 1893, I picked up an instrument brought out in 1863 by RL Teale. This instrument* (Fig. 1.9) *consists of a glass cannula, on one end of which is attached a silver tip……at the other end….is a rubber tube, into which is inserted a mouth piece*". "*The suction method was used by Teale, Bowman, Lawson and others in England*".

The Philadelphia ophthalmologist, Harold Scheie (1909–1990) [16], developed lens aspiration to a fine art, using a 19 gauge thin-walled needle with an oval tip, washing the cataract out by a to-and-fro movement of the syringe handle.

Meanwhile, in Washington DC, Parks and Hiles, using meticulous technique were aspirating through an 18 gauge needle attached to a glass syringe part-filled with saline [17]. Both groups obtained good results despite the prevalence of rubella at that time.

1.10 Further Mechanisation-Microscopes, Vitrectomy Machines Etc

As a trainee ophthalmologist in 1973, I was told not to waste time operating with the surgical microscope because, where I was likely to end up practising, would be unlikely to afford such fads. What started as a fad in the 1970s, often using an angled microscope borrowed from a friendly otolaryngologist, developed soon into mainstream, spawning an industry and vastly improving surgical techniques. Their use is now mandatory all over the world to achieve even routine modern surgery.

The advent of suction-cutting machines designed originally for posterior segment work brought profound changes to the management of congenital cataract and particularly those with substantial membranes and fibrous elements such as Persistent Fetal Vasculature. Together with refined intraocular scissors, forceps and diathermy, the management of many types of congenital cataract widened considerably and became more safe and successful. These machines became smaller-bored, suction methods more refined and controllable and lensectomy became the standard operation in developed countries, despite often precluding the later use of IOLs due to the lack of sufficient support from the posterior capsule.

1.11 Optical Correction of Aphakia

Spectacles have been the mainstay of optical correction of aphakia, where it was applied, for centuries. And a very practical, inexpensive, low risk and adaptable treatment it still is, except for some of the optical or cosmetic effects!

Contact lenses (CLs) were routine in countries with national health systems and for children of wealthy parents in countries without national health systems from the early 1970s. However, a large proportion of children fitted with CLs were unable to wear them well as their parents lacked the skills or time to manage them. The great improvements in IOL design and other technical and surgical techniques, together with critical appraisal of results via national studies, especially in the United Stated and United Kingdom, has led to their widespread use in carefully selected cases, even in infancy.

In 1957, Rosengren observed [18] "….*At the eye clinic in Gothenburg they had treated a little boy of 1½ years….After discission and resorption of the cataract in the left eye a plastic lens was implanted. The original technique according to Ridley could not be used in this case; instead a lens was implanted in the anterior chamber according to Dannheim……. It was supported by two suture loops, which when inserted bent easily and passed into the anterior chamber. There they straightened up, supporting the lens as two arches*".

Early adventures in intraocular Lens (IOL) use in children sought to exploit their use as a neat alternative to contact lenses and spectacles as the primary correction of aphakia. Some of the more discerning ophthalmologists would combine the IOL with spectacles (or, indeed, contact lenses) for more perfect focus. The early operators may have been unaware how difficult it was to insert a standard IOL into an infant's eye. Many of the results were unpublished and alternatives such as epikeratophakia were used for a while. However, with the improvements in IOL materials and design, surgical equipment and techniques, IOLs have become acceptable and safe for most cases at ever younger ages as this book will expound.

1.12 Amblyopia and the Post-amblyopia Era of Management

The understanding of the importance of amblyopia in the management of congenital cataract has been the key to obtaining consistent good results.

Mackenzie (1830) [19] asked "*In cases of congenital cataract, ought the operation to be delayed till the patient has attained an age sufficient to enable him to give his assent or ought it to be practised in infancy*?" He wasted no words in replying to his own question: "*The answer decidedly is to operate in infancy*." Although he felt there were surgical reasons, due to tissue changes that made later surgery more precise but "*If the operation is delayed, the eyes, having no distinct perception of external objects, acquire such an inveterate habit of rolling, that for a long time after the pupil has been cleared by an operation, no voluntary effort can control this irregular motion*". Saunders [20] seemed, in addition, to be aware that it was something related to early vision, not to the eye movements per se. "*The retina too, by a law common to all the structures of the animal body, for want of being exercised, fades in power*". His greatest success came with surgery between 18 months and 4 years.

Gibson [7] wrote "*I have been in the habit of operating, for ten years, upon subjects of all ages; although I prefer an infant, from half a year, to a year or two old*." (his punctuation)

Most surgeons were probably more concerned with the problems in small unanaesthetised babies, than with the optimal time for visual development. Treacher Collins' suggestions [21] in 1908 were more technical: "*.. wait until the child is 10 months before operating. At an earlier age, the cornea is so small and the anterior chamber so shallow that the necessary instrumentation cannot be so satisfactorily carried out as in a more fully developed eye*".

Juler [22], in 1921, published 21 children, 18 with good records, where traumatic unilateral cataract had been treated and followed for (mostly many) years. No eyes that became cataractous after 5 years developed 6/60 vision."… *there is such a disease as amblyopia from disuse, that affects the eyes of children up to the age of six years, that it does not attack eyes after the age of seven, that it is not merely a standing still of the development of the retina or certain cerebral associations, but that it causes a real retrogression of the effective power of the retinal impulse on the consciousness, after the macula has reached an age at which central vision of 6/6 is normally present*".

Broendstrup [23] noted the nineteenth century views, that amblyopia only develops before 6 or 7 years of age although in some views, citing the Viennese, Klein, only developed before 3 years of age. He noted perceptively that not just the cataract but also the aphakia alone may be 'ambliopiogenic'. There were no details of refraction or near correction, nor of any occlusion of the dominant eye.

Nutt [9], in 1957 thought "*Uniocular cataracts are better left untreated, except for cosmetic reasons.........the visual result is always bad... the chances are that the affected eye is abnormal in some other respect.......there is no chance of binocular single vision*". Of his 12 cases of unilateral cataract in which vision was measurable, the best was 2/60. In bilateral cases, excluding lamellar cataracts which mostly did well, the best vision in any eye attained was 6/18.

From 34,600 cases in a practice, Prudhommeaux [24] found 166 cases of congenital cataract of which 65 were operated. 17 were unilaterals: all got good light perception or less. "*Il faut alors poser la question: doit-on pourquoi opérer les cataracts congénitales unilatérales?*" ("*We must then ask the question: why should we operate unilateral congenital cataracts?*")

Deweese [25], in Memphis TN described 133 patients with CCs. "*Also operation for monocular cataracts to obtain good visual acuity does not seem justified even though the vision in the eye with cataract is less than 20/50*". "*The visual results were much poorer if surgery was performed before the age of two and one-half years; therefore operation should be postponed until after this whenever possible*".

In a case report, von Noorden et al. [26] described a case where the first eye was operated at 3/12, the other at 4.5/12. Contact lenses were fitted 2 weeks later. "*There has been a marked decrease in the amplitude and frequency of nystagmus when the contact lenses are worn, nystagmus increases when the contact lenses are removed*". "*We believe that surgery for complete congenital cataracts...... should be performed as early in life as the diagnosis is made. This should be followed by immediate aphakic correction to prevent deprivation amblyopia*". "*It may be well worth while a trial to aspirate a unilateral mature congenital cataract (that is not accompanied by other anomalies) within the first days of life to be followed by immediate contact lens correction*" However in their three children with unilateral congenital cataract, the acuity achieved was no better than 10/200.

Frey et al. [27] in Washington DC, influenced in their management by the then recent amblyopia studies of Hubel and Wiesel, operated on 21 idiopathic unilateral congenital cataracts. The operated eye was fitted with a contact lens which was worn for up to 12 h daily. Occlusion of the phakic eye was attempted. Three of the youngest at surgery, with good contact lens wear but unspecified occlusion achieved 20/40 or better. They wrote: "*...the dictum of extreme conservatism in the management of monocular cataracts in children needs to be re-evaluated*".

A group in London noted [28] "*.....early treatment and optical correction are essential for the management of these patients, since the effects of deprivation start at about 4 months of age....*" They also described 23 cases of unilateral congenital cataract [29], "*....correction before 4 months of age produces less visual loss but we cannot specify the function within this period.*"

Creig Hoyt [30] and his colleagues in San Francisco, described eight neonates with total monocular cataract treated with surgery, occlusion and contact lenses. Five developed VAs of LogMAR 0.18 (6/9, 20/30, 0.67), three with LogMAR 0.6 (6/24, 20/80, 0.25). These were *spectacular* results that confirmed that amblyopia was the most important cause of poor results in the management of congenital cataract.

Initially treated with scepticism, these practice-changing results were confirmed by others, notably by Birch and Stager [31]. Forty-five children diagnosed with unilateral congenital cataract at 1–10 days old and treated with a combination of surgery, contact lens fitting and occlusion. 82 % also had surgery for strabismus. None had congenital malformations or infections. Only patients with 75–95 % of the recommended patching were included. Acuity declined with age and intervention before 6 weeks of age minimised the effects of visual deprivation.

So it became incontrovertible that the management of amblyopia was the major goal of surgery for congenital cataract. Having defined the goal, and proved a successful treatment, much brilliant work around the world has been lavished on this deserving group of children with significant improvement in visual prognosis and reduction in complications that will be outlined in this book.

References

1. Goerig M, Bacon D, van Zundert A. Carl Koller, cocaine, and local anesthesia: some less known and forgotten facts. Reg Anesth Pain Med. 2012;37: 318–24.
2. Mackenzie W. A practical treatise on the diseases of the eye. 4th ed. London: Longman, Brown, Green and Longmans; 1854.
3. Saunders JC. A treatise on some practical points relating to the diseases of the eye. London: Longman, Hurst, Rees, Orme and Brown, Paternoster Row; 1816.
4. Guthrie GJ. A treatise on the operations for the Formation of an Artificial Pupil; in which the morbid states of the eye requiring them, are considered and the mode of performing the operation, adapted to each peculiar case, fully explained. Published London; 1819.
5. Lascaratos J, Marketos S. A historical outline of Greek ophthalmology from the Hellenistic period up to the establishment of the first universities. Doc Ophthalmol. 1988;68:157–69.
6. Pott P. Remarks on the Cataract in: the Chirurgical Works of Percival Pott FRS and surgeon to St Bartholomew's Hospital. London; 1775. p. 705–724.
7. Gibson B. Practical observations on the formation of an artificial pupil in several deranged states of the eye. Cadell & Davies in the Strand; London; 1811. p. 1–153.
8. Zeigler SL. Complete discussion of the lens by the V-shaped method. JAMA. 1921;77:1100–1.
9. Nutt AB. The surgical treatment of congenital cataract. Trans Ophthalmol Soc UK. 1957;77:39–57.
10. Smith H. The treatment of Cataract. Illustrations by Derrick T Vail. Calcutta: Pub Thacker, Spink & Co; 1910. p. 121.
11. Daviel J. Sur une nouvelle méthode de guérir la cataract par l'extraction du cristalin. Memoires de L'Academie Royale de Chirurgie: Sur les Concretions Calculeuses de la Matrice. 337–354. Pub. Theophile Barrois Le Jeune, Paris 1787.
12. Alexander GF. The immediate removal of congenital cataracts. Trans Ophthalmol Soc UK. 1928;48:94–107.
13. Smith H. The treatment of Cataract. Calcutta: Pub Thacker, Spink & Co; 1910. p. 121.
14. Teale TP. On extraction of soft cataract by suction. Lancet. 1864;ii:348–50.
15. Dean FW. Cataracts: operation for congenital and Juvenile. Trans Amer Acad Ophthalmol Otolaryngol. 1926;31:261–70.
16. Scheie HG, Rubinstein RA, Kent RB. Aspiration of congenital or soft cataracts: further experience. Am J Ophthalmol. 1967;63:3–8.
17. Parks MM, Hiles DA. Management of infantile cataracts. Am J Ophthalmol. 1967;63:10–9.
18. Rosengren B in discussion of Nutt AB Trans Ophthalmol Soc UK. 1957;77:54.
19. Mackenzie W. A practical treatise on the diseases of the eye. 1st ed. London: Pub. Longman, Rees, Orme, Brown & Green; 1830. p. 596.
20. Saunders JC. A treatise on some practical aspects relating to diseases of the Eye. 2nd ed. London: Longman, Hurst, Rees, Orme and Browne; 1816. p. 175–94.
21. Collins ET. Developmental deformities of the crystalline lens. Ophthalmoscope. 1908;6:577–583 and 663–676.
22. Juler F. Amblyopia from disuse. Visual acuity after traumatic cataract in children. Trans Ophthalmol Soc UK. 1921;41:129–39.
23. Broendstrup P. Amblyopia ex anopsia in infantile cataract. Acta Ophthalmol. 1944;22:52–71.
24. Prudhommeaux MP. Le résultat obtenu après operation pour cataracte congénitale. Bull Soc Ophtalmol Fr. 1962;62:383–430.
25. Deweese MW. A survey of the surgical treatment of congenital cataracts. Am J Ophthalmol. 1962;53:853–7.
26. Von Noorden GK, Ryan SJ, Maumenee AE. Management of congenital cataracts. Trans Am Acad Ophthalmol Otol. 1969;74:352–9.
27. Frey T, Friendly D, Wyatt D. Re-evaluation of monocular cataracts in children. Am J Ophthalmol. 1973;76:381–8.
28. Taylor D, Vaegan, Morris JA, Rodgers JE, Warland J. Amblyopia in bilateral infantile and juvenile cataract. Trans Ophthal Soc UK. 1979;99:170–5.
29. Vaegan, Taylor D. Critical period for deprivation amblyopia in children. Trans Ophthal Soc UK. 1979;99:432–9.
30. Beller R, Hoyt CS, Marg E, Odom JV. Good visual function after neonatal surgery for congenital monocular cataracts. Am J Ophthalmol. 1981;91:559–65.
31. Birch EE, Stager DR. The critical period for surgical treatment of dense congenital unilateral cataract. Invest Ophthalmol Vis Sci. 1996;37:1532–8.

Epidemiology of Congenital Cataract

2

Ameenat Lola Solebo and Jugnoo Sangeeta Rahi

2.1 Introduction

Epidemiology, the basic science of clinical medicine, is best defined as 'the study of the distribution and determinants of disease frequency in man'. Here the term 'disease' is often limited to 'congenital cataract'. However, it is more correctly translated to congenital cataract **and** blindness or visual impairment due to congenital cataract rather than just to the disorder per se. The different branches of epidemiology guide all aspects of management, from planning prevention strategies at a population level through to helping to involve families of treated children in judging how best to assess a 'good' outcome.

With regards to congenital cataract, the objectives of epidemiology (Fig. 2.1) are to:

- determine the burden of congenital cataract and cataract related blindness/visual impairment
- study the natural history
- identify the underlying causes/aetiological factors, including the causes of associated visual impairment/blindness
- inform the development of, and evaluate, preventive and therapeutic measures from the level of the individual to population based policies

Whilst most clinicians are familiar with classical observational and interventional epidemiology, the field has evolved to include fields such as lifecourse epidemiology, genetic epidemiology and health services research:

- lifecourse epidemiology – the study of physical and social hazards during gestation and childhood (and later life) that affect disease risk and health outcomes in later life. It aims to 'identify the underlying biological, behavioural and psychosocial processes that operate across the life span' [1]
- genetic epidemiology – the study of the interactions between genetic and environmental determinants of disease and health outcomes
- health services research – the study of the accessibility, quality, and cost-effectiveness of health care services, with a focus on patient experiences and reported outcomes

A.L. Solebo, PhD, FRCOphth (✉) • J.S. Rahi, PhD, FRCOphth
Lifecourse Epidemiology and Biostatistics Section, Population, Policy and Practice Programme, UCL Institute of Child Health/Great Ormond Street Hospital and Institute of Ophthalmology UCL/ Moorfields Eye Hospital, London WC1N 1EH, UK

Great Ormond Street Hospital Biomedical Research Centre, London, UK

Moorfields Eye Hospital Biomedical Research Centre, London, UK

Ulverscroft Vision Research Group, London, UK
e-mail: a.solebo@ucl.ac.uk; j.rahi@ucl.ac.uk

I.C. Lloyd, S.R. Lambert (eds.), *Congenital Cataract*, DOI 10.1007/978-3-319-27848-3_2

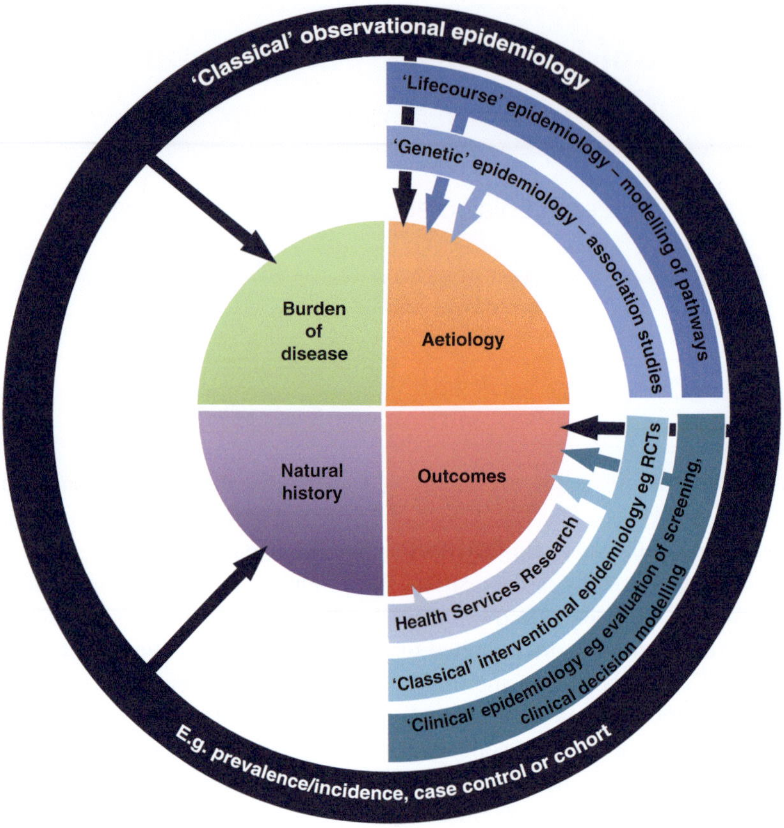

Fig. 2.1 The objectives of epidemiology in understanding and managing disease processes

2.1.1 Methodological Challenges to Epidemiological Research in Congenital Cataract

The challenges include limiting misclassification bias, selection bias and confounding, and lack of statistical power to determine the role of chance. These are of particular importance when undertaking research into a 'rare' disorder (one with a prevalence of less than 5 in 10,000 of the population). The greatest challenge of any study into a rare disease is the creation of a study population which is representative of the total population at risk.

Chance When a disease is uncommon, it can be a challenge to obtain a sufficiently large sample size. Studies with small numbers of children are prone to chance findings (i.e. false positive findings or type I error). Small sample sizes may also result in failure to achieve statistical significance for even potentially large effects (i.e. false negative findings, or type II errors).

Selection Bias: Misclassification and Varying Definitions of Disorders and Outcomes The misclassification of non-diseased/non-affected individuals as diseased/affected (or vice versa) has a profound effect on the subsequent analysis.

The differing definitions of congenital cataract include:

- Any lens opacity present at birth
- Any lens opacity newly diagnosed in the first year of age, particularly if associated with another structural ocular anomaly or congenital systemic disorder (also known as 'congenital/infantile cataract'). This definition is the most robust, on the basis that unless the

examination occurred at birth it is difficult to exclude a congenital onset of lens opacity.

As well as the example of the differing definitions of congenital cataract, associated or secondary conditions such as microphthalmia, or glaucoma following cataract surgery have been defined in numerous ways in the existing literature.

Selection Bias Heterogeneity of Study Populations Children with congenital and infantile cataract form a varied group, and the populations investigated within the literature reflect this heterogeneity and compounds the problems of non-standard case definition. The resultant case mix adversely impacts on attempts to compare the findings of different studies and on the generalisablity of individual study findings. Additionally, risk factor profiles for the development of different outcomes may not be appropriately dealt with at analysis.

Confounding Investigations of potential associations must also consider the issue of confounding. The challenge is to determine the independent effect of one variable on the risk of a particular outcome once other variables have been taken into account, as well as the direction and size of effect one variable has on another variable's association with the risk of the outcome.

The hierarchy of evidence (reflecting the hierarchy of study methodology) can be used to consider the strength of the evidence from epidemiological research into congenital cataract. Methods used in the study types at the "top" of the hierarchy are more likely to minimise bias and confounding (Table 2.1). But, most importantly, methodology needs to be both appropriate to the research question and ethical. For example, to investigate a risk factor for disease, a cohort or case control approach would be adopted rather than an interventional trial exposing individuals to the risk factor.

Thus, the hierarchy is not an inflexible construct, as a 'higher' category of study methodology does not guarantee study quality. For example, a poorly conducted randomised trial will be less robust than a well conducted cohort study with multivariable analysis to account for confounding.

2.2 The Burden of Congenital Cataract

Despite being an uncommon condition, congenital and infantile cataract remains a significant cause of childhood visual impairment worldwide and one of the most common causes of *preventable* childhood severe visual impairment or blindness [17]. Its prominence relative to the many other conditions which impact on children's eyes and vision is explained by a combination of factors. Firstly, limited understanding of aetiology for a significant proportion hampers prevention, and presently there is no effective treatment for cataract due to monogenetic disease other than genetic counselling. Secondly, there are obstacles to prompt and effective management for affected children in resource poor settings. Thirdly, there has been a greater success in reducing the impact of the other causes of childhood blindness, for example corneal opacity disorders caused by measles and or vitamin A deficiency.

Determination of the true global burden of congenital/infantile cataract, particularly in the context of the limited health care infrastructure common to lower and middle income settings, is made difficult by the methodological challenges of population based research on rare conditions. Investigations of the country specific prevalence of paediatric disorders tend to derive estimates using the denominator of school groups or health centres rather than whole populations, as the latter are less easily accessible for research purposes. This leads to under representation of children from groups existing outside formal health care or administrative structures. These are also the children most vulnerable to adverse outcomes from health and developmental disorders, leading to both under representation of blindness/visual

Table 2.1 Levels of evidence [25]

Level of evidence	Outcomes investigated	Study methodology
1 (highest level)	Natural history	Systematic review of inception cohort studies
	Treatment benefits	Systematic review of randomised trials
	Treatment harms	
	Rare treatment harms	Systematic review of case control studies or studies revealing dramatic effects
2	Natural history	Inception cohort study
	Treatment benefits	Randomised trial or observational study with dramatic effect
	Treatment harms	Systematic review of nested case control or dramatic effect
	Rare treatment harms	Randomised trial or observational study with dramatic effect
3	Natural history	Cohort or control arm of randomised trial
	Treatment benefits	Non randomised controlled cohort / follow up study
	Treatment harms	
4	Natural history	Systematic review of case-series
	Treatment benefits	Systematic review of case-control studies, historically controlled studies
	Treatment harms	Case-control studies, historically controlled studies
5 (lowest level)	Natural history	Opinion without explicit critical appraisal, based on limited/undocumented experience, or
	Treatment benefits	
	Treatment harms	based on mechanisms

impairment due to cataract, and selection bias within investigations of outcome.

2.2.1 Prevalence and Incidence

The prevalence of a disorder is the proportion of a defined population affected by the disorder at any time point, whereas the incidence is the number of new cases ('incident cases') added to the existing pool over a defined time period. The cumulative incidence, also described as the cumulative risk, is the incidence rate (or risk of diagnosis for the individual) over a specified period of time, which may be the whole lifetime of the individual. For example the childhood cumulative incidence or risk of cataract would be the rate of diagnosis of new paediatric cases within a defined population, equating to the risk of being diagnosed with cataract by 18 years of age.

Ascertaining Incident Cases Reports from newborn screening programmes or national anomaly registers in industrialised settings can provide some information on the frequency of occurrence of a congenital disorder such as cataract. A North American study, using a national non-statutory birth anomaly reporting system to ascertain cases, estimated the incidence of disease at 2.03 per 10,000 births [3] whilst the discharge diagnoses entered into Denmark's statutory National Register of Patients (NRP) were used to estimate the cumulative incidence amongst Danish children at 5.2 per 10,000 by 16 years old [15]. Another more recent European study involving the non-statutory Swedish National Cataract Register, established in 2006 with an aim to standardize management and improve outcomes, reported an incidence of significant cataract (defined as 'cataract requiring surgery') of 1.9 per 10,000 live births [21]. However non statutory systems are by their nature open to under ascertainment of cases, and even systems which compel reporting have been found to under report the number of children with congenital cataract [36]. A British population based study using active surveillance, an approach which has been shown to have a higher case ascertainment than the formal statutory clinical reporting process [28, 36] estimated the incidence of cataract in the first year of life at 2.5 per 10,000 (95 % confidence interval 2.1–2.9), with a cumulative incidence of congenital and infantile cataract in the first 5 years of life of 4 per 10,000 [27]. Active surveillance is the monitoring of an entire population at risk [18], in which there is not only the identification of cases but also confirmation of the *absence* of cases, thus providing a more precise estimation of frequency.

In 1997 it was estimated that the number of children across the world born each year with congenital cataract was 20–40,000, with a worldwide prevalence of between 1 and 4 affected children per 10,000 [10] The proportion of affected children may be as high as 1.5 per 1000 in low-income countries with high under five mortality rates. In high-income countries with lower under five mortality rates, however, the prevalence is around 0.3 per 1000 children [12]. The estimates of prevalence and incidence of congenital and infantile cataract are sensitive to the overall health and survival of the paediatric population, the socio-economic developmental status of the region as well as the existing organisation in place for the detection of early life vision and eye disorders.

2.2.2 The Burden of Congenital Cataract Blindness

Childhood visual impairment (vision in the better eye worse than 0.48 logMAR or 6/18 Snellen according to World Health Organisation taxonomy), severe visual impairment (vision worse than 1.0 or 6/60) and blindness (worse than 1.3 or 3/60) impact on society as well as the individual through the cost of medical and social support for the child and the adult she becomes, as well as the loss of potential employment related income. It has been estimated that over 21 % of the world's blind children owe their impairment to cataract, with lens related disease coming second to retinal disorders as the most common cause of blindness [17]. The wide range in the proportion of 'blind school' students with cataract (Fig. 2.2) reflects the variation in the frequency and causes of visual impairment across the world. In 1997, the global estimate was 15 % [10], but the relative importance of childhood cataract as a cause of blindness has grown as the pattern of the causes of childhood blindness has changed, with, in particular, successes in the programmes of vitamin A supplementation and measles immunization in reducing the impact of childhood corneal opacity [7, 17, 38]. Whilst we lack the contemporaneous data needed to definitively state the true proportion of childhood cataract related blindness, it is reasonable to assume that congenital and infantile cataract is one of the most common causes of preventable childhood visual impairment in many settings [11].

2.3 Natural History

Congenital and infantile cataract can lead to a lifelong burden of blindness if

- visually significant opacity is untreated
- there is a delay in treatment
- there is failure to institute effective post operative visual rehabilitation to address sensory deprivation amblyopia
- there are co-existent ocular or systemic disorders capable of causing impairment
- iatrogenic conditions such as secondary glaucoma (of which there is a life-long risk) develop following surgery.

In a setting where population based neonatal and or infant eye screening programmes and health service infrastructure allow early diagnosis and prompt treatment, surgery can prevent visual impairment in approximately a third of children with bilateral cataract. However, in the long term a third of these children may nevertheless be severely visual impaired or blind despite, or because of surgery [5].

Compared with those with bilateral cataract, children with unilateral disease generally experience worse visual outcomes in the operated eye. Post operatively, between a third and a half

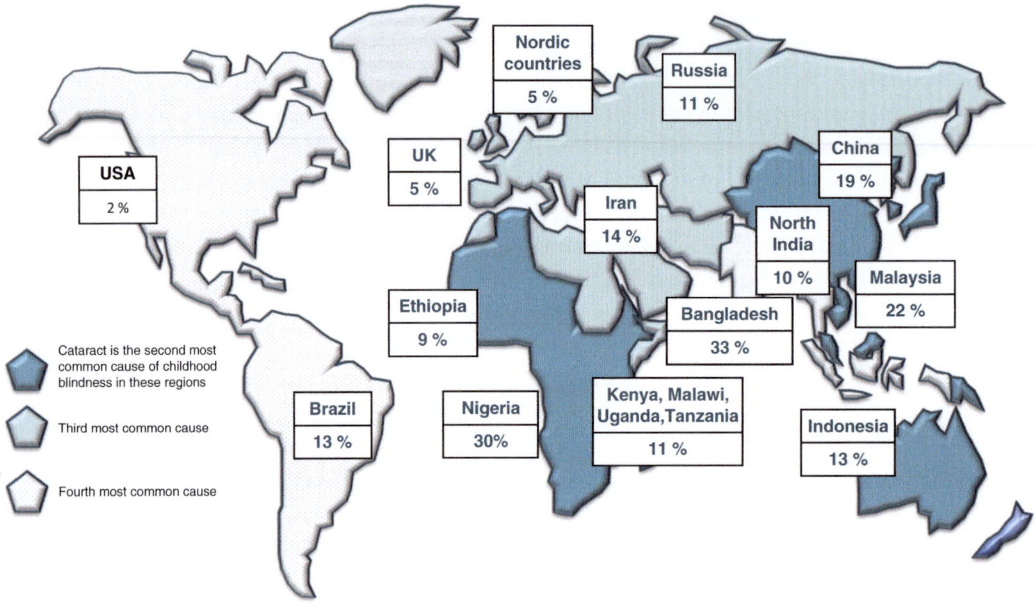

Fig. 2.2 Congenital cataract as a proportion of childhood blindness – regional estimates [2, 9, 14, 16, 22, 30, 31, 33, 37]

of children will have severely impaired vision or worse, and moderate to severe visual impairment in the operated eye is the usual outcome [5].

2.4 Aetiology of Congenital Cataract

The epidemiological approach can help to disentangle the multiple causal mechanisms behind congenital cataract. A cause, or 'an event, condition or characteristic which precedes a disease and without which the disease would not have occurred' can be inferred, with caution, from associations discovered through epidemiological observation studies. These studies can examine the difference between those with and without congenital cataract (case–control approach), working retrospectively in order to discover how the prenatal environment differed for those with and without congenital cataract, or they can instead observe a population prior to the occurrence of cataract, watching prospectively to understand the difference between 'cases' and the general population. The latter approach (a cohort study) is often impractical in the study of a rare disorder. Critically, the difference lies at the 'point of sampling', rather than in any inherent difference in terms of quality of methodology.

2.4.1 Causes in Higher Income Countries

The underlying aetiologies differ for bilateral and unilateral cataract. Hereditary disease accounts for half of bilateral cataract but less than a tenth of unilateral disease in industrialised countries [29], although with increased access to complex genetic testing approaches, the contribution of monogenic disease is increasingly recognised [13]. Bilateral cataract is also a feature of non-inherited genetic disorders, the most common being trisomy 21 or Down's syndrome [15, 29], although the relative proportion of this may change if improvements in prenatal testing continue to reduce the incidence of affected live births of children with trisomy 21 [6]. Aetiology is not known (idiopathic disease) in the great majority of unilateral cataract cases (90 %), and a third of bilateral cataract (Table 2.2) [20, 29].

Environmental, infectious and genetic causes have been proposed, and whilst it is likely that more than one factor is at play, to date the only independent associated factor consistently identified is low birth weight: the odds of being diagnosed with bilateral cataract may be as much as 13 times higher for babies born weighing less than 1500 g (OR 6, 95 % CI 2.2–16.3) [26]. The association is also seen for unilateral cataract and for those weighing under 2500 g at birth. Low birth weight is itself a reliable indicator of the general health of the child and the gestational environment, and is influenced by pre and post conceptual genetic and environmental factors. The association between congenital and infantile cataract and low birth weight within a population is therefore broadly in harmony with the association of the disease with under five mortality rates.

The co-existence of persistent fetal vasculature, or PFV, with unilateral cataract is increasingly recognised to be more common than previously thought. PFV is a spectrum of clinical features caused by failure of the normal regression or apoptosis of the intraocular fetal vasculature. As some features of PFV may only be visible during removal of the cataractous lens, and studies which recruit children undergoing surgery report higher rates of occurrence. A prospective Austrian study of 31 children aged 0–15 years old undergoing surgery for unilateral cataract reported that all were affected by some degree of persistent vasculature [23], whilst PFV was found in over half of all cases of operated unilateral cataract (n = 91) in a recent national epidemiological study [35]. An improved understanding of the mechanisms at play in this developmental disorder may in the future provide clues as to the aetiology of idiopathic unilateral congenital and infantile cataract.

Table 2.2 Causes of congenital/infantile cataract in order of decreasing incidence in higher income settings

I. Idiopathic cataract with or without associated ocular disorder
II. Hereditary cataract without associated systemic disorder
Autosomal dominant, autosomal recessive, or X-linked
III. Hereditary or sporadic genetic cataract with associated systemic disorder (including chromosomal disease)
E.g.: Trisomy 21, oculo-renal disorder of Lowe
IV. Prenatal biological or environmental exposure
E.g.: prenatal rubella

Adapted from Rahi and Dezateux [29]

2.4.2 The Global Pattern

Clinical services such as serology and genetic testing in many countries are under developed, making it impossible to determine with any certainty the causes of congenital and infantile cataract in these settings. It is possible, however, to describe the likely drivers of disease. Whilst intrauterine insult to ocular development through infectious agents is now an uncommon cause of congenital cataract in industrialised countries due to the success of childhood immunisation programmes [7, 19] these agents remain an important preventable cause of childhood cataract globally. Congenital rubella syndrome is responsible for a fifth of childhood cataract in Southern India, although, as seen in industrialised nations, for the majority of children with cataract in this region the cause is unknown [8]. Genetic disease is also a common cause of early life cataract globally, with consanguineous marriage, relatively common in several states across the globe, contributing to the incidence of congenital anomalies such as cataract [19].

2.5 Outcomes: Preventing Cataract, Preventing Blindness

Reducing the global burden of childhood cataract blindness has been the aim of several international programmes. The largest of these, Vision 2020, an international multi-agency initiative, is led by the WHO and aims to reduce ‘avoidable’ visual impairment through improved prevention, treatment and rehabilitation. There is some evidence of a reduction in childhood blindness due to the gains made in the prevention of corneal disease [38].

As with any prevention programme, the prevention of blindness due to congenital or infantile cataract has three aims: preventing incident cases from occurring (primary prevention), preventing incident cases from resulting in blindness for the child (secondary prevention), and preventing cataract related blindness from adversely impacting on the life of the child (tertiary prevention).

2.5.1 Preventing Cataract: Primary Prevention

Primary prevention of cataract blindness involves genetic counselling of families affected by monogenic disease, counselling of mothers of children with Trisomy 21, and immunisation programmes to prevent the occurrence of maternal gestational rubella infection. Improvements in next-generation DNA sequencing technologies may identify a genetic basis for many of the currently 'undetermined' cases [13], providing a possible focus for future research into targeted genetic therapies. Currently, however, as the majority of congenital and infantile cataract is of unknown aetiology, and as the majority of cases occur in countries unable to provide genetic testing on a wide basis, the scope for primary prevention is limited and secondary and tertiary strategies play the main role.

2.5.2 Preventing Cataract Blindness: Secondary Prevention

As irreversible dense sensory deprivation amblyopia can be established within weeks, early detection and early treatment is key in the prevention of blindness due congenital and infantile cataract.

Detection and Diagnosis Although prenatal and ultrasound and MRI diagnosis of cataract is possible [4], there is no evidence on the sensitivity or specificity of the prenatal radiological diagnosis of cataract. Thus, the earliest time that visually significant cataract can be excluded reliably is postnatally. The detection of cataract is the main driver behind the baby and infant (ages 0–4 months) vision screening programmes which currently exist in all but three of the European Union member states [34]. The importance of early (first weeks of life) detection is reflected by the UK Department of Health's formal inclusion of the red reflex test within the neonatal and 6 week postpartum infant health checks [24]. Children with a positive family history or with a systemic diagnosis known to be associated with congenital/infantile cataract may also benefit from ophthalmic review to ensure the absence of cataract. In nations which do not have infant vision or ocular anomaly screening programmes, diagnosis of cataract tends to occur later, by which time visual impairment is often already established [38]. This is a particular issue for populations with limited parental awareness of the milestones of childhood visual development, or limited access to health care services (Table 2.3).

Table 2.3 Barriers to the prompt diagnosis and effective management of congenital and infantile cataract

Lack of a population based screening programme
Lack of awareness among families, community, or primary care practitioners of the necessity of urgent intervention
Lack of training for health practitioners in red reflex detection
Geographical and financial barriers to accessing care provision
Competing demand for resources within a family unit (e.g. the prioritisation of the health of male children)
Shortage of suitably trained paediatric ophthalmologists, orthoptics, optometrists, anaesthetists and nurses
Shortage of appropriate tertiary health centres or other centres capable of providing integrated care
Lack of awareness among families, community, or care practitioners of the necessity of post operative refractive correction or amblyopia therapy, or of the necessity of lifelong surveillance for post operative complications

Adapted from World Health Organization 2007 [38]

Treatment Appropriate and effective surgical intervention and post-operative visual rehabilitation (refractive correction and penalisation therapies for amblyopia) are essential. The WHO has recommended that surgical intervention occurs within tertiary eye care centres with dedicated children's services and post operative follow up in these centres or provided by secondary care services (Courtright et al. 2015). In many developed nations, adult cataract surgical outcomes are maintained through standardisation of practice, ongoing audit processes, and targeted surgical training. These processes are much more difficult to achieve for paediatric cataract services. The heterogeneity of congenital and infantile cataract phenotype and the wide range of associated systemic disorders are barriers to standardisation of practice. Another barrier is the absence of consensus about best practice e.g. the role of artificial intraocular lenses, where the balance lies between decreasing post-operative glaucoma risk and increasing risk of dense amblyopia with regards to the timing of surgical intervention in the first weeks of life, and whether surgery should be limited to higher volume tertiary teams. This fragmentation of care is seen despite the existence of strong infrastructures, such as the UK's National Health Service, which are capable of maintaining multi-centre clinical networks. There are also insufficient numbers of trained paediatric ophthalmologists in many industrialized countries [19, 38], although these nations are well served when contrasted with the startling shortage of paediatric eye professionals in most low-income countries [19, 38], where almost a third of doctors in training plan on working abroad [32].

2.5.3 Tertiary Prevention

Once a child has developed visual impairment or blindness due to cataract, management will involve minimising the limitations imposed on the child and their family. A multidisciplinary approach is necessary to support the child's personal development, with continued specialist ophthalmic input, provision of low vision care, special and specific educational support, and habitation and mobility training to assist activities of daily living. Similar obstacles to those which prevent prompt diagnosis and treatment are at play in the failure to ensure a good quality of life for the individual blind secondary to congenital or infantile cataract, or at least a quality of life compared to others within that community. These obstacles are compounded by the paucity of appropriately trained ancillary support specialists and the scarcity of resources.

2.6 Summary

Congenital and infantile cataract is responsible for a fifth of the world's blind children despite its treatable nature. It is thus an important cause of avoidable childhood visual disability. Despite differing methodologies, the data from the few whole population studies in higher income countries show some agreement, with an annual incidence of 2–3 cases per 10,000 live births and a cumulative annual incidence of 2–6 newly diagnosed cases per 10,000 in the first 18 years of life. Frequency can generally be anticipated to be higher in middle and low income countries. International variance in the frequency of the disorder reflect the global patterns of the overall health and survival of children as well as the socio-economic developmental status of and health infrastructure within the regions in question.

Epidemiological research underpins the management of congenital cataract, informing practice at both population level e.g. screening and service planning, and child level e.g. prognostication and clinical decision making. As the majority of cases are due to as yet undetermined causes, secondary prevention approaches (surgical and optical rehabilitation), and epidemiological investigation and assessment of these approaches, are key to reducing the burden of childhood cataract blindness.

References

1. Ben-Shlomo Y, Kuh D. A life course approach to chronic disease epidemiology: conceptual models, empirical challenges and interdisciplinary perspectives. Int J Epidemiol. 2002;31(2):285–93.
2. Bhattacharjee H, Das K, Borah RR, Guha K, Gogate P, Purukayastha S, Gilbert C. Causes of childhood blindness in the northeastern states of India. Indian J Ophthalmol. 2008;56(6):495–9.
3. Bhatti TR, Dott M, Yoon PW, Moore CA, Gambrell D, Rasmussen SA. Descriptive epidemiology of infantile cataracts in metropolitan Atlanta, GA, 1968–1998. Arch Pediatr Adolesc Med. 2003;157(4):341–7.
4. Brohnstein M, Zimmer E, Gershoni-Baruch R. First- and second-trimester diagnosis of fetal ocular defects and associated anomalies: report of eight cases. Obstet Gynecol. 1991;77(3):443.
5. Chak M, Wade A, Rahi JS. Long-term visual acuity and its predictors after surgery for congenital cataract: findings of the British congenital cataract study. Invest Ophthalmol Vis Sci. 2006;47(10):4262–9.
6. Cocchi G, Gualdi S, Bower C, Halliday J, Jonsson B, Myrelid A, Mastroiacovo P, Amar E, Bakker MK, Correa A, Doray B, Melve KK, Koshnood B, Landau D, Mutchinick OM, Pierini A, Ritvanen A, Ruddock V, Scarano G, Sibbald B, Sipek A, Tenconi R, Tucker D, Anneren G. International trends of Down syndrome 1993–2004: births in relation to maternal age and terminations of pregnancies. Birth Defects Res A Clin Mol Teratol. 2010;88(6):474–9.
7. Courtright P, Hutchinson AK, Lewallen S. Visual impairment in children in middle- and lower-income countries. Arch Dis Child. 2011;96(12):1129–34.
8. Eckstein MB, Foster A, Gilbert CE. Causes of childhood blindness in Sri Lanka: results from children attending six schools for the blind. Br J Ophthalmol. 1995;79(7):633–6.
9. Ezegwui IR, Umeh RE, Ezepue UF. Causes of childhood blindness: results from schools for the blind in south eastern Nigeria. Br J Ophthalmol. 2003;87(1):20–3.
10. Foster A, Gilbert C, Rahi J. Epidemiology of cataract in childhood: a global perspective. J Cataract Refract Surg. 1997;23 Suppl 1:601–4.
11. Gilbert C, Foster A. Childhood blindness in the context of VISION 2020: the right to sight. Bull World Health Organ. 2001;79:227–32.
12. Gilbert CE, Anderton L, Dandona L, Foster A. Prevalence of visual impairment in children: a review of available data. Ophthalmic Epidemiol. 1999;6(1):73–82.
13. Gillespie RL, O'Sullivan J, Ashworth J, Bhaskar S, Williams S, Biswas S, Kehdi E, Ramsden SC, Clayton-Smith J, Black GC, Lloyd IC. Personalized diagnosis and management of congenital cataract by next-generation sequencing. Ophthalmology. 2014;121(11):2124–37.
14. Gogate P, Deshpande M, Sudrik S, Taras S, Kishore H, Gilbert C. Changing pattern of childhood blindness in Maharashtra, India. Br J Ophthalmol. 2007;91(1):8–12.
15. Haargaard B, Wohlfahrt J, Fledelius HC, Rosenberg T, Melbye M. A nationwide Danish study of 1027 cases of congenital/infantile cataracts: etiological and clinical classifications. Ophthalmology. 2004;111(12):2292–8.
16. Kello AB, Gilbert C. Causes of severe visual impairment and blindness in children in schools for the blind in Ethiopia. Br J Ophthalmol. 2003;87(5):526–30.
17. Kong L, Fry M, Al-Samarraie M, Gilbert C, Steinkuller PG. An update on progress and the changing epidemiology of causes of childhood blindness worldwide. JAAPOS. 2012;16(6):501–7.
18. Langmuir AD. The surveillance of communicable diseases of national importance. New Engl J Med. 1963;268:182–92.
19. Lenhart PD, Courtright P, Wilson ME, Lewallen S, Taylor DS, Ventura MC, Bowman R, Woodward L, Ditta LC, Kruger S, Haddad D, El SN, Rai SK, Bailey T, Lambert SR. Global challenges in the management of congenital cataract: proceedings of the 4th International Congenital Cataract Symposium held on March 7, 2014, New York, New York. JAAPOS. 2015;19(2):e1–8.
20. Lim Z, Rubab S, Chan YH, Levin AV. Pediatric cataract: the toronto experience -etiology. Am J Ophthalmol. 2010;149(6):887–92.
21. Magnusson G, Bizjajeva S, Haargaard B, Lundstrom M, Nystrom A, Tornqvist K. Congenital cataract screening in maternity wards is effective: evaluation of the Paediatric Cataract Register of Sweden. Acta Paediatr. 2013;102(3):263–7.
22. Muhit MA, Shah SP, Gilbert CE, Foster A. Causes of severe visual impairment and blindness in Bangladesh: a study of 1935 children. Br J Ophthalmol. 2007;91(8):1000–4.
23. Mullner-Eidenbock A, Amon M, Moser E, Klebermass N. Persistent fetal vasculature and minimal fetal vascular remnants. A frequent cause of unilateral congenital cataracts. Ophthalmology. 2004;111(5):906–13.
24. NHS UK National Screening Committee. Newborn and infant physical examination. 2008.
25. OCEBM Levels of Evidence Working Group. The Oxford 2011 levels of evidence. Oxford: Centre for Evidence-Based Medicine; 2011.
26. Prakalapakorn SG, Rasmussen SA, Lambert SR, Honein MA. Assessment of risk factors for infantile cataracts using a case–control study: National Birth Defects Prevention Study, 2000–2004. Ophthalmology. 2010;117(8):1500–5.
27. Rahi JS, Botting B. Ascertainment of children with congenital cataract through the National Congenital Anomaly System in England and Wales. Br J Ophthalmol. 2001;85(9):1049–51.
28. Rahi JS, Dezateux C. Capture-recapture analysis of ascertainment by active surveillance in the British Congenital Cataract Study. Invest Ophthalmol Vis Sci. 1999;40(1):236–9.
29. Rahi JS, Dezateux C. Congenital and infantile cataract in the United Kingdom: underlying or associated factors. British Congenital Cataract Interest Group. Invest Ophthalmol Vis Sci. 2000;41(8):2108–14.

30. Reddy SC, Tan BC. Causes of childhood blindness in Malaysia: results from a national study of blind school students. Int Ophthalmol. 2001;24(1):53–9.
31. Rosenberg T, Flage T, Hansen E, Riise R, Rudanko SL, Viggosson G, Tornqvist K. Incidence of registered visual impairment in the Nordic child population. Br J Ophthalmol. 1996;80(1):49–53.
32. Silvestri DM, Blevins M, Afzal AR, Andrews B, Derbew M, Kaur S, Mipando M, Mkony CA, Mwachaka PM, Ranjit N, Vermund S. Medical and nursing students' intentions to work abroad or in rural areas: a cross-sectional survey in Asia and Africa. Bull World Health Organ. 2014;92(10):750–9.
33. Sitorus RS, Abidin MS, Prihartono J. Causes and temporal trends of childhood blindness in Indonesia: study at schools for the blind in Java. Br J Ophthalmol. 2007;91(9):1109–13.
34. Sloot F, Hoeve HL, de Kroon ML, Goedegebure A, Carlton J, Griffiths HJ, Simonsz HJ. Inventory of current EU paediatric vision and hearing screening programmes. J Med Screen. 2015;22(2):55–64.
35. Solebo AL, Russell-Eggitt I, Cumberland PM, Rahi JS. Risks and outcomes associated with primary intraocular lens implantation in children under 2 years of age: the IoLunder2 cohort study. Br J Ophthalmol. 2015;99(11):1471–6. doi:10.1136/bjophthalmol-2014-306394.
36. Solebo AL, Russell-Eggitt I, Rahi JS. Accuracy of routine data on paediatric cataract in the UK compared to active surveillance: lessons from the IOLu2 study. Br J Ophthalmol. 2013;97(6):757–9.
37. Titiyal JS, Pal N, Murthy GV, Gupta SK, Tandon R, Vajpayee RB, Gilbert CE. Causes and temporal trends of blindness and severe visual impairment in children in schools for the blind in North India. Br J Ophthalmol. 2003;87(8):941–5.
38. World Health Organization 2007, Global initiative for the elimination of avoidable blindness: action plan 2006–2011. ISBN 978 92 4 159588 9. URL: http://www.who.int/blindness/Vision2020_report.pdf. Accessed Aug 2011.

Part II

Preoperative Assessment

3 The Role of Molecular Genetics in the Assessment of Children with Congenital Cataract

Rachel L. Gillespie and Graeme C.M. Black

3.1 What Are the Macrostructure and Microanatomy of the Lens?

The vertebrate lens has three main anatomical structures: nuclear and cortical lens fibres, a subcapsular lens epithelium, and the lens capsule. Lens fibre cells account for over 95 % of the total lens volume [1]. Lens fibres form a highly organized, radially layered and tightly packaged arrangement that is critical for transparency and light transmission. Further, the hexagonal shape of individual lens fibres, with two broad faces on the apical and basal surfaces and four short faces laterally, is important for tissue integrity, physiological stress resistance and lens metabolism [2]. Similarly, fibre membrane protrusions known as microplicae, are integral for securing immediately adjacent cells together so as to prevent tissue damage, lens deformation, and fibre disorganization during accommodation and biological stress conditions [3]. An epithelial cell layer surrounds the lens fibres on the anterior surface and the entire structure is enclosed the lens capsule; a multifunctional basement membrane serving mechanical, physical, protective, nutritional and inductive roles that are integral to the survival of lens cells and their protein contents (reviewed in [4]). The aqueous and vitreous humors bathe the anterior and posterior surfaces, respectively, supplying nutrients, ions and water by diffusion across the semi-permeable membrane of the lens capsule [5].

Primary lens fibres, formed early in development, are concentrated at the centre of the structure, within the 'foetal nucleus'. Secondary lens fibres extend antero-posteriorly from a mitotic niche just below the lens equator, encircling the primary fibres until the cell tips meet and interlock at the lens sutures [6]. Secondary fibres are continually added throughout life, although at a reducing rate with increasing age, and are constantly migrating from the germinative zone within the lens epithelium towards the centre of the lens. In this way, the age of a fibre cell can be determined from its position within the structure; older cells are concentrated more centrally and closer to the nucleus of the sphere. Intracellular organelles such as mitochondria and nuclei have a higher refractive index (RI) than cell cytoplasm and if present would cause light scattering. During lens formation, primary fibre cells rapidly degrade their entire organelle contents and this process continues in secondary fibre cells; during migration from the outer cortex in to the lens core, concurrent organelle elimination follows terminal differentiation [7, 8]. This process is synchronized such that an

R.L. Gillespie, PhD • G.C.M. Black, DPhil, FRCOphth (✉)
Manchester Centre for Genomic Medicine, Genomic Medicine, The University of Manchester, St Mary's Hospital, Oxford Road, Manchester M13 9WL, UK
e-mail: rachel.gillespie@manchester.ac.uk; graeme.black@manchester.ac.uk

I.C. Lloyd, S.R. Lambert (eds.), *Congenital Cataract*, DOI 10.1007/978-3-319-27848-3_3

'organelle free zone' is created in the centre of the lens, within what is the pupillary space. Accordingly, in the absence of cellular turnover, each fibre cell and its protein contents has a lifelong role within the lenticular mass.

Disruption of any of the embryonic processes responsible for the development of the lens may result in a range of congenital lenticular abnormalities (Table 3.1). Rare, developmental defects include those affecting shape (lenticonus, lentiglobus, coloboma), position (ectopia lentis) and size (microspherophakia, congenital aphakia). However, cataract is the most common pathology of the lens. Further, as correct development of the lens is an important prerequisite for the successful development of the anterior segment of the eye, a degenerate lens may be unable to provide the molecular signals [9, 10] or structural support for the development of the components of the anterior chamber [11]. In this way, a primary defect of the lens may give rise to secondary developmental abnormalities such as microcornea, and anterior segment mesenchymal dysgenesis (ASMD).

3.2 How Is Lens Transparency Established and Maintained?

The lens has the highest protein concentration of any tissue within the human body, accounting for 38 % of its total wet weight [14]. Protein concentration is not uniform; higher concentrations exist in the lens nucleus creating a high refractive index (RI). A gradient of protein concentration, and corresponding RI, corrects for the ellipsoid shape of the lens and allows accurate light focussing across the entire structure. The cytoplasm of lens cells contains high concentrations (~0.2–0.4 g ml^{-1}) of crystallin proteins. Lens crystallins are polydisperse and exist in a dense, short-range spatial order that does not alter with the increasing protein concentration range seen from the lens cortex, to the nucleus [14]. It is this specialized arrangement that allows crystallins to exist at high concentration whilst establishing a high level of transparency and protein stability, and to ensure the longevity of these proteins in the absence of cell turn-over, a vascular supply or innervation. There are two main families of crystallin proteins that exist in the human lens; the βγ-crystallin superfamily that function as structural proteins and the α-crystallins, which function both as structural proteins and as molecular chaperones. As chaperones, α-crystallins recognize and bind non-native and unfolded proteins to prevent accumulation as insoluble light scattering aggregates [15]. The beaded filament of the vertebrate lens is important for establishing the precise cellular architecture that is also critical for transparency. It has been suggested that the beaded filament may facilitate lens protein stability by providing a scaffold for, and thereby optimizing, protein chaperone function [16]. As a form of intermediate filament, the beaded filament may also support tissue integrity during the mechanical stresses of accommodation [17]. Within the human lens, the beaded filament assembles by the binding of BFSP1 (filensin) with BFSP2 (phakinin) [18].

The lens is a non-passive tissue. Since organelle degradation alters the physiology of lens fibre cells – to leave them incapable of generating energy and replacing damaged proteins – lens homeostasis is critical. Within the lens, a specialized internal microcirculatory system exists that delivers essential nutrients throughout the lens mass, whilst maintaining constant cellular volume and preserving tissue architecture. The vertebrate lens relies on the surrounding eye components to provide the nutrients it requires-the aqueous humor is fundamental in this, supplying the lens with metabolites such as glucose and amino acids at the anterior surface. It is also thought that the anterior lens epithelium is proactive in the take up of these molecules and ions for their subsequent diffusion in to the peripheral fibre cells [19]. The microcirculatory current travels through the lens via gap junctions comprised of connexin proteins that are present in the cell membranes of lens fibres. Gap junctions create an intracellular pathway, connecting cells at the surface of the lens mass with central cells. They are responsible for electrically coupling the anterior epithelial cells [20] and for the circulation of nutrients and ions throughout fibres

Table 3.1 Lens abnormalities and developmental defects of the eye resulting from abnormal lens development

	Abnormality	Description	Structures involved	Pathogenesis	Associated gene
Transparency	Cataract	Opacity of the lens	Lens only	Protein misfolding, denaturation and/or loss of solubility	Numerous – see [12]
	Peter's Anomaly	Incomplete separation of the cornea and the lens	Lens and cornea	Failed separation of the LV from the SE	PAX6, FOXC1, PITX2, CYP1B1, FOXE3, PAX6, MAF
Shape	Lenticonus	Conical projection of either the anterior or posterior lens surface and may cause localised cataract	Lens only	Possibly a secondary defect to a thin lens capsule. Often associated with PHPV	COL4A3, COL4A5, COL4A5, TDRD7
	Lentiglobus	Anterior or posterior bulging of the lens that is more spherical in shape than lenticonus			
	Coloboma	Scalloped edge or indentation of the lens. Lens opacities can frequently be found in the same region		Failure in zonular development	Numerous – see [13]
Position	*Ectopia lentis*	Dislocation of the lens	Lens and zonular fibres	Due to defects in the microfibrils of the ciliary zonule- usually asymmetrical excess of laxity or breakage of zonular fibres	ADAMTSL4, ADAMTS10, FBN1, LTBP2
	Subluxation	Partial dislocation			
	Phacodonesis	Vibration of the lens upon eye/head movement			ADAMTS17, LTBP2
Size	Microphakia	Small lens	Lens only	Abnormal degree of contact between OV and SE during lens development	HMX1, LMXB1, RAB3GAP1
	Microspherophakia	Small, spherical lens		As above and impeded/arrested secondary fibre development	LTBP2, ADAMTS17
	Congenital aphakia	Absence of lens		Unsuccessful induction of the embryonic surface ectoderm in forming the lens placode and vesicle	FOXE3
Development	ASD	Developmental abnormality of anterior structures	Structures within the anterior segment	ASD due to defective lens development usually occurs as a result of failed molecular signalling and/or structural support from the lens for development of other components of the anterior segment. Frequently results in cataract plus microphakia, microcornea, and/or microphthalmia	FOXE3, PXDN, HMX1, PITX3, PAX6, OTX2, SIX6, VSX2, LTBP2, miR184, MAF, GJA8, CRYGD, CRYGC, CRYAA, CRYBB3, CRYBB2, CRYBB1, CRYBA4 (See also [13])

LV lens vesicle, *SE* surface ectoderm, *PHPV* persistent hypoplastic primary vitreous, *OV* optic vesicle, *ASD* anterior segment dysgenesis

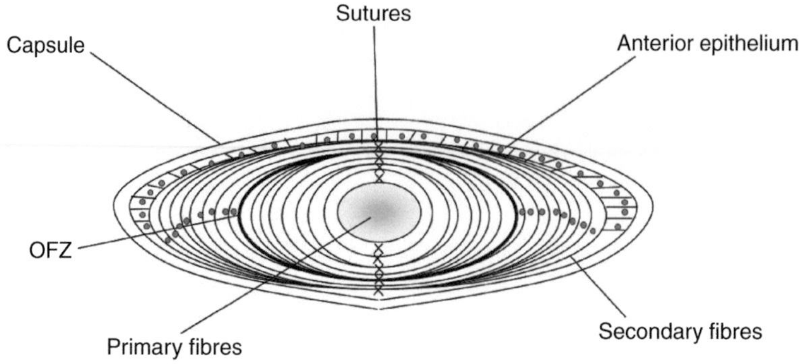

Fig. 3.1 Schematic diagram of the lens

of the lens mass, and the removal of metabolic waste products [21]. Water is circulated through membrane channels comprised of aquaporin 1 (AQP1) in lens epithelial cells [22], and major intrinsic protein (MIP) in fibre cells [23]. The breakdown of glucose by anaerobic metabolism is the main source of energy for both growth and homeostasis in the lens. Uptake of glucose from the aqueous humour appears to be mediated by the glucose transporter, GLUT1 in the lens epithelium, for circulation throughout the structure. Lens fibre cell membranes are incredibly cholesterol saturated such that bilayers form to create areas of pure cholesterol [24] that are thought to facilitate lens transparency by smoothing and maintaining the physical properties of cell membranes to prevent light scattering [25, 26]. The importance of cholesterol in the maintenance of lens clarity is apparent from genetic or therapeutic inhibition of cholesterol biosynthesis which leads to cataractogenesis [27].

Disruption of lens protein function can lead to cataract and other serious developmental abnormalities as highlighted in Table 3.2. A summary of the structural components of the lens and the features that establish and maintain its transparency can be found in Table 3.3.

3.3 What Constitutes the Formation of Cataracts in Children?

Lens opacities develop when the short-range order of crystallin protein is disturbed or the highly regular cellular organisation is disrupted, leading to fluctuation of protein density throughout the dimensions of the lens and resulting in regional differences in protein concentration [28]. At a molecular level, this may occur as a result of protein misfolding, instability or insolubility, leading to aggregation and altered interactions of proteins. Alterations in the homeostatic mechanisms or the physiological environment of the lens may indirectly impact upon crystallin proteins and also lead to cataractogenesis.

Aberrant protein folding results in the development of cataract when the accumulation of damage occurs at a faster rate than the lens chaperone α-crystallin, can manage, resulting in the formation of protein aggregates [28]. α-crystallin can identify partially or fully unfolded protein and segregate it, thus preventing its accumulative aggregation [29]. This mechanism is sufficient in the maintenance of lens clarity over an individual's lifetime, where protein damage only accrues gradually with age. However, mutation of any one of the highly expressed lens crystallins will result in rapidly accumulating protein damage that is likely to overwhelm the chaperoning system [30]. Likewise, mutation of α-crystallin may reduce or abolish chaperone function, also resulting in the accumulation of damaged crystallin proteins [31]. In young fibre cells of the lens cortex, physiological stress caused by the accumulation of damaged protein can prevent differentiation in to mature fibre cells [32]. Therefore, crystallin mutations can cause cataract as a result of aberrant protein folding and where the effect is particularly detrimental to the developing lens, may also cause anterior segment defects such as microphthalmia and microcornea secondary to microphakia (Fig. 3.2).

Table 3.2 Details of lens proteins associated with non-syndromic congenital cataract, their function, respective disease mode of inheritance and phenotypes

Protein	Gene locus	Mode of inheritance	Function	Reported cataract morphologies	Additional phenotype(s)
FOXE3	1p32	AD/AR	Forkhead box-containing transcription factor involved in lens specification, the closure of the OV and its detachment from the SE	Cerulean	Microphthalmia, sclerocornea, microcornea, optic disc coloboma, dysplastic irides, Peter's anomaly, glaucoma, aphakia
EPHA2	1p36.13	AD/AR	Ephrin receptor	Nuclear, cortical, posterior polar, zonular	Persistent foetal vasculature
GJA8	1q21.1	AD/AR	Gap junction protein for small molecule and ion transport	Nuclear, Total, Pulverulent, Y-sutural, Posterior subcapsular, diffuse, lamellar	Microcornea, glaucoma, myopia
CRYGD	2q33.3	AD	Structural cytoplasmic lens protein	Punctate progressive, coralliform, nuclear, lamellar, cerulean, aceuleiform, anterior polar, posterior polar	Microcornea
PXDN	2p25.3	AR	Encodes peroxidasin and has a role in cell adhesion to the ECM		Microphthalmia, microcornea, sclerocornea, developmental glaucoma, ASD
CRYGC	2q33.3	AD	Structural cytoplasmic lens protein	Zonular, pulverulent, nuclear, lamellar	Microphthalmia, microcornea, glaucoma, iris atrophy, corneal opacity, myopia
CRYGB	2q33.3	AD	Structural cytoplasmic lens protein	Anterior polar, lamellar	–
CRYBA2	2q35	AD	Structural cytoplasmic lens protein	Multifocal	Myopia, glaucoma, eccentric pupil
FYCO1	3p21.31	AR	Autophagosome trafficking	Nuclear	–
BFSP2	3q22.1	AD/AR	Combines with BFSP1 to form the beaded filament which establishes cellular architecture, provides a scaffold for protein chaperone function and supports tissue integrity during mechanical stress	Cortical, nuclear, Y-sutural, lamellar	Myopia
CRYGS	3q27.3	AD	Structural cytoplasmic lens protein	Cortical progressive, sutural, lamellar, nuclear	–

(continued)

Table 3.2 (continued)

Protein	Gene locus	Mode of inheritance	Function	Reported cataract morphologies	Additional phenotype(s)
VIM	10p13	AD	Intermediate filament protein that links the beaded filament to the plasma membrane of lens fibre cells	Pulverulent	–
PITX3	10q25	AD/AR	Homeobox-containing transcription factor that directly targets *FOXE3*; is involved in lens fibre cell proliferation and differentiation, and the regulation of crystallin expression	Progressive, posterior polar, posterior subcapsular	ASMD, microphthalmia, microcornia, sclerocornea, Perter's anomaly
PAX6	11p13	AD	Paired-box-containing transcription factor and 'master regulator of eye development'; involved in lens specification and development, optic fissure closure, and the regulation of crystallin gene expression		Aniridia, iris and foveal hypoplasia, corneal abnormalities, glaucoma
CRYAB	11q23.1	AD	Structural cytoplasmic lens protein, molecular chaperone, cellular proteostasis (retina), cell death regulation, multispan transmembrane protein folding, cytoskeletal remodelling, and Z-disc support (skeletal muscle)	Nuclear, posterior polar, lamellar	Myofibrillar myopathy, cardiomyopathy
MIP	12q13	AD	Lens fiber membrane channel protein for water transport and forms adhesion complex in combination with LIM2.	Cerulean, lamellar, punctate, Y-sutural, total, posterior polar	Myopia
GJA3	13q12.11	AD	Gap junction protein for small molecule and ion transport	Nuclear, pulverulent, posterior polar, total, cortical, lamellar, coralliform, punctate	–
OTX2	14q22.3	AD	Homeobox-containing transcription factor involved in embryonic rostral patterning, brain development, lens specification, and rod cell differentiation in the retina		Microphthalmia and pattern dystrophy of the retina

Table 3.2 (continued)

Protein	Gene locus	Mode of inheritance	Function	Reported cataract morphologies	Additional phenotype(s)
SIX6	14q23.1	AR	Homeobox and SIX-domain-containing transcription factor involved in forebrain patterning, lens induction, and regulation of lens cell proliferation, specification and development		Microphthalmia
VSX2	14q24.3	AR	Homeobox-containing transcription factor involved in cell proliferation during eye development, and specification, development and maintenance of the neural retina.		Microphthalmia, anophthalmia, iris coloboma
LTBP2	14q24.3	AR	Exact role unknown but highly expressed in the trabecular meshwork and ciliary processes		Congenital glaucoma, microspherophakia, ectopia lentis
MiR184	15q25.1	AD	Involved in corneal lineage specification but role in the lens is unknown	Anterior polar	Endothelial dystrophy, stromal thinning, keratoconus, iris hypoplasia
HSF4	16q21	AD/AR	Heat-shock transcription factor: regulates fibroblast growth factor, γ-crystallin and beaded filament expression during lens growth and development	Cortical, total, lamellar, sutural, nuclear	–
MAF	16q23.2	AD	bZIP domain-containing transcription factor involved in lens fibre cell differentiation and regulation of crystallin expression	Nuclear, cerulean, lamellar, pulverulent, posterior polar	Peters anomaly, myopia, microcornea, iris coloboma
CRYBA1	17q11.2	AD	Structural cytoplasmic lens protein	Nuclear, lamellar, pulverulent, Y-sutural, cortical	–
LIM2	19q13.4	AR	Combines with MIP to form robust adhesion complexes in mature lens fibre cells	Cortical, sutural	–

(continued)

Table 3.2 (continued)

Protein	Gene locus	Mode of inheritance	Function	Reported cataract morphologies	Additional phenotype(s)
BFSP1	20p12.1	AD/AR	Combines with BFSP2 to form the beaded filament which establishes cellular architecture, provides a scaffold for protein chaperone function and supports tissue integrity during mechanical stress	Cortical progressive, nuclear	–
CRYAA	21q22.3	AD/AR	Structural cytoplasmic lens protein and molecular chaperone	Nuclear, lamellar, posterior polar, anterior polar, Y-sutural, disc-like membranous	Microcornea, iris coloboma, glaucoma, crneal opacity
CRYBB3	22q11.23	AD/AR	Structural cytoplasmic lens protein	Nuclear, cortical	Microcornea
CRYBB2	22q11.23	AD	Structural cytoplasmic lens protein and function of the hippocampal network	Posterior subcapsular, cerulean, total, nuclear, disc-like membranous, lamellar, progressive polymorphic	Microcornea
CRYBB1	22q12.1	AD/AR	Structural cytoplasmic lens protein	Nuclear, pulverulent, progressive cortical	Glaucoma, microcornea
CRYBA4	22q12.1	AD	Structural cytoplasmic lens protein	Nuclear, lamellar	Microcornea, microphthalmia

RI refractive index, *OFZ* organelle free zone, *MIP* major intrinsic protein, *LIM2* lens intrinsic membrane protein, *AQP1* aquaporin 1

Cataract can also occur in the absence of protein misfolding. Within lens fibres, extremely soluble and stable crystallin proteins exist at high concentration. They are tightly and regularly packaged in a highly ordered manner to create an even protein distribution [28]. Given that crystallins also vary in size, they are said to exist in polydisperse, short-range order. To achieve this arrangement, crystallins display repulsive charges on their protein surface [33]. Crystallin mutations that alter protein surface charges lead to altered interactions and reduced solubility that cannot be resolved by the α-crystallin chaperone [34, 35]. Such alterations are disruptive to the normal short-range protein order and subsequently result in the co-existence of pockets of high and low protein concentration. Protein-rich areas have a higher refractive index than protein-poor areas of the lens, thus causing light scattering that appears as opacity within the lens [36].

3.4 What are the Aetiological and Genetic Bases of Paediatric Cataract?

3.4.1 Incidence and Epidemiology

Congenital cataract has a calculated incidence of 1 per 10,000 live births in the UK, increasing to approximately 3.5 per 10,000 cases for childhood cataract [37]. Global estimates of congenital and childhood cataract are 1–6 per 10,000 in developed countries and 5–15 per 10,000 in developing countries [38], making cataract the leading cause

Table 3.3 Summary of the structural components of the lens and the factors that contribute to and maintain its transparency

			Function	*Key gene(s)/protein(s) and/or molecules*
Structural Components		Fibre cells	Constitute >95 % of lens volume. Organisation facilitates transparency and tissue integrity	FGF, BMP, Wnt/PCP, TGF signalling Crystallins, HSF3, PAX6, PITX3, PROX1, SOX1, SOX2 and C-MAF
		Lens epithelium	Proliferation, differentiation and appendage of secondary fibre cells, uptake of nutrients from aqueous humour for homeostasis	Wnt/Notch signalling, E-cadherin, FOXE3, AP2α, PROX1, SOX1, C-MAF, YAP1
		Lens capsule	Uptake of nutrients, ions, water from aqueous and vitreous humours, protects protein contents of the lens, and provides structural/mechanical support to the mass	Integrins, collagen IV, collagen XVIII, laminin, fibronectin, matrix metalloproteinases
		Microplicae	Locks neighbouring fibre cells together to maintain structural integrity and prevent damage during lens accommodation	Cholesterol
			Mechanism	
Features for Transparency	Structural	Organelle degradation	Cellular organelles have a higher RI than the cytoplasm of lens cells, causing light scatter. Organelle degradation is synchronized upon terminal differentiation of lens fibre cells such that an OFZ is created at the centre of the lens, within the pupillary space	Tryptophan, DNase-IIβ, calpains
		Protein concentration	Extremely high concentrations of crystallin proteins exist in dense, short-range spatial order within the cytoplasm of lens cells. Protein concentration is higher in the centre of the lens compared with the periphery, to correct for its ellipsoid shape	Crystallins
		Beaded filament	Establishes cellular architecture and possibly provides a scaffold for protein chaperone function	BFSP1, BFSP2, α-crystallin, vimentin
		Molecular chaperones	In the absence of protein turn-over, small heat-shock protein, α-crystallin, recognizes and binds non-native and/or unfolded proteins to prevent accumulation in to light scattering aggregates.	CRYAA and CRYAB (α-crystallin)

(continued)

Table 3.3 (continued)

	Structural & Homeostatic	Lipids & cholesterol	Lens fibre cell membranes are highly saturated with cholesterol and sphingolipids which are thought to smooth cell membranes, promote cell stability during accommodation, and maintain physical, physiological and homeostatic properties of lens fibres	Dihydrosphingomyelin, sphingolipids, cholesterol
		Adhesive junctions	Adherens junction proteins are expressed in lens epithelial and fibre cell membranes and possibly maintain structural stability of fibres during lens development. MIP and LIM2 are also thought to form an adhesion complex that is unique to the lens that is important to organelle eliminated, mature fibre cells	N-cadherin, E-cadherin, MIP, LIM2
		Lens capsule	Basement membrane surrounding the lens that helps shape the lens curvature during accommodation, promotes cell migration, differentiation and survival, protects the contents of the lens from the immune system, and is involved in the passive exchange of metabolic substrates and waste products in and out of the lens	(See above)
	Homeostatic	Gap junctions	A network of intercellular channels for the transport of ions and small molecules throughout the lens mass for growth, development and maintenance of the lens and its contents	GJA8 (connexin 50), GJA3 (connexin 46), GJA1 (connexin 43)
		Water channels	Membrane channels are integral for the circulation of water throughout the lens mass	AQP1, MIP
		Anaerobic glycolysis	Uptake of glucose from the aqueous humour appears to be mediated by GLUT1, a glucose transporter that is highly expressed in the lens epithelium. The breakdown of glucose by anaerobic metabolism is the main source of energy for growth and maintenance of the lens	SLC2A1 (GLUT1), SLC2A3 (GLUT3)

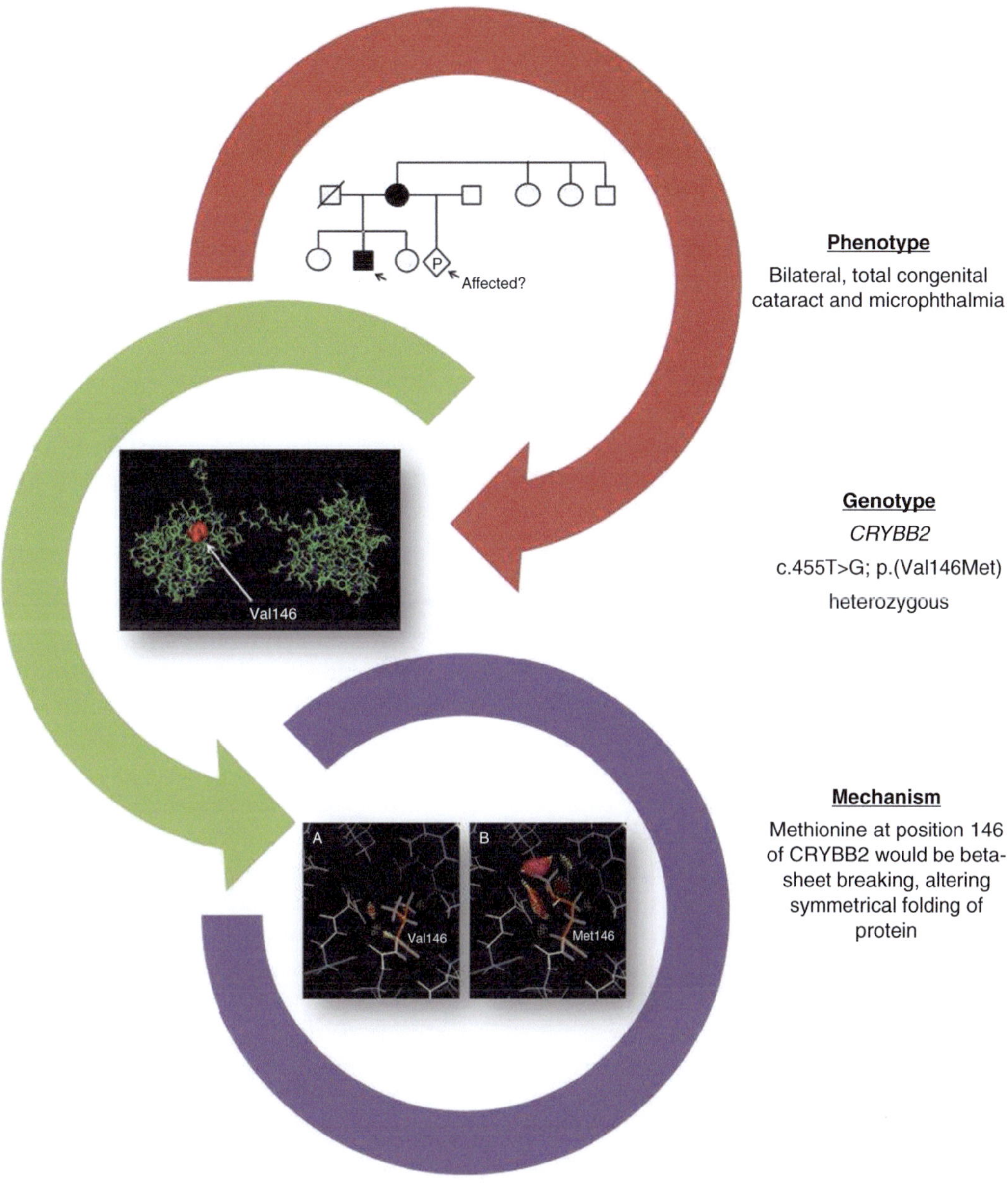

Fig. 3.2 Protein modelling to estimate variant mechanism pathogenicity: Identification of a variant that is predicted to be highly damaging to CRYBB2 protein structure in a family an autosomal dominant cataract and microphthalmia phenotype

of treatable blindness in children [37]. Causes of cataract in children include trauma, maternal TORCHS (toxoplasmosis, rubella, cytomegalovirus, herpes simplex and syphilis) infection (accounting for approximately 1 % of cases [39]), and intrauterine exposure to drugs or radiation. A large portion of paediatric cataracts are attributable to genetic variants or mutations, and in the majority of cases are inherited in a Mendelian fashion. Whilst the vast majority of unilateral cataract cases are idiopathic, it is estimated that 25–50 % of bilateral congenital and childhood cataract cases have a genetic basis [40, 41]. However, this is likely to be an underestimate since a number of apparently idiopathic cases will represent *de novo* dominant or recessive mutations [42]. Inherited cataracts can be grouped in to four main categories: (1) Isolated or non-syndromic cataracts; (2) Cataracts with extra-lenticular abnormalities; (3) Cataracts manifesting as a feature of a multi-system condition; (4) Cataracts presenting as a manifestation of an inborn-error of metabolism.

3.4.2 Genetic Aetiology

Inherited paediatric cataract can occur as a result of chromosomal rearrangements (Jamieson et al. 2007), trisomies (Down, Patau, Edwards syndromes); recurrent deletions (5p, 18q, 18p); triplet repeat disorders (e.g.- myotonic dystrophy [43]); mitochondrial disorders (e.g.- cytochrome C oxidase deficiency caused by MTCO1, [44]); loss of heterozygosity (e.g.- neurofibromatosis type 2 [45]) and microduplications/deletions [46, 47]. However, cataracts are most frequently caused by single nucleotide variations. Non-synonymous missense variants, single nucleotide base pair changes that alter an amino acid sequence, account for the vast majority of cataract-causing mutations in children. Since missense variants can have a variable effect on the function of the encoded protein of a gene, pathogenicity is difficult to assign in the absence of experimental evidence [48]. Congenital and childhood cataract is further complicated by extreme genetic heterogeneity. Mutations in over 100 genes have been associated with all types of the condition. Non-syndromic cataract, that is estimated to account for 70 % of inherited paediatric cataract cases [39], has been associated with around 25 genes, to date (Table 3.2). There are many more genes associated with syndromes that feature cataracts as an early manifestation (Table 3.4) [49]. Here, phenotypic ambiguity, overlap and complexity can preclude disease recognition and diagnosis.

Cataract morphology and location has traditionally been used to try to estimate the underlying mutated gene. However, there is no single cataract morphology associated with mutations in one specific gene. In fact, there are several reports of various cataract morphologies resulting from the same genetic mutation in different families (phenotypic heterogeneity), and contrarily- there are reports of the same morphology in association with different mutations in the same gene (locus heterogeneity) [50, 51]. Cataract-causing mutations can also display variable expressivity (i.e.- individuals with the same genetic mutation present with varying degrees of disease severity) [52, 53]. However, for some cataract-syndromes, the presence of particular cataract morphologies may facilitate a clinical diagnosis of a syndromic condition. For example, the very rare 'oil droplet on water' cataract morphology is strongly associated with the metabolic disorder, galactosemia [54], whilst white 'sunflower' cataracts are associated with Wilson disease [55].

3.4.2.1 Genetic Aetiology of Non-syndromic Cataract

Non-syndromic congenital cataract is most commonly inherited as an autosomal dominant trait with high penetrance. However, autosomal recessive forms are seen more frequently in communities where parental consanguinity is prevalent, although they are not exclusive to these populations. Genes implicated thus far mainly encode major lens proteins, and the majority of pathogenic mutations result in direct alteration of protein conformation, stability and/or solubility (Table 3.2). Other mutations affect fibre cell differentiation or organization, cell or membrane integrity, or solute, water and/or nutrient transport. In addition, if a genetic mutation is seriously detrimental to the growth and development of the lens, it may be unable to support the formation of components of the anterior chamber [56]. In this way, disruption of lens development can result in malformation of other eye structures, and so cataract can present alongside additional ocular developmental defects. Autosomal dominant cataract frequently occurs in conjunction with microphthalmia, microcornea and anterior segment mesenchymal dysgenesis (ASMD) [41].

Historically, owing to technological limitations and expense, cataract-causing mutations have been investigated on a case-by-case basis with reports detailing genetic findings from cases

Table 3.4 Examples of systemic conditions associated with congenital and childhood cataract

	Syndrome	Phenotype	Gene symbol
Renal/Genitourinary	Peters-plus	CC	*B3GALTL*
		Corneal opacities	
		ASD	
		Facial clefting	
		Brachydactyly	
		Short stature	
		Rhizomelia	
		Hypospadias	
		Hydronephrosis	
		Kidney and ureteral duplication	
	Smith-Lemli-Opitz	Cataract	*DHCR7*
		Microcephaly	
		Learning difficulties	
		Hypotonia	
		Cryptochidism	
		Hypospadias	
		Renal agenesis	
		Cystic kidney	
	Lowe Syndrome	CC	*OCRL1*
		Microphthalmia	
		Glaucoma	
		Hearing loss	
		Short stature	
		Cryptorchidism	
		Proximal renal tubular acidosis	
		Renal fanconi	
		Joint hypermobility	
Central nervous system	Warburg- MICRO syndrome	CC	*RAB3GAP1*
		Microcephaly	*RAB3GAP2*
		Microphthalmia	*RAB18*
		Microcornea	*TBC1D20*
		Optic Atrophy	
		Cortical dysplasia	
		Severe mental retardation	
		Spastic diplegia	
		Hypogonadism	
	Martsolf syndrome	CC	*RAB3GAP2*
		Microphthalmia	
		Brachycephaly/microcephaly	
		Severe mental retardation	
		Cryptochidism	
		Short stature	

(continued)

Table 3.4 (continued)

	Syndrome	Phenotype	Gene symbol
	Marinesco-Sjogren	CC	*SIL1*
		Microcephaly	
		Short stature	
		Severe myopathy/hypotonia	
		Skeletal deformaties	
		Muscle weakness/atrophy	
		Psychomotor/mental retardation	
		Cerebellar ataxia	
		Spasticity	
		Cerebellar atrophy	
	Cerebro-oculo-facial-skeletal (COFS)	Cataracts	*ERCC6*
		Microphthalmia	
		Microcephaly	
		Micrognathia	
		Arthrogryposis	
		Kyphoscoliosis	
		Contractures	
		Mental retardation	
		Absent motor development	
		Cerebella hypoplasia	
	Hallermann-Streiff syndrome	Cataracts	*GJA1*
		Microphthalmia	
		Iris coloboma	
		Brachycephaly	
		Microcephaly	
		Scaphocephaly	
		High arched palate	
		Thin Lips	
		Dental anomalies	
		Recurrent pulmonary infections	
		Cryptochidism	
		Skeletal abnormalities (Skull, spine, limbs and hands)	
		Telangiectasia	
		Hypotrichosis	
		Tonic-clonic seizures	
Cranio-mandibulo-facial	Nance Horan syndrome	Congenital cataracts (males)	*NHS*
		Mild sutural opacities (females)	
		Microcornea	
		Microphthalmia	
		Large anteverted pinnae	
		Prominent nose	
		'Screwdriver' shaped incisors	
		Tapered premolar and molar cusps	
		Behavioural problems	
		Autism	

Table 3.4 (continued)

	Syndrome	Phenotype	Gene symbol
	Brancio-oculo-facial syndrome	Cataract	*TFAP2A*
		Microphthalmia	
		Coloboma (iris and/or retinal)	
		Microcephaly	
		Micrognathia	
		Ear malformation	
		Facial clefting	
		Renal agenesis	
		Cystic kidneys	
		Skeletal abnormalities (Skull, spine, hands)	
		Skin sensitivity and cysts	
		Mental retardation	
		Agenesis of the cerebellar vermis	
	Cockayne Syndrome	Cataract	*ERCC8*
		Optic atrophy	*ERCC6*
		Corneal opacities	
		Delayed dentition and abnormalities	
		Cardiac arrhythmia and hypertension	
		Hetatosplenomegaly	
		Cutaneous photosensitivity	
		Mental retardation	
		Seizures	
		Cerebral atrophy	
		Ataxia and neuropathy	
Dermatological	Nail-patella Syndrome	Cataract	*LMX1B*
		Microcornea	
		Keratoconis	
		Oral clefting	
		Hypoplasia of the sternum	
		Scoliosis	
		Skeletal abnormalities	
		Abnormal/slow/absent nail growth	
		Muscle aplasia	
	Werner Syndrome	Cataracts	*RECQL2*
		Retinal degeneration	
		Short/stocky stature	
		Beaked nose	
		Scleroderma-like skin	
		Subcutaneous calcification	
		Skin ulcerations	
		Osteosarcoma	

(continued)

Table 3.4 (continued)

	Syndrome	Phenotype	Gene symbol
	Rhizomelic Chondroplasia Punctata	CC	*PEX7*
		Sensorineural deafness	*AGPS*
		Oral clefting	*GNPAT*
		Microcephaly	
		Coronal clefting of vertebrae	
		Kyphoscoliosis	
		Contractures	
		Rhizomelic limb shortening	
		Ichthyosis	
		Seizures	
		Mental retardation	
Skeletal	Stickler Syndrome	Cataracts	*COL2A1*
		Retinal detachment	*COL11A1*
		Sensorineural hearing loss	
		Scoliosis	
		Kyphosis	
		Platyspondyly	
		Arachnodactyly	
		Arthropathy	
	Craniolenticulosutural dysplasia	Cataract	*SEC23A*
		Optic atrophy	
		Macrocephaly with frontal bossing	
		Mild facial dysmorphism	
		Delayed dentition	
		Cryptochidism	
		Joint laxity	
		Osteopenia	
		Scoliosis	
		Skull ossification	
		Brittle/coarse/sparse hair	
	Homocystinuria	Cataract	*CBS*
		Ectopia lentis	
		High palate	
		Extra dentition	
		Cardiovascular problems	
		Kyphoscoliosis	
		Arachnodactyly	
		Hypopigmentation (skin/hair)	
		Seizures	
		Mental retardation	
		Behavioural problems	

Table 3.4 (continued)

	Syndrome	Phenotype	Gene symbol
Metabolic	Galactosaemia	Cataract	*GALT*
		Hepatomegaly	
		Decreased liver function and cirrhosis	
		Failure to thirive	
		Mental retardation (if untreated)	
		Hemolytic anemia	
	Cerebrotendinous xanthomatosis	Juvenile cataract	*CYP27A1*
		Infantile chronic diarrhea	
		Tendon xanthoma	
		Premature atherosclerosis	
		Neurological deterioration	
		Peripheral neuropathy	

of familial cataract. In this way, estimations of gene mutation frequencies are difficult to make. Mutations in crystallin genes are believed to account for as many as 50 % of paediatric cataract cases [41], with the majority of reported mutations appearing to be non-synonymous missense variants that act in a dominant negative manner. Of the 13 crystallin genes known to be expressed in the human lens, 12 have thus far been associated with cataract- *CRYAA*, *CRYAB*, *CRYBA1*, *CRYBA2*, *CRYBA4*, *CRYBB1*, *CRYBB2*, and *CRYBB3*, *CRYGB*, *CRYGC*, *CRYGD*, and *CRYGS*. The accumulation of denatured crystallin proteins is known have a detrimental effect the differentiation of fibre cells [32], subsequently affecting growth and development of the lens. As such, crystallin mutations are often associated with microphakia, microphthalmia, and microcornea in addition to cataract. *CRYAB* is the only crystallin expressed at substantial levels outside of the lens, with expression identified in the heart, retina, brain and striated muscle. Correspondingly, *CRYAB* mutations have also been reported to cause cardiomyopathy or myofibrillar myopathy with or without cataract [57–60]. Numerous mutations have also been identified in lens specific connexin genes, *GJA3* and *GJA8*, which are estimated to be the second most frequent cause of inherited cataract in children. As with the crystallins, connexin mutations are also thought to act in a dominant negative manner. Connexin mutations are frequently reported in association with nuclear cataracts caused by the build-up of calcium in the centre of the lens as a consequence of the loss of the lens microcirculatory system [61]. Mutations in transcription factors such as PAX6, *FOXE3*, *PITX3* and *MAF* are known to cause congenital cataract in association with anterior segment defects representing the true pleiotropic effect of the genes when mutated.

3.4.2.2 Genetic Aetiology of Syndromic Cataract

Syndromic cataract is an umbrella term for a broad range of hereditary multisystem disorders that feature cataract as manifestation (Table 3.4); each is considered to be a very rare but lifelong health burden. The overall proportion of paediatric cataract cases suggested to be attributable to syndromic disease is between 11.4–15 % [41, 62]; with Down syndrome estimated to be the most frequent cause [39]. As opposed to non-syndromic forms, there are several X-linked and numerous recessive causes of syndromic cataracts. X-linked conditions featuring cataract include Nance Horan syndrome and Lowe syndrome. In each case, hemizygous males are affected by cataracts and extra-ocular manifestations, whilst obligate carrier females present with Y-sutural (NHS) or spoke-like (OCRL) lens opacities where only a portion of lens fibre cells are affected, owing to the lyonization effect of X-activation [63].

3.5 What Is the Current Care Pathway for Children with Inherited Cataract?

Congenital and childhood cataract remains an important yet difficult condition to diagnose and manage. Increased understanding of the visual system, and the latent and sensitive periods of visual development has led to better visual outcomes in paediatric cataract patients owing to improved comprehension of the impact of surgical timing, techniques and post-operative rehabilitation [64, 65]. Although prompt observation of cataract is a crucial aspect of the care of these patients, determining the precise underlying cause of opacities presenting in children is equally significant. This remains challenging, however, and is often hindered by the absence of a standardised paediatric cataract care pathway within healthcare institutions.

First and foremost, an integrated ophthalmological and systemic review is required to distinguish the subtype (i.e.- non-syndromic versus syndromic). Standard paediatric work-up involves TORCH screening, basic blood tests (e.g.- full blood count, thyroid and liver function tests, and calcium profiling), analysis of reducing substances in the urine to determine levels of galactose and glucose, and karyotyping to detect chromosomal aberrations. Various studies have raised questions over the effectiveness of such testing, particularly of TORCH screening which has repeatedly been demonstrated to be unreliable, inconsistent, open to misinterpretation and unduly expensive considering its low pick-up (and false negative) rate [66–70]. Evidence for the poor diagnostic yield of this approach to diagnosis comes from large, population-based studies; a study of 1027 Danish children found bilateral cataracts were of unknown aetiology in 50 % of cases [39], corroborating the findings of an earlier UK based study that stated 61 % of bilateral paediatric cataracts were idiopathic in a cohort of 248 children [37].

Assessment by a geneticist may follow initial ophthalmological examination, where a detailed family history will also be taken, along with information regarding antenatal, perinatal and postnatal health [71]. Given the extensive number of possible disorders underlying the development of congenital or childhood cataract [49], the route to precise diagnosis of the underlying genetic cause can be complex with input required from multiple medical specialities in addition to ophthalmology and genetics, including dysmorphology, neurology, metabolics, and orthopaedics [64]. Clinically, numerous diagnostic investigations may be pursued to identify physiological, haematological, or metabolic causes. Upon the identification of additional phenotypic manifestations, more specialised diagnostic tests may be conducted to build or confirm a working clinical hypothesis such as array comparative genomic hybridisation (aCGH), fluorescence *in situ* hybridisation (FISH), plasma sterol analysis or gene screening. Systemic investigations such as magnetic resonance imaging (MRI) may be used for the characterization of anatomical, neurological and skeletal abnormalities that may facilitate, but rarely define, a diagnosis. The traditional diagnostic pathway is illustrated in Fig. 3.3.

Traditional genetic testing is used as a means of confirming a working diagnosis, established by clinical assessment [49]. Findings from clinical investigations are used to develop a working hypothesis regarding the underlying disease and to direct genetic testing to a single or small number of relevant genes. However, conditions of extreme genetic and phenotypic heterogeneity, such as paediatric cataract, are difficult to diagnose by Sanger sequencing [72], which has been the long-standing, prevailing means of genetic diagnosis for over three decades. Phenotypic ambiguity and/or complexity in dysmorphic and developmentally delayed infants preclude disease recognition that is further hindered by weak genotype-phenotype correlations, particularly for cases of suspected non-syndromic cataract. The yield of traditional sequencing approaches is an additional limitation of this diagnostic strategy, in particular as throughput remains low owing to practicality and analytical drawbacks.

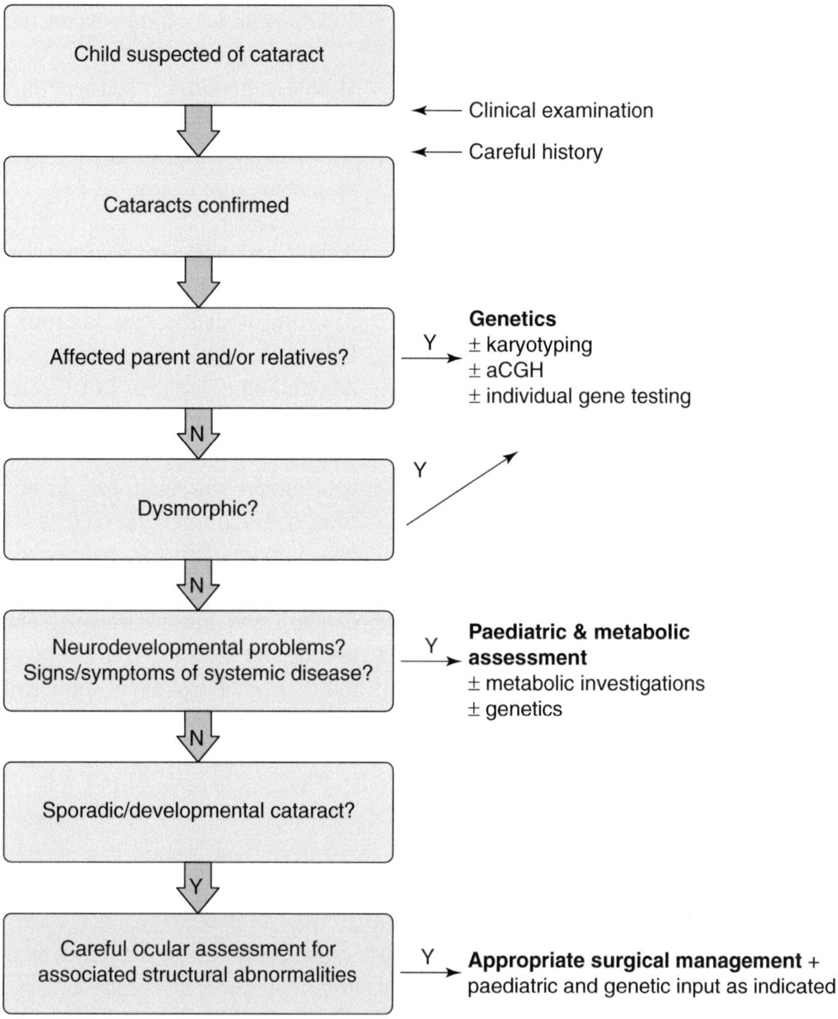

Fig. 3.3 Schematic diagram of traditional diagnostic pathway for paediatric cataract (Modified from Gillespie et al. [73])

3.6 How Can Inherited Paediatric Cataract Be Diagnosed Using Genomic Medicine Approaches?

The advent of next generation sequencing (NGS) in 2005 revolutionised DNA sequencing [74, 75], enabling the sequence content of an entire genome to be analysed in a single experiment. Rapid improvements in sequencing chemistry and bioinformatics means that NGS is now a robust and relatively inexpensive technique for generating thousands to millions of parallel sequencing reactions, to accurately and quickly screen large amounts of DNA at reduced price on a cost per nucleotide basis, when compared to standard Sanger sequencing methods. Creating a new paradigm for the diagnosis of human disease, the impact of these advanced sequencing technologies on human genetics cannot be understated, proving particularly useful in the diagnosis of human heterogeneous monogenic disease. Allowing diagnosis irrespective of disease recognition, atypical or complex phenotypes and suspected mode of inheritance, this is extending access to genetic testing for many more patients and their families. Different approaches exist and are adopted according to laboratory setting (i.e. – clinical diagnostic versus research laboratories):

(i) **'Targeted' NGS strategies**. Selective capture of genomic regions of interest was developed as an intermediate solution to the initial expense of whole genome sequencing; requiring much less sequencing, reducing data output, data storage requirements and total cost, this was a much more sustainable routine approach to human disease diagnosis [76, 77]. Such targeted approaches include:
   (a) Disease-targeted gene panels: Designed to target only genomic regions of interest, such as genes associated with a particular disease, phenotypic feature, or developmental pathway. Sequencing analysis yields only disease relevant information, greatly facilitating interpretability of the data-set and reducing the risk of unexpected findings.
   (b) Whole exome sequencing (WES): Protein coding genes comprise approximately 2 % of the entire human genome and variations in these regions are thought to account for as many as 85 % cases of inherited disease. WES is a powerful means of diagnosing genetic disease and for identifying novel disease genes [78]. WES can identify tens of thousands of variants post-quality-informatics filtering. Strategic approaches to experimental design and data filtering can greatly assist variant prioritization [79]. WES strategies based on family history, presumed mode of inheritance and experimental approach can reduce the number of variants for consideration, up to 95 % in some scenarios [79]. However, such a comprehensive analysis carries the possibility of incidental findings, adding complexity to analysis, reporting and results delivery. It is possible to limit bioinformatics analysis to a subset of genes associated with the phenotypic manifestations presenting in the patient tested – this can be used to offset the analytical drawbacks of WES.

(ii) **Whole genome sequencing (WGS)**. Undoubtedly the most comprehensive and unbiased approach to investigating the cause of human monogenic disease, WGS offers the advantage that both coding and non-coding variants are detected in the same experiment. WGS does not require capture-based methods that can be prone to bias and failure. However, understanding of the role of non-coding components of the genome such as transcriptional enhancers and splicing regulatory elements [80], and their impact on gene expression relative to phenotypic variation, is still in its infancy. Consequently, data interpretation remains challenging, while significant drawbacks remain with regards to expense and practicalities of data manageability and storage. The use of WGS in the delineation of the role of genic and non-genic susceptibility loci in heterogeneous disease [81] and its potential clinical applications are fast becoming obvious [82–84].

Next generation sequencing approaches to the diagnosis of paediatric cataract have proven highly successful. A disease-targeted panel approach, focussing sequencing at 115 genes associated with all forms of paediatric cataract (i.e.- non-syndromic, syndromic and metabolic), achieved an overall pick-up rate of approximately 75 % [73]. This study showed that cataract-targeted NGS can accurately and efficiently identify known, rare, and novel variants underlying non-syndromic and syndromic forms of the disease. Interestingly, in a number of cases, genetic findings revealed unsuspected, rare syndromic forms of the condition demonstrating the significant clinical utility of the test [73]. Other studies have used WES 'virtual panel' approaches with mutation detection rates ranging from 36 to 50 %, with differences likely to variations in patient selection criteria, disparities in patient cohort sizes, and almost certainly the number and variety of genes selected for analysis by NGS [85–87]. Regardless of the specific approach, the application of genomics in the diagnosis of paediatric cataract has been demonstrated to have

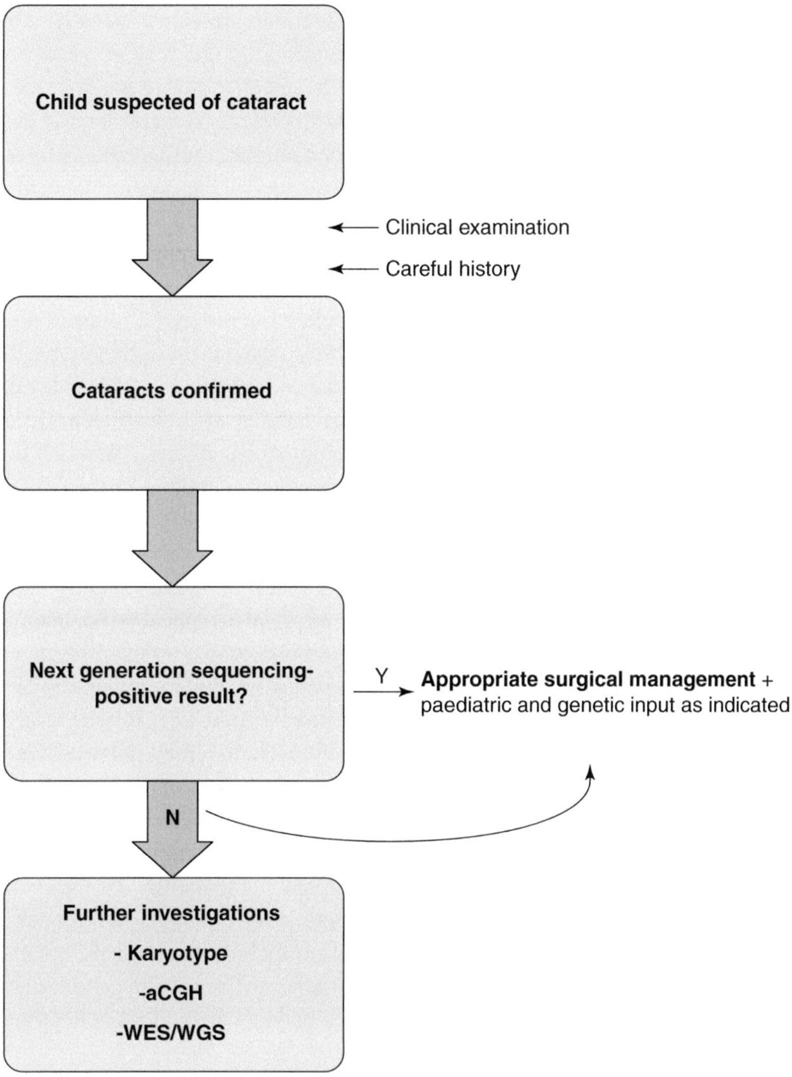

Fig. 3.4 Schematic diagram of the newly proposed diagnostic pathway for paediatric cataract; incorporating next generation sequencing (NGS) as the frontline means of diagnosis creates a more efficient and effective diagnostic process when compared to the traditional pathway (Fig. 3.3) (Modified from Gillespie et al. [73])

considerable power. Implementation of NGS early in the diagnostic pathway can alter management and improve patient outcomes, attributable to the implementation of a personalised genomic approach to stratified medicine. In a subset of cases, cataract-targeted NGS will delineate individuals with cataract caused by an underlying biochemical defect and a proportion of these individuals will be eligible for preventative treatment (Gillespie et al., 2015, in press) (Fig. 3.4).

3.7 What Is the Benefit of a Precise Molecular Diagnosis in Paediatric Cataract?

The evidence is now accumulating to augur an era of genomic ophthalmology. The increased understanding of the mutational basis of inherited ophthalmic disease provides insight into molecular mechanisms, streamlines clinical care, extends access to genetic testing, and improves patient outcomes. Delineation of the precise cause of paediatric cataract first defines the subtype of the condition and hence

- Refines a working clinical hypothesis.
- Allows delineation of inheritance patterns, allowing accurate risk estimations for family members and future pregnancies.
- Provides more accurate prognosis, particularly important for neurodegenerative conditions, such as, Warburg MICRO syndrome.

Identification of a syndromic condition can direct disease-specific monitoring and management, and may lead to the initiation of treatment, for example- Losartan treatment in Marfan syndrome [88]. For a particular subset of congenital and childhood cataract patients, timely identification of the precise mutation underlying cataract presentation is arguably more critical. A number of rare metabolic conditions, for which cataract is an early manifestation, are amenable to preventative treatment or dietary management. Such conditions may be associated with complex developmental and/or multi-systemic features that are difficult to define or may not become apparent until a later age. Here, examples include: dietary avoidance of glucose in GLUT1 deficiency [89]; exclusion of galactose from the diet of individuals with galactosaemia [90]; chenodeoxycholic acid treatment of cerebrotendinous xanthomatosis [91]. NGS has been shown to efficiently and accurately diagnose such disorders, allowing early disease intervention where possible [73].

The identification of the precise genetic mutation facilitates accurate genetic counselling, providing families with information about their condition and ongoing support following diagnosis [92, 93]. Such 'all-inclusive' sequencing approaches of the genomic era have made genetic testing applicable to many more patients and are delivering positive results to a larger proportion of those tested. It is important to note that this has meant that consent protocols have also been altered and that the availability of effective post-test counselling is key. Molecular diagnosis of inherited paediatric cataract patients is also of considerable research benefit allowing better understanding the role of gene and protein in health and disease. Increasing the spectrum of known deleterious and tolerated genetic variants in cataract genes will enable delineation of novel variants as disease-causing or benign, thus serving to facilitate data interpretation in clinical scenarios [48]. Screening increased numbers of patients for mutations in known genes is leading to better definition of clinical phenotypes and enabling characterisation of atypical and complex disease manifestations. This is leading to a better understanding of cataractogenesis and associated developmental disease, and is facilitating the development of novel therapies [94–96].

Ophthalmology – and specifically the care of children with congenital cataract – has provided a strong model for demonstrating the advantageous use of detailed phenotypic data and genomic information to dissect the molecular mechanisms and pathways underpinning ocular development and disease [97, 98]. Research in this area has largely been driven by the need for disease stratification to facilitate an individualized approach to patient care with the aim of improving clinical outcomes by the implementation of personalised medicine. Targeted-NGS has rapidly been embraced for the diagnosis of heterogeneous eye disease, including paediatric cataract, and is an exemplar of the use of genomic information to guide patient care and tailor treatment [73].

References

1. Bassnett S, Shi Y, Vrensen GF. Biological glass: structural determinants of eye lens transparency. Philos Trans R Soc Lond B Biol Sci. 2011;366(1568):1250–64. Epub 2011/03/16.
2. Shi Y, Barton K, De Maria A, Petrash JM, Shiels A, Bassnett S. The stratified syncytium of the vertebrate lens. J Cell Sci. 2009;122(Pt 10):1607–15. Epub 2009/04/30.
3. Blankenship T, Bradshaw L, Shibata B, Fitzgerald P. Structural specializations emerging late in mouse lens fiber cell differentiation. Invest Ophthalmol Vis Sci. 2007;48(7):3269–76. Epub 2007/06/27.
4. Danysh BP, Duncan MK. The lens capsule. Exp Eye Res. 2009;88(2):151–64. Epub 2008/09/09.
5. Dahm R, van Marle J, Quinlan RA, Prescott AR, Vrensen GF. Homeostasis in the vertebrate lens:

mechanisms of solute exchange. Philos Trans R Soc Lond B Biol Sci. 2011;366(1568):1265–77. Epub 2011/03/16.
6. Lovicu FJ, McAvoy JW. Growth factor regulation of lens development. Dev Biol. 2005;280(1):1–14. Epub 2005/03/16.
7. Bassnett S. On the mechanism of organelle degradation in the vertebrate lens. Exp Eye Res. 2009;88(2): 133–9. Epub 2008/10/09.
8. Vrensen GF, Graw J, De Wolf A. Nuclear breakdown during terminal differentiation of primary lens fibres in mice: a transmission electron microscopic study. Exp Eye Res. 1991;52(6):647–59. Epub 1991/06/01.
9. Thut CJ, Rountree RB, Hwa M, Kingsley DM. A large-scale in situ screen provides molecular evidence for the induction of eye anterior segment structures by the developing lens. Dev Biol. 2001;231(1):63–76.
10. Zhao SL, Chen Q, Hung FC, Overbeek PA. BMP signaling is required for development of the ciliary body. Development. 2002;129(19):4435–42.
11. Idrees F, Vaideanu D, Fraser SG, Sowden JC, Khaw PT. A review of anterior segment dysgeneses. Surv Ophthalmol. 2006;51(3):213–31. Epub 2006/04/29.
12. Shiels A, Hejtmancik JF. Genetics of human cataract. Clin Genet. 2013;84(2):120–7. Epub 2013/05/08.
13. Williamson KA, FitzPatrick DR. The genetic architecture of microphthalmia, anophthalmia and coloboma. Eur J Med Genet. 2014;57(8):369–80. Epub 2014/05/27.
14. Delaye M, Tardieu A. Short-range order of crystallin proteins accounts for eye lens transparency. Nature. 1983;302(5907):415–7. Epub 1983/03/06.
15. Horwitz J, Emmons T, Takemoto L. The ability of lens alpha crystallin to protect against heat-induced aggregation is age-dependent. Curr Eye Res. 1992;11(8):817–22. Epub 1992/08/01.
16. Song S, Landsbury A, Dahm R, Liu Y, Zhang Q, Quinlan RA. Functions of the intermediate filament cytoskeleton in the eye lens. J Clin Invest. 2009; 119(7):1837–48. Epub 2009/07/10.
17. Kim S, Coulombe PA. Intermediate filament scaffolds fulfill mechanical, organizational, and signaling functions in the cytoplasm. Genes Dev. 2007;21(13):1581–97.
18. Carter JM, Hutcheson AM, Quinlan RA. In vitro studies on the assembly properties of the lens proteins CP49, CP115: coassembly with alpha-crystallin but not with vimentin. Exp Eye Res. 1995;60(2):181–92. Epub 1995/02/01.
19. Mathias RT, Kistler J, Donaldson P. The lens circulation. J Membr Biol. 2007;216(1):1–16. Epub 2007/06/15.
20. Rae JL, Kuszak JR. The electrical coupling of epithelium and fibers in the frog lens. Exp Eye Res. 1983;36(3):317–26. Epub 1983/03/01.
21. Piatigorsky J. Intracellular ions, protein metabolism, and cataract formation. Curr Top Eye Res. 1980;3:1–39. Epub 1980/01/01.
22. Patil RV, Saito I, Yang X, Wax MB. Expression of aquaporins in the rat ocular tissue. Exp Eye Res. 1997;64(2):203–9. Epub 1997/02/01.
23. Varadaraj K, Kushmerick C, Baldo GJ, Bassnett S, Shiels A, Mathias RT. The role of MIP in lens fiber cell membrane transport. J Membr Biol. 1999;170(3):191–203. Epub 1999/08/12.
24. Jacob RF, Cenedella RJ, Mason RP. Direct evidence for immiscible cholesterol domains in human ocular lens fiber cell plasma membranes. J Biol Chem. 1999;274(44):31613–8. Epub 1999/10/26.
25. Plesnar E, Subczynski WK, Pasenkiewicz-Gierula M. Saturation with cholesterol increases vertical order and smoothes the surface of the phosphatidylcholine bilayer: a molecular simulation study. Biochim Biophys Acta. 2012;1818(3):520–9. Epub 2011/11/09.
26. Subczynski WK, Raguz M, Widomska J, Mainali L, Konovalov A. Functions of cholesterol and the cholesterol bilayer domain specific to the fiber-cell plasma membrane of the eye lens. J Membr Biol. 2012;245(1):51–68. Epub 2011/12/31.
27. de Vries AC, Cohen LH. Different effects of the hypolipidemic drugs pravastatin and lovastatin on the cholesterol biosynthesis of the human ocular lens in organ culture and on the cholesterol content of the rat lens in vivo. Biochim Biophys Acta. 1993;1167(1):63–9. Epub 1993/03/17.
28. Bloemendal H, de Jong W, Jaenicke R, Lubsen NH, Slingsby C, Tardieu A. Ageing and vision: structure, stability and function of lens crystallins. Prog Biophys Mol Biol. 2004;86(3):407–85. Epub 2004/08/11.
29. Horwitz J. Alpha-crystallin can function as a molecular chaperone. Proc Natl Acad Sci U S A. 1992;89(21):10449–53. Epub 1992/11/01.
30. Csermely P. A nonconventional role of molecular chaperones: involvement in the cytoarchitecture. News Physiol Sci Int J Physiol Prod Jointly Int Union Physiol Sci Am Physiol Soc. 2001;16:123–6. Epub 2001/07/10.
31. Derham BK, Harding JJ. Alpha-crystallin as a molecular chaperone. Prog Retin Eye Res. 1999;18(4):463–509. Epub 1999/04/27.
32. Sandilands A, Hutcheson AM, Long HA, Prescott AR, Vrensen G, Loster J, et al. Altered aggregation properties of mutant gamma-crystallins cause inherited cataract. EMBO J. 2002;21(22):6005–14. Epub 2002/11/12.
33. Veretout F, Delaye M, Tardieu A. Molecular basis of eye lens transparency. Osmotic pressure and X-ray analysis of alpha-crystallin solutions. J Mol Biol. 1989;205(4):713–28. Epub 1989/02/20.
34. Heon E, Priston M, Schorderet DF, Billingsley GD, Girard PO, Lubsen N, et al. The gamma-crystallins and human cataracts: a puzzle made clearer. Am J Hum Genet. 1999;65(5):1261–7. Epub 1999/10/16.
35. Kmoch S, Brynda J, Asfaw B, Bezouska K, Novak P, Rezacova P, et al. Link between a novel human gammaD-crystallin allele and a unique cataract phenotype explained by protein crystallography. Hum Mol Genet. 2000;9(12):1779–86. Epub 2000/08/01.
36. Moreau KL, King JA. Protein misfolding and aggregation in cataract disease and prospects for prevention. Trends Mol Med. 2012;18(5):273–82. Epub 2012/04/24.

37. Rahi JS, Dezateux C. British Congenital Cataract Interest G. Measuring and interpreting the incidence of congenital ocular anomalies: lessons from a national study of congenital cataract in the UK. Invest Ophthalmol Vis Sci. 2001;42(7):1444–8. Epub 2001/05/31.
38. Apple DJ, Ram J, Foster A, Peng Q. Elimination of cataract blindness: a global perspective entering the new millenium. Surv Ophthalmol. 2000;45 Suppl 1:S1–196. Epub 2001/04/09.
39. Haargaard B, Wohlfahrt J, Fledelius HC, Rosenberg T, Melbye M. A nationwide Danish study of 1027 cases of congenital/infantile cataracts: etiological and clinical classifications. Ophthalmology. 2004;111(12): 2292–8. Epub 2004/12/08.
40. Francis PJ, Moore AT. Genetics of childhood cataract. Curr Opin Ophthalmol. 2004;15(1):10–5. Epub 2004/01/27.
41. Hejtmancik JF. Congenital cataracts and their molecular genetics. Semin Cell Dev Biol. 2008;19(2):134–49. Epub 2007/11/24.
42. Wirth MG, Russell-Eggitt IM, Craig JE, Elder JE, Mackey DA. Aetiology of congenital and paediatric cataract in an Australian population. Br J Ophthalmol. 2002;86(7):782–6. Epub 2002/06/27.
43. Voermans NC, Erasmus CE, Ockeloen CW, van Engelen BG, Eggink CA. Primary cataract as a key to recognition of myotonic dystrophy type 1. Eur J Ophthalmol. 2015. Epub 2015/02/07.
44. Debray FG, Seneca S, Gonce M, Vancampenhaut K, Bianchi E, Boemer F, et al. Mitochondrial encephalomyopathy with cytochrome c oxidase deficiency caused by a novel mutation in the MTCO1 gene. Mitochondrion. 2014;17:101–5. Epub 2014/06/24.
45. Evans DG, Huson SM, Donnai D, Neary W, Blair V, Newton V, et al. A genetic study of type 2 neurofibromatosis in the United Kingdom. II. Guidelines for genetic counselling. J Med Genet. 1992;29(12):847–52. Epub 1992/12/01.
46. Cordovez JA, Capasso J, Lingao MD, Sadagopan KA, Spaeth GL, Wasserman BN, et al. Ocular manifestations of 22q11.2 microduplication. Ophthalmology. 2014;121(1):392–8. Epub 2013/08/27.
47. Martinez-Frias ML, Ocejo-Vinyals JG, Arteaga R, Martinez-Fernandez ML, Macdonald A, Perez-Belmonte E, et al. Interstitial deletion 14q22.3-q23.2: genotype-phenotype correlation. Am J Med Genet A. 2014;164A(3):639–47. Epub 2013/12/21.
48. MacArthur DG, Manolio TA, Dimmock DP, Rehm HL, Shendure J, Abecasis GR, et al. Guidelines for investigating causality of sequence variants in human disease. Nature. 2014;508(7497):469–76. Epub 2014/04/25.
49. Trumler AA. Evaluation of pediatric cataracts and systemic disorders. Curr Opin Ophthalmol. 2011;22(5):365–79. Epub 2011/08/13.
50. Ionides A, Francis P, Berry V, Mackay D, Bhattacharya S, Shiels A, et al. Clinical and genetic heterogeneity in autosomal dominant cataract. Br J Ophthalmol. 1999;83(7):802–8. Epub 1999/06/25.
51. Deng H, Yuan LM. Molecular genetics of congenital nuclear cataract. Eur J Med Genet. 2014;57(2–3): 113–22.
52. Eiberg H, Lund AM, Warburg M, Rosenberg T. Assignment of congenital cataract Volkmann type (CCV) to chromosome 1p36. Hum Genet. 1995;96(1):33–8. Epub 1995/07/01.
53. Burdon KP, McKay JD, Sale MM, Russell-Eggitt IM, Mackey DA, Wirth MG, et al. Mutations in a novel gene, NHS, cause the pleiotropic effects of Nance-Horan syndrome, including severe congenital cataract, dental anomalies, and mental retardation. Am J Hum Genet. 2003;73(5):1120–30. Epub 2003/10/18.
54. Wijburg MT, Wenniger-Prick LJ, Bosch AM, Visser G, Bams-Mengerink A. Bilateral cataract in childhood years: always an indication for screening on a metabolic disorder. Nederlands tijdschrift voor geneeskunde. 2008;152(11):632–6. Epub 2008/04/16. Bilateraal cataract op de kinderleeftijd: altijd een indicatie voor aanvullend onderzoek naar stofwisselingsziekten.
55. Cairns JE, Williams HP, Walshe JM. "Sunflower cataract" in Wilson's disease. Br Med J. 1969;3(5662):95–6. Epub 1969/07/12.
56. Kuszak JR, Zoltoski RK, Sivertson C. Fibre cell organization in crystalline lenses. Exp Eye Res. 2004;78(3):673–87. Epub 2004/04/27.
57. Vicart P, Caron A, Guicheney P, Li Z, Prevost MC, Faure A, et al. A missense mutation in the alphaB-crystallin chaperone gene causes a desmin-related myopathy. Nat Genet. 1998;20(1):92–5. Epub 1998/09/10.
58. Selcen D, Engel AG. Myofibrillar myopathy caused by novel dominant negative alpha B-crystallin mutations. Ann Neurol. 2003;54(6):804–10. Epub 2003/12/19.
59. Inagaki N, Hayashi T, Arimura T, Koga Y, Takahashi M, Shibata H, et al. Alpha B-crystallin mutation in dilated cardiomyopathy. Biochem Biophys Res Commun. 2006;342(2):379–86. Epub 2006/02/18.
60. van der Smagt JJ, Vink A, Kirkels JH, Nelen M, ter Heide H, Molenschot MM, et al. Congenital posterior pole cataract and adult onset dilating cardiomyopathy: expanding the phenotype of alphaB-crystallinopathies. Clin Genet. 2014;85(4):381–5. Epub 2013/04/18.
61. Gao J, Sun X, Martinez-Wittinghan FJ, Gong X, White TW, Mathias RT. Connections between connexins, calcium, and cataracts in the lens. J Gen Physiol. 2004;124(4):289–300. Epub 2004/09/29.
62. Lim Z, Rubab S, Chan YH, Levin AV. Pediatric cataract: the Toronto experience-etiology. Am J Ophthalmol. 2010;149(6):887–92. Epub 2010/05/01.
63. Lyon MF. Gene action in the X-chromosome of the mouse (Mus musculus L.). Nature. 1961;190:372–3. Epub 1961/04/22.
64. Lloyd IC, Goss-Sampson M, Jeffrey BG, Kriss A, Russell-Eggitt I, Taylor D. Neonatal cataract: aetiology, pathogenesis and management. Eye. 1992;6(Pt 2):184–96. Epub 1992/01/01.

65. Chan WH, Biswas S, Ashworth JL, Lloyd IC. Congenital and infantile cataract: aetiology and management. Eur J Pediatr. 2012;171(4):625–30. Epub 2012/03/03.
66. Abdel-Fattah SA, Bhat A, Illanes S, Bartha JL, Carrington D. TORCH test for fetal medicine indications: only CMV is necessary in the United Kingdom. Prenat Diagn. 2005;25(11):1028–31. Epub 2005/10/19.
67. Garland SM, Gilbert GL. Investigation of congenital infection–the TORCH screen is not a legitimate test. Paediatric Infectious Diseases Group of the Australasian Society for Infectious Diseases. Med J Aust. 1993;159(5):346–8. Epub 1993/09/06.
68. Khan NA, Kazzi SN. Yield and costs of screening growth-retarded infants for torch infections. Am J Perinatol. 2000;17(3):131–5. Epub 2000/09/30.
69. Yamamoto R, Ishii K, Shimada M, Hayashi S, Hidaka N, Nakayama M, et al. Significance of maternal screening for toxoplasmosis, rubella, cytomegalovirus and herpes simplex virus infection in cases of fetal growth restriction. J Obstet Gynaecol Res. 2013;39(3):653–7. Epub 2012/10/31.
70. van der Weiden S, de Jong EP, Te Pas AB, Middeldorp JM, Vossen AC, Rijken M, et al. Is routine TORCH screening and urine CMV culture warranted in small for gestational age neonates? Early Hum Dev. 2011;87(2):103–7. Epub 2010/12/15.
71. Lloyd IC, Ashworth J, Biswas S, Abadi RV. Advances in the management of congenital and infantile cataract. Eye. 2007;21(10):1301–9. Epub 2007/10/05.
72. Sanger F, Nicklen S, Coulson AR. DNA sequencing with chain-terminating inhibitors. Proc Natl Acad Sci U S A. 1977;74(12):5463–7. Epub 1977/12/01.
73. Gillespie RL, O'Sullivan J, Ashworth J, Bhaskar S, Williams S, Biswas S, et al. Personalized diagnosis and management of congenital cataract by next-generation sequencing. Ophthalmology. 2014;121(11): 2124–37.e1–2. Epub 2014/08/26.
74. Shendure J, Porreca GJ, Reppas NB, Lin X, McCutcheon JP, Rosenbaum AM, et al. Accurate multiplex polony sequencing of an evolved bacterial genome. Science. 2005;309(5741):1728–32. Epub 2005/08/06.
75. Margulies M, Egholm M, Altman WE, Attiya S, Bader JS, Bemben LA, et al. Genome sequencing in microfabricated high-density picolitre reactors. Nature. 2005;437(7057):376–80. Epub 2005/08/02.
76. Rehm HL. Disease-targeted sequencing: a cornerstone in the clinic. Nat Rev Genet. 2013;14(4):295–300.
77. Mamanova L, Coffey AJ, Scott CE, Kozarewa I, Turner EH, Kumar A, et al. Target-enrichment strategies for next-generation sequencing. Nat Methods. 2010;7(2):111–8. Epub 2010/01/30.
78. Bamshad MJ, Ng SB, Bigham AW, Tabor HK, Emond MJ, Nickerson DA, et al. Exome sequencing as a tool for Mendelian disease gene discovery. Nat Rev Genet. 2011;12(11):745–55. Epub 2011/09/29.
79. Gilissen C, Hoischen A, Brunner HG, Veltman JA. Disease gene identification strategies for exome sequencing. Eur J Hum Genet EJHG. 2012;20(5):490–7. Epub 2012/01/20.
80. Patwardhan RP, Hiatt JB, Witten DM, Kim MJ, Smith RP, May D, et al. Massively parallel functional dissection of mammalian enhancers in vivo. Nat Biotechnol. 2012;30(3):265–70. Epub 2012/03/01.
81. Yuen RK, Thiruvahindrapuram B, Merico D, Walker S, Tammimies K, Hoang N, et al. Whole-genome sequencing of quartet families with autism spectrum disorder. Nat Med. 2015;21(2):185–91. Epub 2015/01/27.
82. Feero WG, Guttmacher AE. Genomics, personalized medicine, and pediatrics. Acad Pediatr. 2014;14(1): 14–22. Epub 2013/12/29.
83. Balasubramanian S. Decoding genomes. Biochem Soc Trans. 2015;43(1):1–5. Epub 2015/01/27.
84. Drmanac R, Peters BA, Church GM, Reid CA, Xu X. Accurate whole genome sequencing as the ultimate genetic test. Clin Chem. 2015;61(1):305–6. Epub 2014/12/07.
85. Reis LM, Tyler RC, Muheisen S, Raggio V, Salviati L, Han DP, et al. Whole exome sequencing in dominant cataract identifies a new causative factor, CRYBA2, and a variety of novel alleles in known genes. Hum Genet. 2013;132(7):761–70. Epub 2013/03/20.
86. Mackay DS, Bennett TM, Culican SM, Shiels A. Exome sequencing identifies novel and recurrent mutations in GJA8 and CRYGD associated with inherited cataract. Hum Genomics. 2014;8(1):19. Epub 2014/11/19.
87. Prokudin I, Simons C, Grigg JR, Storen R, Kumar V, Phua ZY, et al. Exome sequencing in developmental eye disease leads to identification of causal variants in GJA8, CRYGC, PAX6 and CYP1B1. Eur J Hum Genet EJHG. 2014;22(7):907–15. Epub 2013/11/28.
88. Lacro RV, Dietz HC, Wruck LM, Bradley TJ, Colan SD, Devereux RB, et al. Rationale and design of a randomized clinical trial of beta-blocker therapy (atenolol) versus angiotensin II receptor blocker therapy (losartan) in individuals with Marfan syndrome. Am Heart J. 2007;154(4):624–31. Epub 2007/09/26.
89. Klepper J. GLUT1 deficiency syndrome in clinical practice. Epilepsy Res. 2012;100(3):272–7. Epub 2011/03/09.
90. Hudson FP, Ireland JT, Ockenden BG, White-Jones RH. Diagnosis and treatment of galactosaemia. Br Med J. 1954;1(4856):242–5. Epub 1954/01/30.
91. Kuriyama M, Tokimura Y, Fujiyama J, Utatsu Y, Osame M. Treatment of cerebrotendinous xanthomatosis: effects of chenodeoxycholic acid, pravastatin, and combined use. J Neurol Sci. 1994;125(1):22–8. Epub 1994/08/01.
92. Mezer E, Babul-Hirji R, Wise R, Chipman M, DaSilva L, Rowell M, et al. Attitudes regarding predictive testing for retinitis pigmentosa. Ophthalmic Genet. 2007;28(1):9–15. Epub 2007/04/25.
93. Clarke AJ. Managing the ethical challenges of next-generation sequencing in genomic medicine. Br Med Bull. 2014;111(1):17–30. Epub 2014/08/15.
94. Gong B, Zhang LY, Lam DS, Pang CP, Yam GH. Sodium 4-phenylbutyrate ameliorates the effects of cataract-causing mutant gammaD-crystallin in cultured cells. Mol Vis. 2010;16:997–1003. Epub 2010/06/26.

95. Goulet DR, Knee KM, King JA. Inhibition of unfolding and aggregation of lens protein human gamma D crystallin by sodium citrate. Exp Eye Res. 2011;93(4):371–81. Epub 2011/05/24.
96. Knee KM, Goulet DR, Zhang J, Chen B, Chiu W, King JA. The group II chaperonin Mm-Cpn binds and refolds human gammaD crystallin. Protein Sci Publ Protein Soc. 2011;20(1):30–41. Epub 2010/10/29.
97. Gillespie RL, Hall G, Black GC. Genetic testing for inherited ocular disease: delivering on the promise at last? Clin Experiment Ophthalmol. 2014;42(1):65–77. Epub 2013/07/13.
98. Gillespie RL, Lloyd IC, Black GC. The use of autozygosity mapping and next-generation sequencing in understanding anterior segment defects caused by an abnormal development of the lens. Hum Hered. 2014;77(1-4):118–37. Epub 2014/07/26.

Morphology of Congenital Cataracts

4

David G. Morrison

4.1 Introduction

Diagnosis and management of congenital cataracts can be aided by an understanding of cataract morphology and presentation. Smaller opacities may be visually insignificant, and require only serial monitoring, while total opacities may require urgent surgical removal. The appearance and location of the cataract within the lens may provide a clue to the presence of systemic disease or metabolic disorder. A primary decision-making point involves the laterality of lens pathology. In general, unilateral cataracts are idiopathic and will not require systemic work-up. Bilateral cataracts are generally thought to be caused by genetic, metabolic or infectious etiologies; however, idiopathic cases are quite common [1]. Bilateral cataracts without a known pedigree of genetic inheritance require systemic evaluation.

D.G. Morrison, MD
Department of Ophthalmology and Visual Sciences, Vanderbilt University Medical Center Vanderbilt University, 2311 Pierce Avenue, Nashville, TN 37232, USA
e-mail: david.morrison.1@vanderbilt.edu

4.2 Defining Cataract Morphology Through Embryology

Extensive discussion of lens development is covered in Chap. 3. The lens begins to form at around 3 weeks of gestation in the human. Surface ectoderm invaginates into the optic pit to form a lens vesicle. The cells inside the lens vesicle expand to form a sphere. Subsequently, anterior epithelial cells proliferate and elongate to produce lens fibers that deposit around the embryonic nucleus to form the fetal nucleus. The connection of these cells forms the Y sutures that define the front and back portion of the fetal nucleus. The anterior Y suture is facing upwards, while the posterior Y suture is inverted. The space located between the Y sutures is defined after birth as the lens nucleus. Lens epithelium continues to develop, especially in early childhood, creating the lens cortex [2, 3]. It may be possible to estimate the time that a cataract forms with knowledge of lens embryology; however, great variability in presentation of lens opacities exists. Nuclear opacities are likely formed early in the development of the eye, while lamellar or cortical changes likely appear with later insults to the lens. As the continued development of the eye relies on complex interactions of embryonic tissues, many eyes with congenital nuclear cataract are smaller than normal eyes [4].

I.C. Lloyd, S.R. Lambert (eds.), *Congenital Cataract*, DOI 10.1007/978-3-319-27848-3_4

Several authors have proposed classification strategies to describe congenital cataracts [5–7]. For the purposes of this work, we will define cataract morphology by primary location of lens opacity. These will include total cataract, anterior lens opacities (anterior polar cataracts, anterior lenticonus), sectoral/zonular cataracts (lamellar cataract, sutural cataract, nuclear cataract, cortical cataract including diffuse lens opacities such as fleck or oil droplet cataract), posterior cataracts (posterior polar cataract, posterior subcapsular cataract, posterior lenticonus/lentiglobus), and persistent fetal vasculature (PFV).

4.3 Clinical Examination and Timing of Lensectomy

Examining an infant with cataract can be challenging. Visual assessment is generally limited to light reaction or fixing and following behaviors in infants less than 3 months of age. Evaluation of the lens opacity can be performed with portable slit lamp, but meticulous evaluation of lens morphology is not generally possible until the time of surgery with the operating microscope. Red reflex assessment is often performed in clinic to gauge the level of opacity and size of the cataract. Lens opacities greater than 3 mm are generally presumed to be of visual significance [8]. Dilated fundus exam is mandatory to determine if ciliary processes are stretched, or to determine if persistent fetal vasculature (PFV), mass, or retinal detachment are present. Ultrasonography should be performed prior to surgery if the posterior segment cannot be visualized. Finally, structural anterior segment abnormalities may present in conjunction with congenital cataract, and intraocular pressure should be measured. Intraoperative assessment may include corneal diameter and pachymetry assessments, axial length measurements, or gonioscopy.

Timing of lensectomy is critical in congenital cataracts to decrease form deprivation amblyopia. Without visual input, the neural pathways that carry vision rapidly deteriorate. Birch and colleagues have established that a critical period for visual development exists such that the best visual outcomes occur in children having lensectomy before 6 weeks of age for unilateral cataracts [9]. However, glaucoma rates are substantially higher when lensectomy is performed before 4 weeks of age [10]. Thus, many now advocate surgery between 4 and 6 weeks of age if possible.

4.4 Laboratory Assessment of Congenital Cataract

Laboratory assessment of bilateral congenital cataract can be costly and of limited clinical benefit. A complete infant and family history is often the best mechanism to determine what lab tests are needed.

4.4.1 Genetic Evaluation

While many cataracts are inherited, Chap. 3 details that no specific gene defect is associated with one exact lens morphology. It is estimated that 27 % of bilateral cataracts have a known family history [11]. As penetrance can be variable, examination of parents can reveal cataracts that have not been previously recognized. DNA microarray or whole exome sequencing can be performed; however, these tests are at present generally reserved for research purposes.

4.4.2 Infectious Causes

Infectious causes of congenital cataract should be evaluated when appropriate. Intrauterine infections with TORCH infections (toxoplasmosis, rubella, cytomegalovirus, and herpes virus) are highly associated with cataract formation [12–14]. Prenatal varicella infection is also highly associated with cataract formation [15]. A thorough maternal health history is necessary with specific questioning for infections or the presence of rash during pregnancy. A complete physical exam performed by the pediatrician is also needed to determine if systemic manifestation of infection are present. Many of these infants will present with skin lesions, hearing loss, pigmentary retinopathy, or other structural abnormalities that are a hallmark of infection. Due to this, diagnostic evaluation has often been initiated prior to surgery.

4.4.3 Systemic Syndromes

Evaluation of children with systemic syndromes may include karyotype analysis, or specific genetic testing. These tests should be initiated by a medical geneticist or general pediatrician rather than the ophthalmologist. Multiple systemic syndromes have been associated with cataract formation. Diseases with known genetic causes are outlined in Chap. 3. Common associations include Down syndrome [16], Lowe's syndrome [17], and peroxisomal disorders including rhizomelic chondrodysplasia, and Zellwegers syndrome [18].

4.4.4 Metabolic Disorders

Galactosemia is the prototypical example of a metabolic disease that results in cataract formation. This inborn error of metabolism is caused by a defect in galactokinase, galactose-1-phosphate uridyltransferase, or uridine diphosphate 1–4 epimerase. The absence of any of these enzymes causes poor break down of galactose sugars and the accumulation of galactitol within the lens. Water osmotically follows the galactitol into the lens. Hydration of lens fibers disrupts lens clarity. The initial change observed is oil droplet cataract formation in the lens cortex with progression of findings to total opacification of the lens over time. While infants are tested for this condition at birth, some infants may not have received an adequate milk feed with galactose for the test to be positive. Other symptoms of galactosemia include vomiting, and diarrhea. Most infants with galactosemia can be treated with dietary restriction and do not form cataracts [19].

Other common metabolic abnormalities include abnormalities of glucose or calcium metabolism. While infantile diabetes is rare, severe fluctuations of glucose due to maternal diabetes or severe systemic illness may contribute to infantile cataract formation [20, 21]. Abnormal calcium or phosphorus metabolism can be associated with hypoparathyroidism or skeletal diseases such as chondrodysplasia [22, 23].

Laboratory work up for congenital, bilateral cataracts of unknown origin may include: Basic metabolic panel or simple blood glucose, peroxisomal panel (VLCFA+phytanic acid), plasma amino acids, plasma acylcarnitine profile, red blood cell Galactose-1-phosphate, urine for reducing substances and urine amino acids. Infectious work up may include TORCH and varicella titers. Karyotype may be included if trisomy is suspected. Specific tests for an individual patient can be tailored by systemic findings and history (Table 4.1).

4.5 Unilateral Congenital Cataract Morphology

The Infant Aphakia Treatment Study added much to what is known about the morphology of unilateral congenital cataract [24]. The specific morphology of unilateral cataract was reported after expert video review from the 83 treated infants. Results are summarized in Table 4.2. Total cataract and posterior lentiglobus were present in less than 10 % of infants. Fetal nuclear cataracts were the most common form of unilateral cataract, presenting in 54 % of eyes. There was extension of

Table 4.1 Laboratory evaluation of bilateral infantile cataract of unknown origin

Laboratory exam	Diagnosis
Basic metabolic panel, or blood glucose	Hypoglycemia, diabetes mellitus
Peroxisomal panel (VLCFA, phytanic acid)	Perixozomal disorders (chondrodysplasia, zellweger syndrome, refsum disease, neonatal adrenoleukodystrophy)
Plasma amino acids, acylacarnitine profile Urine aminoacids	Lowe's syndrome
Red blood cell Galactose-1-phosphate Urine for reducing substances	Galactosemia
TORCH titres, varicella	Infectious causes
Karyotype	Trisomy
DNA microarray, exome sequencing[a]	Hereditary causes

[a]Generally reserved for research purposes

Table 4.2 Definition and occurrence of individual cataract diagnosis categories among 83 patients from the Infant Aphakia Treatment Study

	Diagnostic categories	Definition	N (% of 83 patients)
1	Entire lens is white	A uniform total white color lens with no red reflex visible even in the periphery of the lens	3 (3.6 %)
2	Lens partially reabsorbed	An appearance of reduced central lens thickness leaving little if any cortex between the central anterior and posterior capsule	7 (8.4 %)
3	Anterior capsular fibrosis	Presence of a dense, white fibrous-appearing opacity adherent to the anterior capsule	5 (6.0 %)
4	Anterior and/or posterior cortical opacity not involving nucleus	Opacity located within any of the cortex peripheral to the "Y" sutures with clear nuclear sparing	21 (25.3 %)
5	Opacity between Y-sutures (fetal nucleus)	Opaque lens material located between the anterior and posterior "Y" sutures	45 (54.2 %)
6	Nuclear opacity extending into surrounding cortex	An opacity appeared to be mostly nuclear but with "riders" spreading into the adjacent cortex or if a predominantly nuclear opacity demonstrated evidence of posterior cortical opacification behind the nucleus that extended towards the posterior capsule without intervening clear cortex	41 (49.4 %)
7	Posterior bowing of posterior lens capsule	Clear video evidence of bowing, such as posterior capsular defects associated with a lentiglobus lens.	4 (4.8 %)
8	Opacity of posterior lens capsule	Presence of opacity of the posterior capsule after the entire cortex had been surgically aspirated	73 (88.0 %)
9	Retrolental membrane with or without visible vessels	An opacity or vascular network on the posterior aspect of the lens that was associated with a fetal remnant and appeared to be distinct from a standard posterior capsular plaque	12 (14.5 %)
10	Patent persistent hyaloid vessel	Appearance of blood within the persistent hyaloid vessel	9 (10.8 %)
11	Non patent persistent hyaloid vessel	Absence of visible blood within the persistent hyaloid vessel	2 (2.4 %)
12	Ciliary processes stretched	Visible stretched ciliary process	2 (2.4 %)

nuclear opacity into posterior cortex in over 90 % of nuclear cataracts. Additionally 100 % of nuclear opacities had a posterior capsular plaque present after lens removal was complete (Fig. 4.1). Cortical cataract was present in 25 % of cases; 76 % of these also had posterior capsular plaque present. Six percent of eye had isolated findings of persistent fetal vasculature, and an additional 16 % had evidence of persistent hyaloid artery in the presence of another cataract form (either nuclear or posterior cortical opacity type).

4.5.1 Minimal Fetal Remnants

The concept of minimal fetal remnants was first introduced by Müllner-Eidenböck [25]. It was hypothesized that all unilateral cataracts resulted from a form of persistent fetal vasculature. In this study, 31 children with unilateral cataract were evaluated for persistent fetal remnants defined as perfused or non-perfused hyaloid remnants, but also including more subtle changes of the posterior lens such as posterior capsular plaque, retrolental membrane, and posterior bowing of lens capsule. All children with unilateral congenital cataract were reported to have changes consistent with classic PFV or minimal fetal remnants. This, in conjunction with IATS data, has led to the concept that PFV may present with a spectrum of severity. Severe cases may include a patent hyaloid remnant, ciliary body stretching, microphthalmia and retinal detachment. In milder forms, a unilateral congenital cataract with a posterior capsular

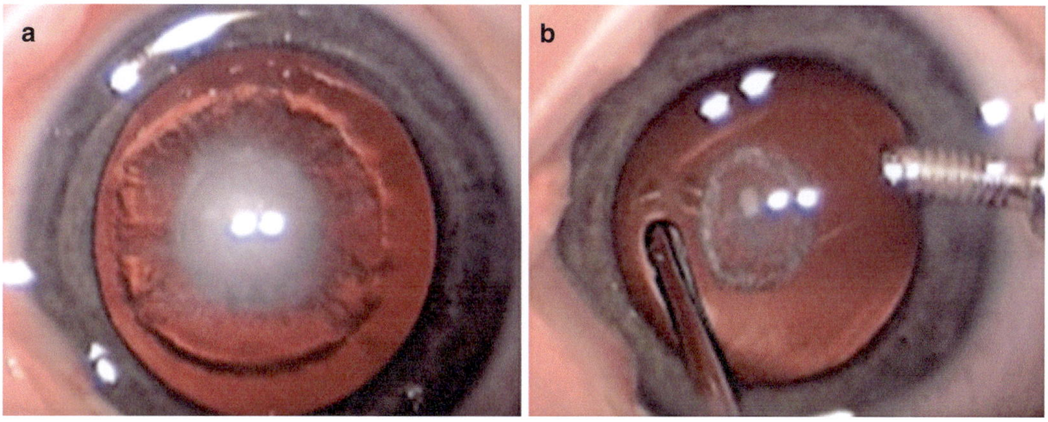

Fig. 4.1 Fetal nuclear cataract prior to surgery (**a**) and posterior capsule plaque visible after lens removal (**b**). Posterior capsular plaque may represent a fetal remnant and common origin of unilateral congenital cataract

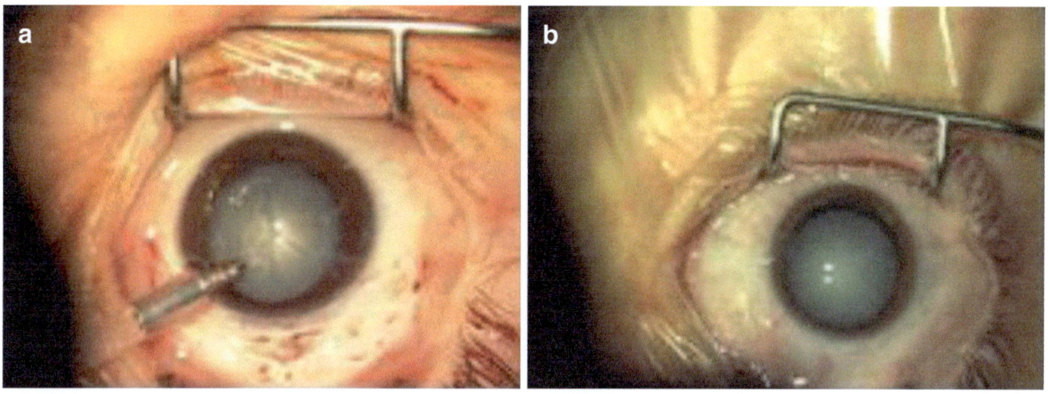

Fig. 4.2 Total cataract in two patients

plaque may be the only evidence of delayed hyaloid dissolution. The theory that many unilateral cataracts may result from a mild form of PFV has not been proven with basic clinical science. However, posterior capsular plaque has been studied in children with bilateral cataracts. As expected, the rate of posterior capsular plaque was much lower at 21 % in bilateral cataract cases [26].

4.6 Bilateral Congenital Cataract Morphology

Total cataract (Fig. 4.2) is the state of having a white lens, and no features of lens architecture beyond capsule able to be differentiated. Several genetic causes of total cataract have been identified. If left untreated, many forms of congenital cataract can progress to total lens opacity. As vision is completely obscured by this type of lens opacity, aggressive surgical intervention is warranted to clear the visual axis.

4.6.1 Anterior Cataracts

Anterior polar cataracts (Fig. 4.3) are lens opacities found on the anterior capsule of the lens. They are generally less than 1 mm in size. They are often hereditary if bilateral, but can occur sporadically in unilateral cases. Pyramidal cataracts are a more severe form of anterior polar cataract where the lens opacity extends forward into the anterior chamber towards the cornea. Pathological study of these specimens reveals these lesions to be composed of fibrous metaplasia of lens epithelium

(Figs. 4.4 and 4.5) [27]. It is likely that this type of opacity develops as a result of incomplete lens vesicle dislocation during emryogenesis. Due to their location, anterior polar cataracts are visible to the naked eye, and are often first noted by the parents. Anterior polar cataracts are not commonly visually significant, but can be associated with refractive error and amblyopia. If surgery is necessary, capsulorrhexis is quite challenging, as the capsule is pulled taught into the lesion. Thus, there is an even greater tendency for the capsule to tear peripherally than in other forms of infantile cataract [1].

Anterior lenticonus is a bulging, or weakening, of the anterior capsule. This type of cataract is quite rare. When present, a child should be examined for Alport's syndrome or Lowe's syndrome.

Other anterior cataracts include anterior plaque cataract (Fig. 4.6). These are commonly secondary to other structural abnormalities of lens development. Anterior plaque cataracts will be discussed in the PFV section. Anterior segment abnormalities such as persistent pupillary membranes often result in small lens opacities at the site of iris adhesion. These lens opacities are not usually significant; however, like anterior polar cataracts, refractive error and amblyopia are common.

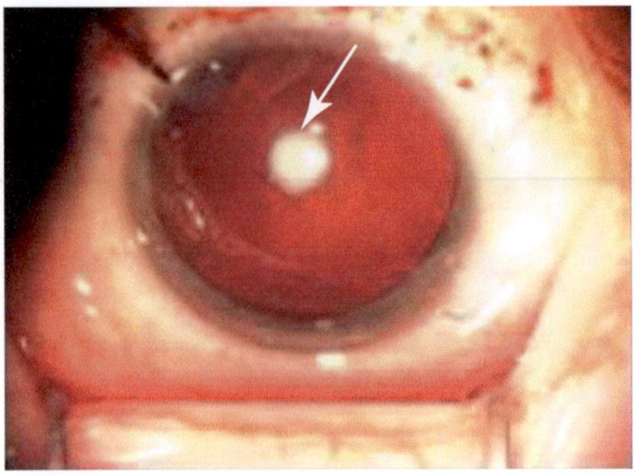

Fig. 4.3 Anterior polar cataract

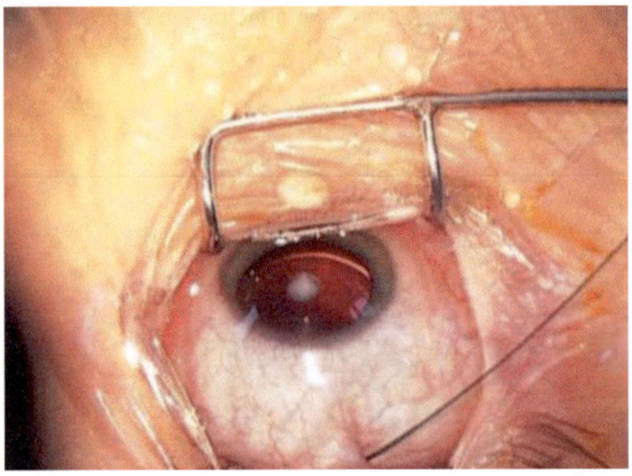

Fig. 4.4 Pyramidal cataract

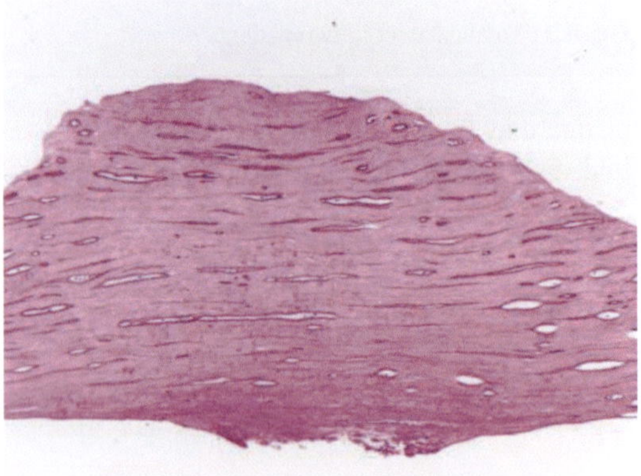

Fig. 4.5 Light microscopy of pyramidal cataract (periodic acid–Schiff, original magnification ×200) microphotograph revealing probable fibrous metaplasia of the lens epithelium

4.6.2 Zonular Cataracts

Lamellar cataracts appear as a fine haze surrounding the border of the fetal nucleus. Lamellar cataracts may be visually insignificant at birth, but can be progressive and visually significant. These generally occur later in fetal development. It is thought that a transient insult impacts the lens, and an opacity forms at the demarcation zone defining the fetal nuclear and the surrounding cortical tissue (Fig. 4.7). This type of opacity is often associated with an autosome dominant inheritance pattern. Examination of primary relatives may alleviate the need for extensive laboratory work up in these cases.

Suture (sutural) cataracts occur within the fetal nuclear anterior or posterior Y sutures. Suture cataracts alone are generally not visually significant, but can occur in conjunction with other forms of visually significant lens opacity such as lamellar opacity.

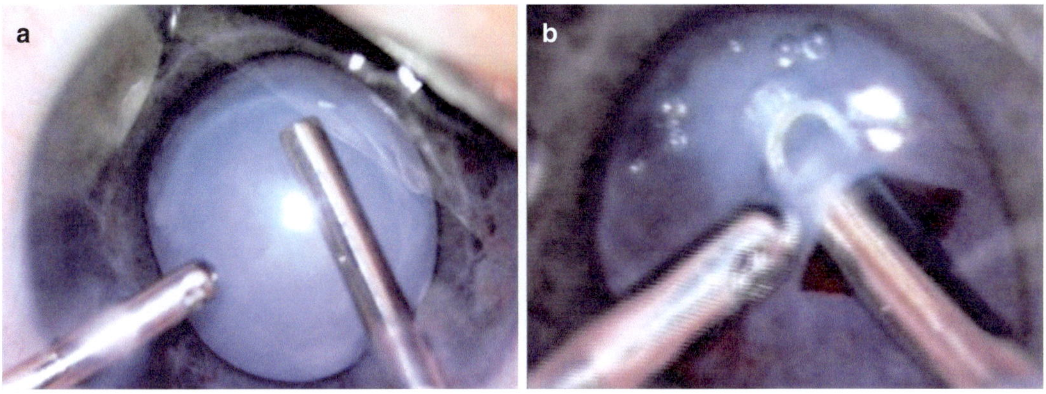

Fig. 4.6 Total cataract (**a**) associated with anterior capsular plaque (**b**), most notable with anterior capsulotomy

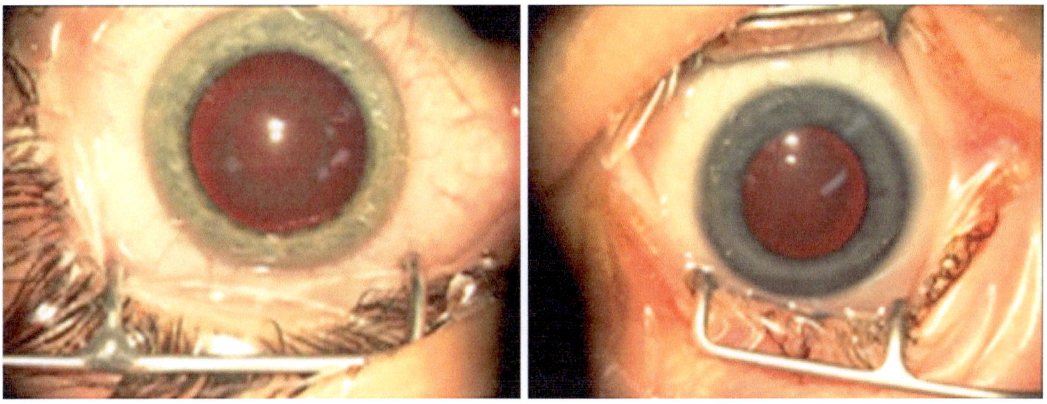

Fig. 4.7 Lamellar cataract with fleck opacities surrounding fetal nucleus

Congenital nuclear cataract is the most common form of unilateral cataract; bilateral nuclear cataracts are common as well. This is an opacity that appears between the Y sutures of the lens. Opacities are generally 3–4 mm in size (roughly the size of the fetal nucleus). It is common for the opacity to extend into the cortex surrounding the nucleus. When this is present, the term cortical rider is used (Fig. 4.8). Multiple inheritance patterns are reported within genetic pedigrees, with autosomal dominant forms being common. Congenital nuclear cataracts are almost always visually significant, and surgical intervention is necessary.

Cortical cataract (Fig. 4.9) changes generally occur late in development, or after birth. Cortical cataracts include isolated lens abnormalities and diffuse lens changes such as oil droplet or fleck cataract. While heritable forms are reported, systemic syndromes are commonly associated with this presentation. Galactosemia is associated with oil droplet cataract formation due to poor metabolic break down of galactose sugars. Fleck cataracts are commonly associated with systemic syndromes such as Down syndrome. Cortical cataracts associated with metabolic diseases are less likely to be visually significant at birth. Milder forms of cortical cataract should be serially monitored for progression.

Posterior subcapsular cataract (PSC) is often seen in children after the use of corticosteroids. However, infantile forms can be present. Autosomal dominant and recessive forms are reported (Fig. 4.10). Systemic syndromes such as neurofibromatosis type 2 are also associated with PSC cataract.

Posterior polar lens opacities are opacities of the posterior cortex and lens capsule. It is likely

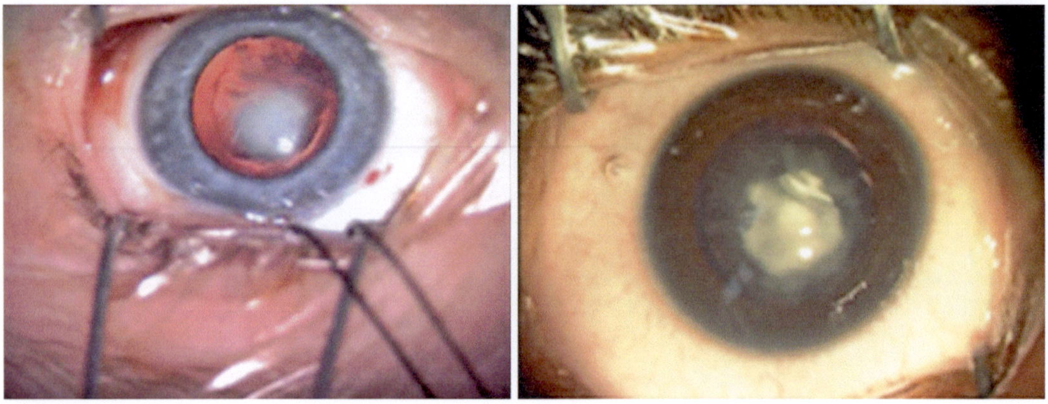

Fig. 4.8 Nuclear cataract with cortical riders present

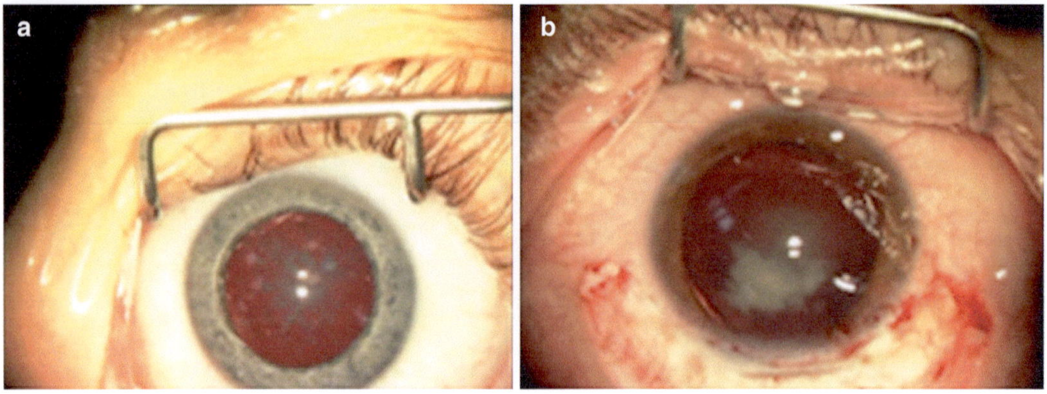

Fig. 4.9 Cortical cataract displaying diffuse fleck opacities (**a**) and sectoral lens changes (**b**)

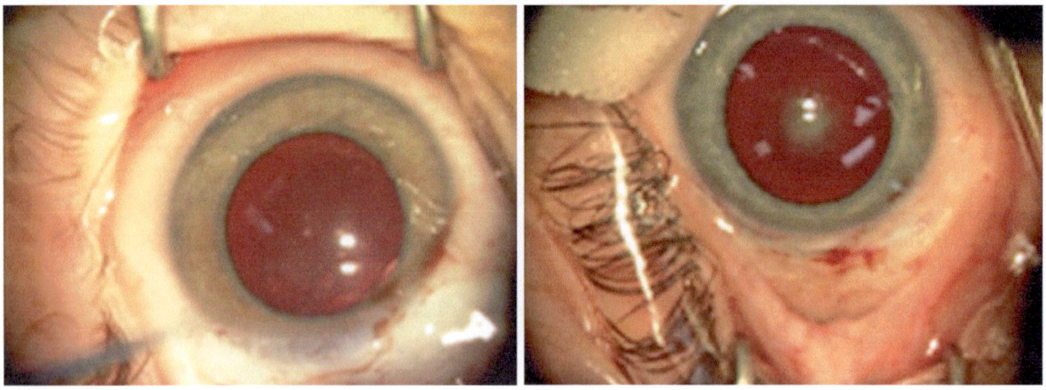

Fig. 4.10 Posterior subcapsular cataract in an infant

that these opacities occur on a spectrum with posterior lentiglobus. Wilson defines posterior polar cataracts as a posterior opacity that initial presents without a posterior bulging of the lens capsule. This is different from lentiglobus in that this type of lens abnormality may initially present with a lens capsule defect, but no opacity [21]. Due to posterior location of this lens opacity, it is

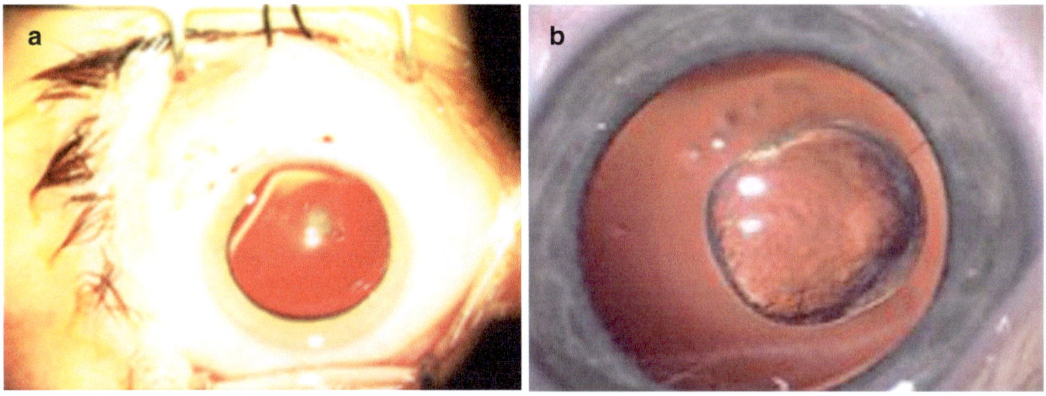

Fig. 4.11 Posterior polar cataract (**a**). Note the wrinkling of posterior capsule present under high illumination. Posterior lentiglobus cataract with hyaloid remnant visible to the right (**b**)

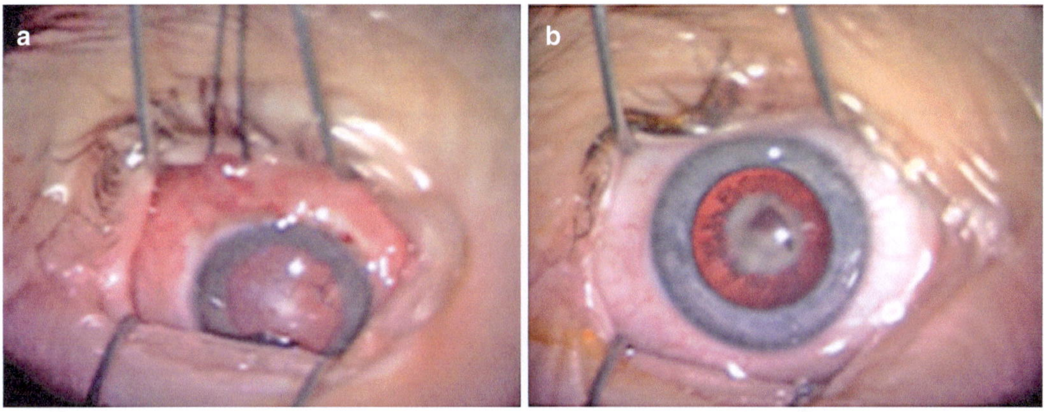

Fig. 4.12 PFV cataracts demonstrating vascularized retrolental membrane with relatively clear lens (**a**), and central nuclear and posterior cortical opacity with intralenticular hemorrhage caused by patent hyaloid artery remnant (**b**)

often visually significant, although the size of the opacity is integral to determining if surgery is necessary (Fig. 4.11).

Posterior lenticonus/lentiglobus refers to a weakness of the posterior capsule of the lens, causing a herniation of the capsule posteriorly into the vitreous cavity (Fig. 4.11). While the capsular abnormality is present from birth, the lens itself may initially remain clear. It is thought that the posterior capsule eventually opens, allowing fluid to infiltrate the lens, thus causing opacity. These cataracts may be visually insignificant at birth, but become opacified in a very brief period. Thus, surgery should be attempted even when the child is older. Autosomal dominant forms of lentiglobus exist, but may occur as sporadic, unilateral cases as well.

Persistent fetal vasculature (PFV) is caused by the presence of a hyaloid artery remnant on the posterior aspect of the lens. The hyaloid artery supplies the anterior segment of the eye during fetal development. After the development of the anterior ciliary circulation, the hyaloid artery regresses. If persistent, this remnant can be perfused or unperfused. It can be associated with anterior or posterior capsular plaque, central nuclear or posterior cortical cataract, and abnormal anterior segment vasculature resembling iris neovascularization. PFV lenses may also have retrolental membranes that exist behind the lens capsule. Often vascularized, this tissue can be quite dense and challenging to remove surgically (Fig. 4.12). It is estimated that fewer than 10 % of cases are bilateral in nature. There are two pedigrees of hereditary PFV reported. One occurred in Korean twins, and a second occurred in multiple members of an Egyptian family [28, 29].

4.6.3 Special Cases

Several additional ocular syndromes may present with congenital cataract in addition to structural abnormalities of the eye. Lens coloboma results from the failure of lens material and zonules to develop in a specific area of the lens. Cataract associated with this type of abnormality can be congenital, but is often developmental. Care should be taken in determining if there is enough zonular stability to support an intraocular lens in these cases. Microspherophakia occurs when zonular development is completely absent. The resultant small, round lens may sublux into the anterior chamber and cause pupillary block [21]. Ectopia lentis et pupillae is a condition associated with ectopic pupil and displaced crystalline lens. It is thought to be autosomal recessive, although a dominant pedigree has been published [30]. Iridogoniodysgenesis is a term describing iris and corneal abnormalities associated with glaucoma, cataract, and lens changes (Fig. 4.13). It is unclear if this condition represents a new genetic diagnosis or a more severe presentation of known abnormalities such as Axenfeld- Reiger syndrome and Peters Anomaly. Anterior segment dysgenesis syndromes have been associated with neural crest cell migration abnormalities caused by PAX6, PITX2, and FOXC1 genes [31].

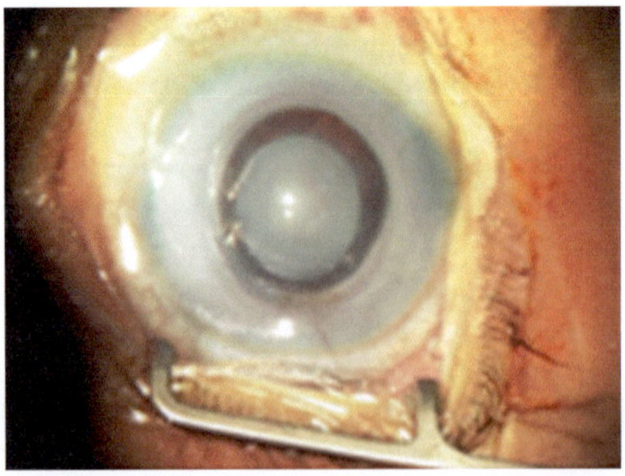

Fig. 4.13 Iridogoniodysgenesis syndrome. Buphthalmos from congenital glaucoma is present and iris is hypoplastic. Lens is small and subluxed into the anterior chamber

References

1. Amaya L, Taylor D, Russell-Eggitt I, et al. The morphology and natural history of childhood cataracts. Surv Ophthalmol. 2003;48:125–44.
2. Zwann J. Fine structure of the developing lens. Int Ophthalmol Clin. 1975;15:39–52.
3. Ozanics V, Jacobiec FA. Prenatal development of the eye and its adnexa. In: Tasman W, editor. Biomedical foundations of ophthalmology. Philadelphia: JB Lippincott & Co; 1993. p. 1–86.
4. Johnson DA, Parks MM. Cataracts in childhood: prognosis and complications. Semin Ophthalmol. 1991;6:201–11.
5. Clapp C. Cataract: its aetiology and treatment. London: Henry Kimpton Press; 1934.
6. Duke-Elder S. The eye. London: Henry Kimpton Press; 1964. p. 715–59.
7. Lambert SR, Drack AV. Infantile cataracts. Surv Ophthalmol. 1996;40(6):427–58.
8. Wright K, Matsumoto E, Edelmann P. Binocular fusion and stereopsis associated with early for monocular congenital cataracts. Am J Ophthalmol. 1992; 114:409–15.
9. Birch EE, Steger DR. The critical period for surgical treatment of dense congenital unilateral cataract. Invest Ophthalmol Vis Sci. 1996;37:1532–8.
10. Vishwanath M, Cheong-Leen R, Taylor D, et al. Is early surgery for congenital cataract a risk factor for glaucoma? Br J Ophthalmol. 2004;88(7):905–10.
11. Rahi JS, Dezateux C. Congenital and infantile cataract in the United Kingdom: underlying or associated factors. Invest Ophthalmol Vis Sci. 2000;41:2108–14.
12. Stagno S, Reynolds DW, Amos CS, et al. Auditory and visual defects resulting from symptomatic and subclinical cytomegalovirus and toxoplasma infections. Pediatrics. 1977;59:669–78.
13. Cotlier E. Congenital rubella cataracts. In: Cotlier E, Lambert SR, Taylor D, editors. Congenital cataracts. Boca Raton: R.G. Landes/CRC; 1994. p. 65–76.
14. Nahmias AJ, Visintine A, Caldwell DR, et al. Eye infections with herpes simplex viruses in neonates. Surv Ophthalmol. 1976;21:100–5.
15. Lambert SR, Taylor D, Kriss A, et al. Ocular manifestations of the congenital Varicella syndrome. Arch Ophthalmol. 1989;107:52–6.
16. Catalano RA. Down syndrome. Surv Ophthalmol. 1990;24:56–63.
17. Tripathi RC, Cibis GW, Tripathi BJ. Pathogenesis of cataracts in patients with Lowe's syndrome. Ophthalmology. 1986;93:1046–51.
18. Kohlschutter A, Bley A, Brockmann K, et al. Leukodystrophies and other genetic metabolic leukodystrophies in children and adults. Brain Dev. 2010; 32(2):82–9.

19. Stambolian D. Galactose and cataract. Surv Ophthalmol. 1988;32:333–49.
20. Merin S, Crawford JS. Hypoglycemia and infantile cataracts. Can J Ophthalmol. 1971;6:495–8.
21. Wilson ME, Trivedi RH, Pandey SK, Johnson JJ. Etiology and morphology of pediatric cataracts. In: Wilson ME, Trivedi RH, editors. Pediatric cataract surgery. Philadelphia: Lippincott Williams & Wilkins; 2014. p. 9–21.
22. Gass JD. The syndrome of keratoconjunctivitis, superficial moniliasis, idiopathic hypoparathyropidism and Addison's disease. Am J Ophthalmol. 1962;54:660.
23. Jones KL. Smith's recognizable patterns of human malformation. Philadelphia: WB Saunders Co; 1976. p. 340.
24. Wilson ME, Trivedi RH, Morrison DG, et al. The Infant Aphakia Treatment Study: evaluation of cataract morphology in eyes with monocular cataracts. J AAPOS. 2011;15:421–6.
25. Mullner-Eidenbock A, Amon M, Moser E, et al. Persistent fetal vasculature and minimal fetal vascular remnants. Ophthalmology. 2004;111:906–13.
26. Morrison DG, Lambert SR, Wilson ME. Posterior capsular plaque in bilateral congenital cataracts. J AAPOS. 2012;16:17–20.
27. Chang TC, Reyes MC, Morrison DG, Albert DM. Anterior polar cataract: a clinical pathological correlation. JAMA Ophthalmol. 2013;131:22.
28. Yu YS, Chang BL. Persistent hyperplastic primary vitreous in male twins. Korean J Ophthalmol. 1997; 11:123–5.
29. Galal AH, Kotoury AI, Azzab AA. Bilateral persistent hyperplastic primary vitreous: an Egyptian family supporting a rare autosomal dominant inheritance. Genet Couns. 2006;17:441–7.
30. Cruysberg JR, Pinckers A. Ectopia lentis et pupillae syndrome in three generations. Br J Ophthalmol. 1995;79(2):135–8.
31. Ito YA, Walter MA. Genomics and anterior segment dysgenesis: a review. Clin Experiment Ophthalmol. 2014;42(1):13–24.

5 Baseline Predictors of Visual Outcome

E. Eugenie Hartmann

Surgical techniques have greatly improved in the last 50 years and the majority of cataract extractions in infant eyes are technically successful [1]. Nonetheless, the treatment of these patients postoperatively, especially those with a unilateral cataract, is intense and arduous for both the clinician and the family. These children require regular monitoring to ensure the proper correction of their refractive error, especially during the first few years when most eye growth occurs. Additionally, in the case of a unilateral congenital cataract (UCC), the untreated eye must be occluded part-time on a consistent basis, to allow neural connections to develop so that a reasonable level of visual function can be obtained. Thus, given the years of impending commitment when confronted with a family whose child has a UCC, any baseline predictors that will elucidate the potential outcome for that child are helpful to provide sufficient motivation for parents to follow the arduous postoperative treatment regimen. The purpose of this chapter is to empirically specify the extent to which baseline characteristics of a patient can be used to predict recognition visual acuity at 4.5 years of age.

E.E. Hartmann, PhD
Department of Vision Sciences, University of Alabama at Birmingham,
42/2 Vestview Circle, Birmingham, AL 35242, USA
e-mail: eehartmann@uab.edu

5.1 Baseline Characteristics

Using data from the Infant Aphakia Treatment Study (IATS), we defined three categories of baseline characteristics that are typically accessible to any clinician [2].

1. Physical characteristics of the cataractous eye;
2. Physiological characteristics of the infant, including age;
3. Sociological characteristics of the family.

The complete set of variables, separated according to these three categories, is listed in Table 5.1 along with summary statistics from the IATS population for each. Characteristics of the treated eye included the type of cataract (mild or possibly developmental, versus other), corneal diameter, average central keratometric power, axial length, intraocular pressure and pupil diameter. Physiological characteristics of the infant included: age at surgery, gestational age at birth, birth weight, sex, race (white versus other), and whether Hispanic. Sociologic characteristics of the participant's family included whether or not the family had private insurance, age of the primary caregiver at the time of surgery, and the highest education level achieved by either mother or father.

Many of the characteristics of the treated eye were restricted by the inclusion and exclusion criteria for the IATS. Thus patients with a corneal diameter <9 mm or an intraocular pressure ≥25 mmHg were automatically excluded. Additionally, patients

I.C. Lloyd, S.R. Lambert (eds.), *Congenital Cataract*, DOI 10.1007/978-3-319-27848-3_5

Table 5.1 Summary statistics for baseline characteristics

Baseline characteristic	# Patients	Summary statistics[a]
Characteristics of treated eye		
Type of cataract (mild/possibly developmental)	114	14 (12 %)
Orthotropic (yes)	108	80 (74 %)
Corneal diameter (mm)	114	10.5 ± 0.7, 9.0–12.5
Average central keratometric power (D)	114	46.4 ± 2.7, 40.1–53.8
Axial length (mm)	101	18.0 ± 1.3, 15.6–21.9
Intraocular pressure (mmHg)	114	12.2 ± 4.9, 3.0–24.0
Pupil diameter (mm)	101	3.3 ± 1.0, 1.0–6.0
Aphakia treatment (IOL)	114	57 (50 %)
Physiological characteristics of infant		
Patient age at surgery (months)	114	1.8 (1.2–3.2), 0.9–6.8
Patient age strata at surgery (49–210 days)	114	64 (56 %)
Gestational age at birth (weeks)	102	38.8 ± 1.3, 36–42
Birth weight (grams)	112	3457 ± 489, 2041–5087
Gender (female)	114	60 (53 %)
Race (white)	114	97 (85 %)
Hispanic (yes)	114	19 (17 %)
Sociological characteristics of family		
Private insurance (yes)	114	70 (61 %)[b]
Primary caregiver age at surgery (years)	111	29.2 ± 5.7, 16.8–41.7
Highest education level of mother or father		
High school graduate or less	111	24 (22 %)
Vocational/some college		40 (36 %)
College graduate		27 (24 %)
Graduate or professional school		20 (18 %)

[a]The values for the summary statistics follow one of the following forms: n (%); mean ± standard deviation, range; median (inter-quartile range), range

[b]The 44 patients without private insurance reported the following insurance coverage: medicaid: 38; self-pay: 2; other: 4

whose cataractous eye had persistent fetal vasculature (PFV) causing stretching of the ciliary processes or tractional detachment of the retina were not eligible. The presence of active uveitis or signs of previous episodes of uveitis, as well as retinal disease or optic nerve disease, that could limit the visual potential of the eye were also exclusion criteria. These are all likely poor prognostic factors, but will not be discussed in this chapter.

We used the 4.5 year recognition visual acuity (VA) data to explore the relationship between baseline variables and later visual outcome. Correlations were determined between each baseline characteristic as a single variable and logMAR VA. The results are shown in Tables 5.2 and 5.3, with statistical analyses from continuous baseline variables listed in Table 5.2 and analyses from categorical variables listed in Table 5.3. We found that only age at the time of surgery and type of health care insurance had any statistically significant relationship with logMAR VA in our sample. Nonetheless, we will initially discuss information obtained about the type of cataract.

5.2 Type of Cataract

The majority of surgeries were videotaped and a total of 83 were available for classification of cataract type [3]. The remaining 31 were classified at the time of surgery by the clinician. Only 14 of the IATS patients had cataracts that were classified as mild or possibly acquired. The range of the acuities measured between the two groups

Table 5.2 Bivariate associations of continuous baseline characteristics and visual acuity at 4.5 years of age

Baseline characteristic	# Patients	Spearman rank correlation coefficient for factor and visual acuity (p-value)
Characteristics of treated eye		
Corneal diameter	112	0.11 (0.27)
Average central keratometric power	112	0.03 (0.79)
Axial length	99	0.15 (0.14)
Intraocular pressure	112	0.07 (0.48)
Pupil diameter	99	0.05 (0.60)
Physiological characteristics of infant		
Patient age at surgery	112	0.19 (0.041)
Gestational age at birth	100	−0.03 (0.78)
Birth weight	110	−0.04 (0.65)
Sociological characteristics of family		
Primary caregiver age at surgery	109	−0.02 (0.87)

was almost identical. This factor plus the low number of mild or possibly acquired cataracts, and the unequal numbers between the two categories most likely explains the lack of significant statistical difference.

5.3 Age at Surgery

We analyzed age at surgery both as a continuous and a categorical variable. Visual acuity at 4.5 years of age was weakly associated with age at surgery for both analyses. When age was considered as a continuous variable, the Spearman rank correlation coefficient was 0.19, P = 0.041. Similarly, when age was examined as a categorical variable, the median visual acuity was significantly better for patients whose surgery occurred earlier rather than later (≤48 days = 0.50 logMAR; ≥49 days = 1.10 logMAR, P = 0.046).

Table 5.3 Bivariate associations of categorical baseline characteristics and visual acuity at 4.5 years of age

Baseline characteristic	# Patients	Visual acuity (logMAR) Median (IQR[a])	p-value[b]
Characteristics of treated eye			
Type of cataract			
Mild/possibly acquired	14	1.15 (0.30–1.60)	0.72
Other	98	0.80 (0.30–1.70)	
Orthotropic			
No	27	1.20 (0.70–1.92)	0.17
Yes	79	0.70 (0.30–1.70)	
Aphakia treatment			
CL	57	0.90 (0.30–1.60)	0.54
IOL	55	0.90 (0.40–1.73)	
Physiological characteristics of infant			
Patient age at surgery			
28–48 days	48	0.50 (0.20–1.55)	0.046
49–210 days	64	1.10 (0.50–1.71)	
Gender			
Female	59	0.70 (0.30–1.40)	0.60
Male	53	1.10 (0.30–1.82)	
Race			
White	95	1.00 (0.30–1.70)	0.82
Non-white	17	0.70 (0.40–1.40)	
Hispanic			
No	94	0.85 (0.30–1.73)	0.89
Yes	18	0.95 (0.30–1.70)	

(continued)

Table 5.3 (continued)

Baseline characteristic	# Patients	Visual acuity (logMAR) Median (IQR[a])	p-value[b]
Sociological characteristics of family			
Private insurance			
No	43	1.40 (0.60–2.22)	0.0004
Yes	69	0.60 (0.30–1.20)	
Highest education level of mother or father			
High graduate or less	23	1.10 (0.50–1.20)	0.19
Vocational/some college	40	0.90 (0.30–2.17)	
College graduate	27	0.70 (0.30–1.20)	
Graduate or professional school	19	0.50 (0.30–1.20)	

[a]*IQR* interquartile range
[b]The p-value for the Wilcoxon rank sum test comparing the medians of two groups or the Kruskall-Wallis test comparing the medians of more than two groups

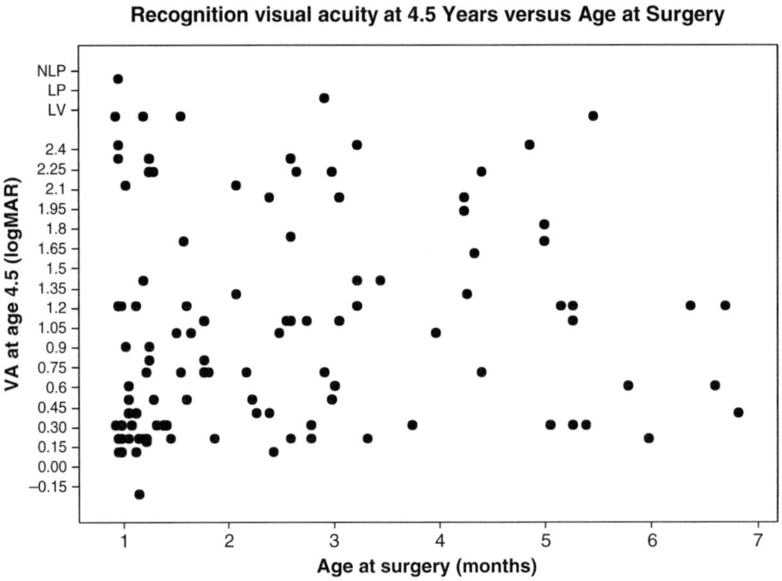

Fig. 5.1 Recognition visual acuity at 4.5 years versus age at surgery

Previous research by Birch and colleagues [4] has demonstrated that the optimal time for initial surgery for a UCC is between 4 and 6 weeks of age. Our data concur with these reports. Nonetheless some of the patients whose surgery occurred later than 48 days were able to achieve a reasonable degree of vision in their treated eye, as can be seen in Fig. 5.1. The implication from this result should not be taken as an endorsement of postponing initial surgery, but rather as an indication that the outcome could still be positive, even if the patient presents later than 6 weeks of age.

5.4 Type of Health Insurance

The only other baseline characteristic that showed an association with visual acuity at age 4.5 years was the type of health insurance available to the family. Patients from families with private insurance had significantly better median visual acuity at 4.5 years age (0.60 vs. 0.1.40 logMAR, P=0.0004).

5.5 Multivariate Analysis

Our next step was to use all baseline characteristic variables in a multivariate analysis. Interestingly enough, a multiple regression analysis of these data demonstrated that the type of health insurance available to the family was the only variable that contributed to the model. Unfortunately, while the association was highly statistically significant (P=0.002), the regression model accounted for only 12 % of the variability, meaning that there are many more influences on visual outcome that we have not yet identified.

It is likely that the type of health insurance coverage held by a family is a stand-in for a measure of socio-economic status (SES) in our population. In a previous report we established that better adherence to occlusion therapy during the first 3 months after surgery was associated with the presence of private health insurance [5]. In addition, closer inspection of the data presented here identifying the association between type of health insurance and all other baseline characteristics demonstrated that families with private health insurance tended to have higher levels of education and caregivers were older. (See Table 5.4)

Table 5.4 Relationship between private insurance and other baseline characteristics

	Private insurance		
Characteristic	No (n=44)	Yes (n=70)	p-value[a]
Characteristics of treated eye			
Type of cataract (mild/possibly developmental)	4 (9 %)	10 (14 %)	0.56
Orthotropic	(n=41) 28 (68 %)	(n=67) 52 (78 %)	0.37
Corneal diameter (mm)	10.4±0.7	10.5±0.8	0.79
Average central keratometric power (D)	45.9±2.5	46.7±2.8	0.15
Axial length (mm)	(n=42) 18.0±1.3	(n=59) 17.9±1.3	0.70
Intraocular pressure (mmHg)	12.2±5.1	12.2±4.8	0.99
Pupil diameter (mm)	(n=43) 3.0±0.8	(n=58) 3.5±1.0	0.016
Aphakia treatment (IOL)	24 (55 %)	33 (47 %)	0.56
Physiological characteristics of infant			
Patient age at surgery (months)	2.1 (1.2–3.1)	1.8 (1.2–3.2)	0.88
Patient age strata at surgery (49–210 days)	26 (59 %)	38 (54 %)	0.70
Gestational age at birth (weeks)	(n=41) 38.9±1.5	(n=61) 38.8±1.1	0.68
Birth weight (grams)	(n=43) 3492±501	(n=69) 3435±484	0.55
Gender (male)	19 (43 %)	41 (59 %)	0.13
Race (white)	36 (81 %)	61 (87 %)	0.43
Hispanic (yes)	12 (27 %)	7 (10 %)	0.021
Sociological characteristics of family			
Primary caregiver age at surgery (years)	(n=41) 26.3±6.3	30.9±4.6	<0.0001
Highest education level of mother or father:	(n=42)	(n=69)	<0.0001
High school graduate or less	19 (45 %)	5 (7 %)	
Vocational/some college	16 (38 %)	24 (35 %)	
College graduate	8 (14 %)	21 (30 %)	
Graduate or professional school	1 (2 %)	19 (28 %)	

Values are n (%), mean ± standard deviation, or median (interquartile range)

[a]p-value for comparing patients with and without private insurance on percentages (fisher's exact test), means (independent groups t test), or medians (Wilcoxon rank sum test)

[b]Maximum education attained by the mother or father

There is an extensive literature demonstrating that poverty and poor health are closely related [6]. In fact, the topic of health disparities is receiving a great deal of attention at national level in the USA, particularly in terms of decreasing this phenomenon. Thus, it is not totally surprising that we found a significant association between type of health insurance available to a family and visual outcome for IATS patients. To the best of our knowledge, the association between visual outcome in children with UCC and the SES of their family as a baseline characteristic, has not been previously reported.

5.6 Discussion

While the association between recognition visual acuity and type of health insurance is highly statistically significant at P=0.0002, only 12% of the variance is accounted for by this factor. Ultimately, this implies that numerous other elements not identifiable at the time of surgery contribute to the final visual outcome. Nonetheless, the clinician can take heed of this evidence and recognize that in the USA, families whose health insurance is other than private, are likely to require additional support in order to obtain an optimal visual outcome for their child. This assistance could be offered through a Social Worker trained to address issues of child behavior and occlusion treatment for amblyopia. It is also highly likely that the extended family's attitudes will influence the parents' acceptance of the required patching regimen. Seeing a young infant in glasses and/or wearing a patch may initially generate an alarming response. However, with suitable education parents can understand that the efforts they are making to adhere to the patching requirement while their child is young may enable their child to be better able to perform activities later in life, e.g. playing sports such as baseball; driving. Finally it is prudent to put additional help in place early in the treatment process.

Justification of the intensive rehabilitation process for a child with a UCC is provided by the frequency of good visual outcomes. Children with significant amblyopia of one eye have been shown to be at higher risk of losing vision in their "normal" other eye later in life [7]. Therefore achieving a reasonable level of visual function in the treated eye can provide them with a "spare" eye and help prevent severe visual impairment should this situation arise.

References

1. Vasavada AR, Praveen MR, Tassignon MJ, Shah SK, Vasavada VA, Vasavada VA, Looveren JV, De Veuster I, Trivedi RH. Posterior capsule management in congenital cataract surgery. J Cataract Refract Surg. 2011;37(1):173–93.
2. Hartmann EE, Lynn MJ, Lambert SR, Infant Aphakia Treatment Study Group. Baseline characteristics of the Infant Aphakia Treatment Study: predicting recognition acuity at 45 years of age. Invest Ophthalmol Vis Sci. 2015;56:388–95.
3. Wilson ME, Trivedi RH, Morrison DG, et al. The Infant Aphakia Treatment Study: evaluation of cataract morphology in eyes with monocular cataracts. J AAPOS. 2011;15:421–6.
4. Birch EE, Stager DR. The critical period for surgical treatment of dense congenital unilateral cataract. Invest Ophthalmol Vis Sci. 1996;37:1532–8.
5. Drews-Botsch CD, Hartmann EE, Celano M, Infant Aphakia Treatment Study Group. Predictors of adherence to occlusion therapy three months after cataract extraction in the Infant Aphakia Treatment Study. J AAPOS. 2012;16(2):150–5.
6. Fiscella K, Williams DR. Health disparities based on socioeconomic inequities: implications for urban health care. Acad Med. 2004;79:1139–47.
7. Rahi JS, Logan S, Timms C, Russell-Eggitt I, Taylor D. Risk, causes, and outcomes of visual impairment after loss of vision in the non-amblyopic eye: a population-based study. Lancet. 2002;360(9333): 597–602.

Part III

Surgical Techniques

6 Anterior Capsulotomy

Ken K. Nischal

6.1 The Pediatric Capsule

The neonatal pediatric lens capsule differs from the infant lens capsule, which differs from the toddler lens capsule, which differs from the child over 4 years of age. This difference is in the elasticity of the capsule. This elasticity can make it difficult to control the shape and direction of any manual rhexis that is attempted unless the surgeon is aware of it. There is good evidence that by making the opening of the anterior capsule slightly smaller than the optic of any intraocular lens that may be placed in the bag, the rate of posterior capsule opacification is reduced [1]. While this is important in adult cataract surgery it becomes less relevant in pediatric cataract surgery since posterior capsulorhexis is often performed in children. However, its importance lies in the fact children will often rub their eyes vigorously and this results in a trampolining effect of the anterior chamber; if the anterior capsulotomy diameter is larger than the optic of the IOL, then this can cause fusion of the anterior and posterior capsules with the inevitable IOL iris capture (see Fig. 6.1). It therefore becomes important to develop techniques that allow reliable and repeatable anterior capsulotomy of the correct size in children. The need for such techniques is greater the younger the child.

K.K. Nischal, MD, FRCOphth
Pediatric Ophthalmology, Strabismus and Adult Motility, Children's Hospital of Pittsburgh of UPMC, University of Pittsburgh, Pittsburgh, PA, USA
e-mail: nischalkk@upmc.edu

6.2 Anterior Capsulotomy Techniques

There are several techniques that have been employed to perform anterior capsulotomy in children. They include

- Vitrectorhexis
- Diathermy
- Plasma blade
- Traditional Manual capsulorhexis
- Foldable template ring
- Two Incision push-pull (TIPP) rhexis
- Femtosecond laser

6.2.1 Vitrectorhexis

In this technique a low aspiration high cut rate is employed to construct an anterior capsular opening. The vitrector port can be employed face down so that the initial cut is employed to break into the capsule and then a smooth circular motion employed to complete the opening. Alternatively after the initial cut is made the port is turned up and the opening made in exactly the same way but now the surgeon has a view of where the cut is being made. A venturi pump is best for this technique because a peristaltic pump

I.C. Lloyd, S.R. Lambert (eds.), *Congenital Cataract*, DOI 10.1007/978-3-319-27848-3_6

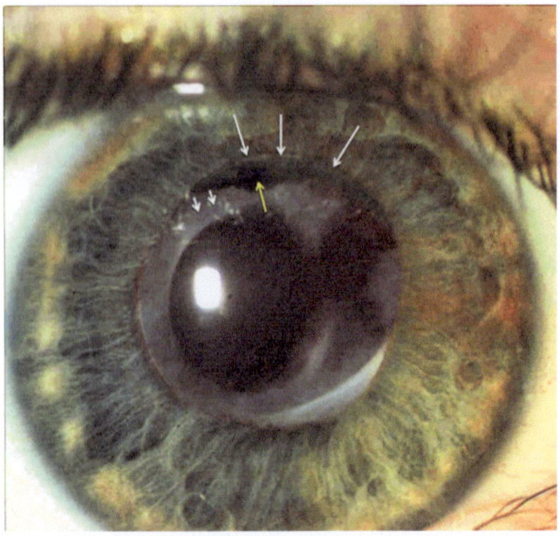

Fig. 6.1 This shows lens iris capture superiorly (*white arrows*); this occurred because the anterior capsulorhexis diameter was larger than that of the optic of the intraocular lens. In these circumstances the anterior capsule edge and the posterior capsule fuse (*short white arrows*) and push the lens forward. When the child rubs his/or her eyes this causes trampolining of the anterior chamber and the lens can move forward also, causing lens iris capture (*long yellow arrow* showing iris behind optic edge, *white arrows*). This can also be seen if an implant is placed in the sulcus

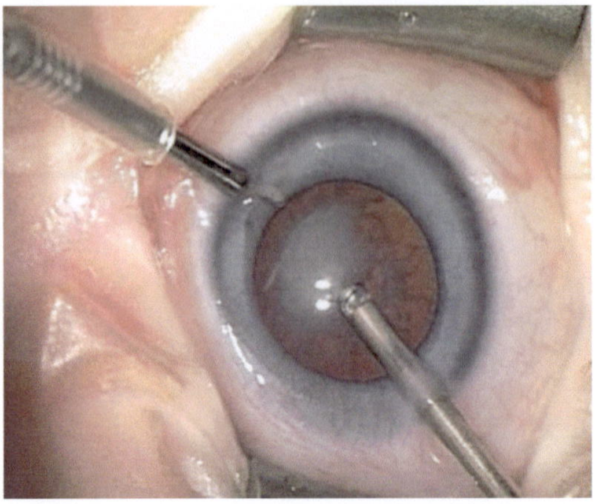

Fig. 6.2 This shows the vitrectorhexis technique. Here there is an anterior chamber maintainer being used and the port of the vitrector has been turned up after breaching the capsule and passing the vitrector under the anterior capsule through the initial breach. A circular motion is used to achieve a round rhexis

relies on occlusion of the port to develop aspiration vacuum, which of course is only momentary given how thin the capsule is. The author preferentially uses this technique when no implant is being used (Fig. 6.2). The reason for this is that there is good evidence that the rhexis edge produced by this method is not as robust as a manual tear [2]. Comparison of mechanized anterior capsulectomy and manual CCC in vitro (18 pairs of postmortem eyes aged 4 days to 16 years) where one eye of each pair had vitrectorhexis, and the other eye manual tear resulted in a radial tear in one of 18 eyes (16 year old eye) with vitrectorhexis but none in the eyes with manual tear.

However, in six eyes (all under 5 years of age), the manual tear could not be successfully continued or completed [3].

Subsequently, a study comparing anterior vitrectorhexis and manual tear in pediatric cataract surgery showed that 19 of 339 eyes (5.6 %) had an anterior capsule tear (in vitrectorhexis group, 12 of 226 eyes (5.3%) and in the manual tear group, 7 of and eyes (6.2%). This study concluded that vitrectorhexis was appropriate for use in children under the age of 6 years [4]. This author's experience is that the younger the child (especially under the age of 1 year) the more robust the vitrectorhexis edge and the more reliable its use when implanting IOLs. If an IOL is not being implanted it is the technique of choice.

Recently authors have described the use of a 23G system to perform the anterior capsulotomy [5]. These authors implanted nine eyes and reported no capsular tears. Theoretically a smaller gauge may well result in a more robust rhexis edge but no studies have looked at this using the 23G system.

6.2.2 Radiofrequency Diathermy

Capsulotomy using radiofrequency diathermy was originally described by Kloti in 1984 [6] and further explored by Gassmann et al. in 1988 [7]. Comer et al. [8] described its use in pediatric cataract surgery for both the anterior and posterior capsule and reported no complications. The use of radiofrequency diathermy, however, has become less and less favorable because the technique predisposes to a higher rate of tags and tears. The idea is to use a diathermy tip to score out the rhexis and then remove the central area.

The problem is that when the capsule is removed there are often tags left behind and again the rhexis edge is not as robust as a manual tear.

6.2.3 Plasma Blade

The plasma blade (also known as the Fugo blade after the inventor) uses pulses of plasma that are generated around its tip to cut and cauterize tissue. The resulting rhexis edge appears to be robust [9]. The advantage of this technique is that it can be used to create an anterior capsulotomy through fibrous tissue e.g. in a traumatic cataract and also other anterior capsular plaques where traditional manual tearing may not be successful. However experience with the plasma blade in pediatric ophthalmology is limited.

6.2.4 Traditional Manual Capsulorhexis

The traditional manual capsulorhexis technique is by far the most popular in the world, mainly because individuals who perform adult cataracts as well as pediatric cataracts perform the majority of the world's pediatric cataracts [10, 11]. The transition from the adult capsule to the pediatric capsule has a definite learning curve. Using a capsulotomy needle is possible but more difficult than using a capsulorhexis forceps. The younger the child, the more elastic the capsule and the more there is curvature of the anterior lens capsule. To counter these two findings, a heavy viscoelastic should be used to hyper inflate the anterior chamber and so flatten the anterior capsule as much as possible Fig. 6.3a). In this way while the capsule may be elastic the surgeon now longer has to worry about the tear running away down the anterior curvature of the lens (see Fig. 6.3a, b, c). The next trick is to starts in the center of the putative rhexis need and makes short tears and re-grasp at the root of the tear so as to have maximum control. It is best to spiral the tear until the desired size is needed. In Fig. 6.3d, The tear is started centrally (#1) and then regrasped for segment #2, and again for segments #3, #4 and #5 and each segment spirals out until the desired size is reached and the rhexis completed by segment #6. Each time the flap is re-grasped it is important to pull to the center of the capsule, as the elasticity of the capsule will give the curvilinear edge desired. If this is not done the edge will tend to tear out and the capsulorhexis will become bigger and bigger. The downside of this technique is that it takes a little while to get used to getting a consistent sized capsulorhexis.

The use of trypan blue to stain the capsule and so be able to see the capsule when there is complete white lens opacity has been shown to immediately physically reduce the elasticity of the human lens capsule after application. This in turn makes the pediatric capsule more stiff and less elastic [12].

6.2.5 Foldable Template Intraocular Ring

One method of ensuring extremely accurately the size of the capsulorhexis has been employed by Tassignon for the use of her 'Bag-in-the-Lens IOL' which demands a very accurate sizing of both the anterior and posterior rhexis. A compressible intraocular ring [13, 14] is placed on the anterior capsule and then the anterior chamber hyper inflated. The rhexis is started centrally again, as described above, but now there is a barrier to prevent the rhexis getting larger or running out. Once the rhexis is completed the ring is removed.

6.2.6 The Two Incision Push Pull Rhexis (T.I.P.P. Rhexis)

Nischal first described this technique in 2002 [15]. The technique entails two stabs being made using an MVR blade, after the anterior chamber has been inflated with a viscoelastic. In this technique it is better not to hyper inflate the eye because the curvature of the anterior lens actually helps to make the rhexis more round. The technique differs depending on the age of the child.

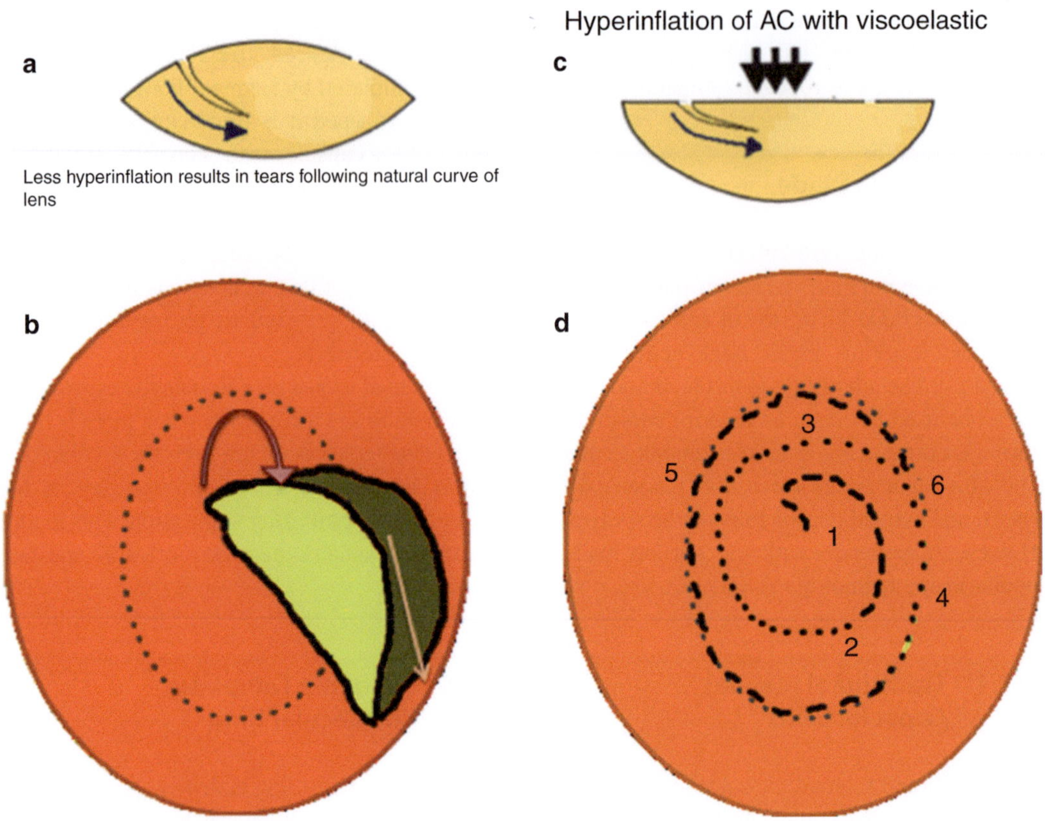

Fig. 6.3 This schematic shows a technique for manual capsulorhexis in children. (**a**) shows that if the anterior chamber is NOT hyper inflated the anterior curvature of the child's eye and the elasticity of the child's capsule can cause the tear to run away towards the equator (*long black curved arrow*). This is shown in (**b**) also. In this figure the *dotted circle* is the target capsulorhexis. The *pink curved arrow* shows where the rhexis was initiated (in the center of the capsule) and the *yellow shaded area* is the flap. The *dark green* is the exposed lens material. The *straight arrow* shows that the tear is running away towards the equator because of the situation shown in (**a**). When the anterior chamber is hyper-inflated, (**c**), control of the rhexis is easier (*long curved black arrow* shows tear is not running to the equator) but the elasticity of capsule must be tackled. One way to do this, is to use a spiraling technique shown in (**d**). The tear is started centrally (*1*) and then regrasped for segment *2*, and again for segments *3*, *4* and *5* and each segment spirals out until the desired size is reached and the rhexis completed by segment *6*. Each time the flap is re-grasped it is important to pull to the center of the capsule, as the elasticity of the capsule will give the curvilinear edge desired

In infants two stabs are made in the anterior capsule the distance between which approximates to the eventual diameter of the rhexis (Figs. 6.4 and 6.5). A caliper can be used to place on the cornea to give the surgeon a guide as to where to place the initial stabs (Fig. 6.4). This author uses an IOL that is 6 mm in diameter so the eventual diameter of the rhexis needs to be 5 mm. The caliper is set at 4.5 mm allowing for a little enlargement if needed. The distal edge of the proximal flap is grasped and the flap pushed to the center of the capsule. Once the tear reaches half way (Figs. 6.4 and 6.5), the flap is released and the proximal edge of the distal flap is grasped and pulled (Figs. 6.4 and 6.5). At this stage one of two things will happen: either the tear formed by pulling the distal flap will be the same size as the initial tear in which cases the two tears can be joined slowly to form a complete rhexis (Figs. 6.4 and 6.5) or the distal tear will be narrower than the initial tear (Fig. 6.5). If this happens one side of the initial flap is grasped and used to complete

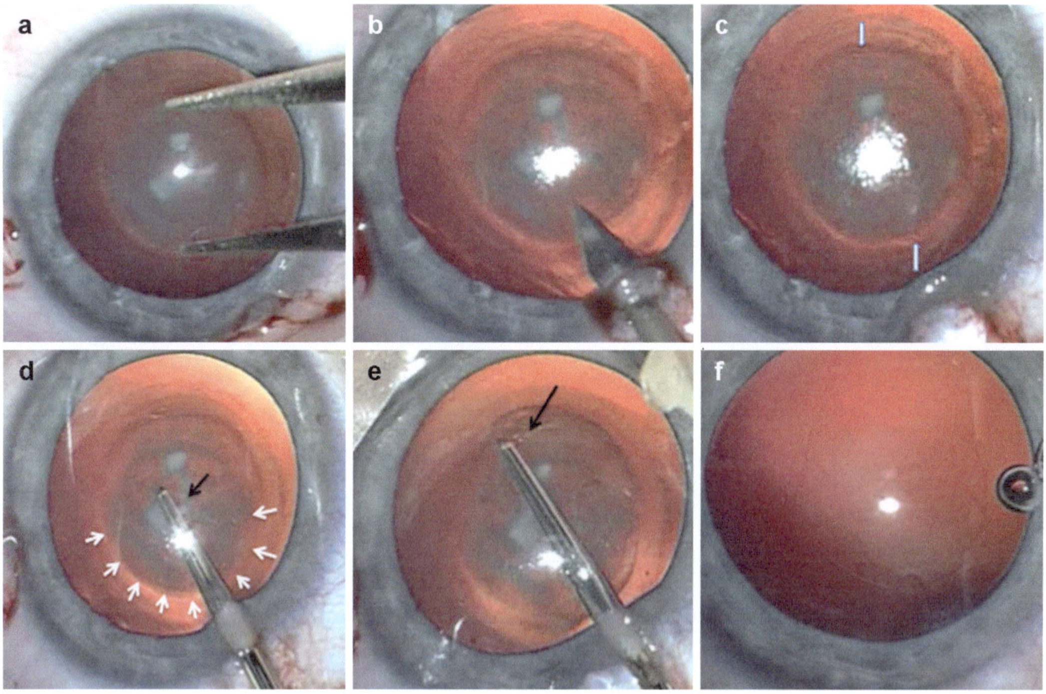

Fig. 6.4 This is a composite of intraoperative pictures of an anterior TIPP rhexis in an infant. (**a**) Shows use of calipers on the cornea to give an estimate where the MVR stabs should be made. (**b**, **c**) Show the stabs being made and completed (**c** *white arrows* show the two stabs). It is very important to remember that the MVR blade is stabbed proximally then withdrawn from the lens (still in the anterior chamber) and then advanced and stabbed distally. This stab must not have any posterior vector force or a 'V' shaped stab will occur. Using intraocular micro forceps the distal flap of the proximal stab is grasped and pushed (**d**, *black arrow*) and a semicircular tear forms (*white arrows* outline the tear). The proximal flap of the distal stab is now grasped and pulled (**e** *black arrow*) to complete the rhexis (**f**). See the schematic in Figs. 6.5 and 6.6 for further technique tips

the rhexis, noting to include the initial distal stab in the rhexis.

In older children after the initial two stabs are made then as the distal flap of the proximal flap is grasped it becomes evident that the tear is going to be too narrow. Under these circumstances it is better to adopt a spiral technique, where the flap is grasped to the left (or right –this is arbitrary) and the flap pushed slightly out and then re-grasped and pulled back towards the center of the capsule. This is repeated until the tear is taken around the distal stab so as to include it in the tear. This is repeated for the proximal flap of the distal stab. (See Fig. 6.6).

Experience with this technique was reported in 2006 [16]. The mean age at operation was 70.21 months (range, 4 weeks-18 years). All eyes had anterior TIPP rhexis and 41 eyes also had posterior TIPP rhexis. While no rhexes were lost during the TIPP technique, four anterior capsular tears were reported, one during irrigation and aspiration and three during rigid lens insertion. No late complications were noted. All eyes had anterior rhexis diameters that were smaller than the optic diameter.

Other authors have reported how this technique can be used when there are large anterior capsular plaques [17] and also a modification of the technique where four stabs have been utilized have also been described [9]. The TIPP rhexis can be used for the posterior capsule as well.

6.2.7 Femtosecond Laser

The advantage is that the elasticity of the pediatric capsule is no longer an issue and the size of the rhexis can be precisely controlled. There are

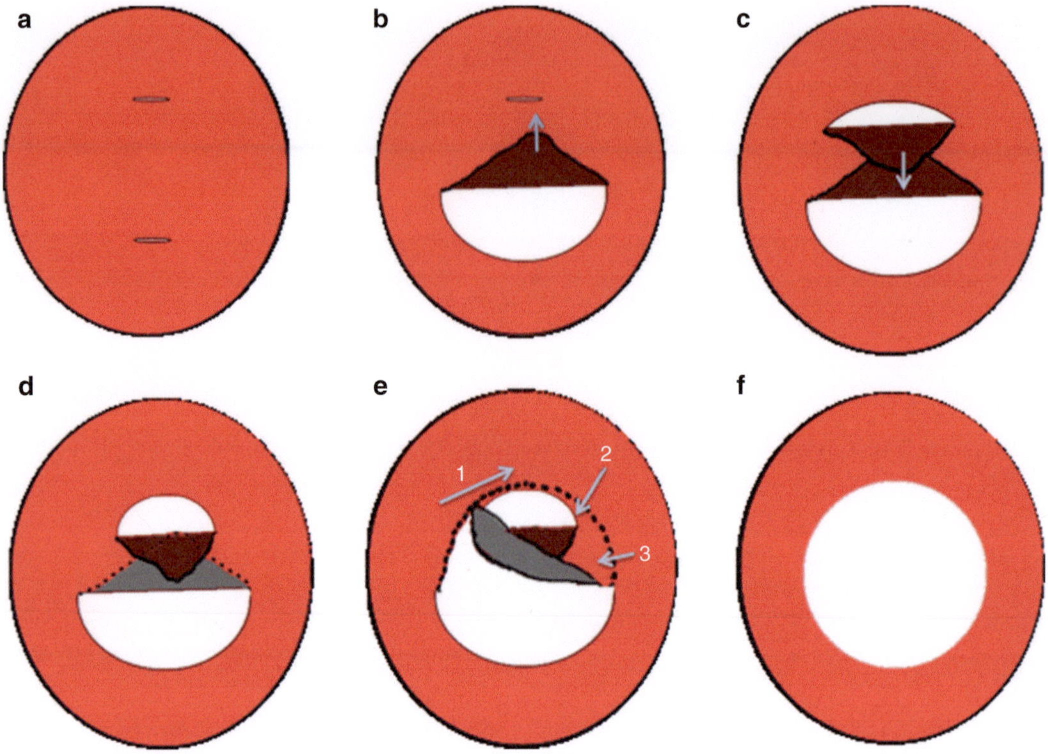

Fig. 6.5 Schematic essentially showing what is happening in Fig. 6.4. Two stabs have been made in (**a**) and the distal flap of the proximal stab is grasped and pushed to the center of the capsule (**b** *blue arrow*). Since the force of the push is to the center of the capsule the vector forces and the elasticity of the capsule cause a semicircular tear forms. The proximal flap of the distal stab is grasped and pulled to the center of the capsule (**c**, *blue arrow*). In infants both tears are often the same size and the two tears can be approximated slowly until a complete rhexis is formed (**f**). Sometimes however, the distal tear (or less commonly the proximal tear) is narrower than the proximal one (or the distal one, **d**)). In this circumstance the flap of the proximal tear (**d** & **e** - *grey shaded area*) is pushed to initially tear out (*#1 blue arrow*) and then pulled back to the center of the capsule (*blue arrows #2 and #3*), so as to include the initial distal stab and complete the rhexis (**f**)

two commercial systems available for femtosecond rhexis, one using optical coherence tomography and the other with off-axis cameras for viewing the capsule during the procedure. This last system allows a better simultaneous posterior capsule view [18]. Dick et al. [19, 20] who have popularized this technique, found that even in younger children there was an unexpected deviation from the target capsular opening diameter, which they were able to account for using an age-dependent correction formula, developed using a linear regression algorithm. This group found that both anterior and posterior capsulotomies could be easily performed with this adjustment. It has been used in a limited number of infant eyes and in this limited cohort it was found to be safe and without complications [20].

At present the cost of the machine limits it's availability.

6.2.8 Special Circumstances

There are always going to be unique circumstances where the surgeon has to use his or her wits to deliver the best result for a child. However there are some instances where there is enough experience in the literature to discuss specific circumstances. This includes cataract surgery when there is a corneal opacity and the view is reduced but not completely lost. Under such circum-

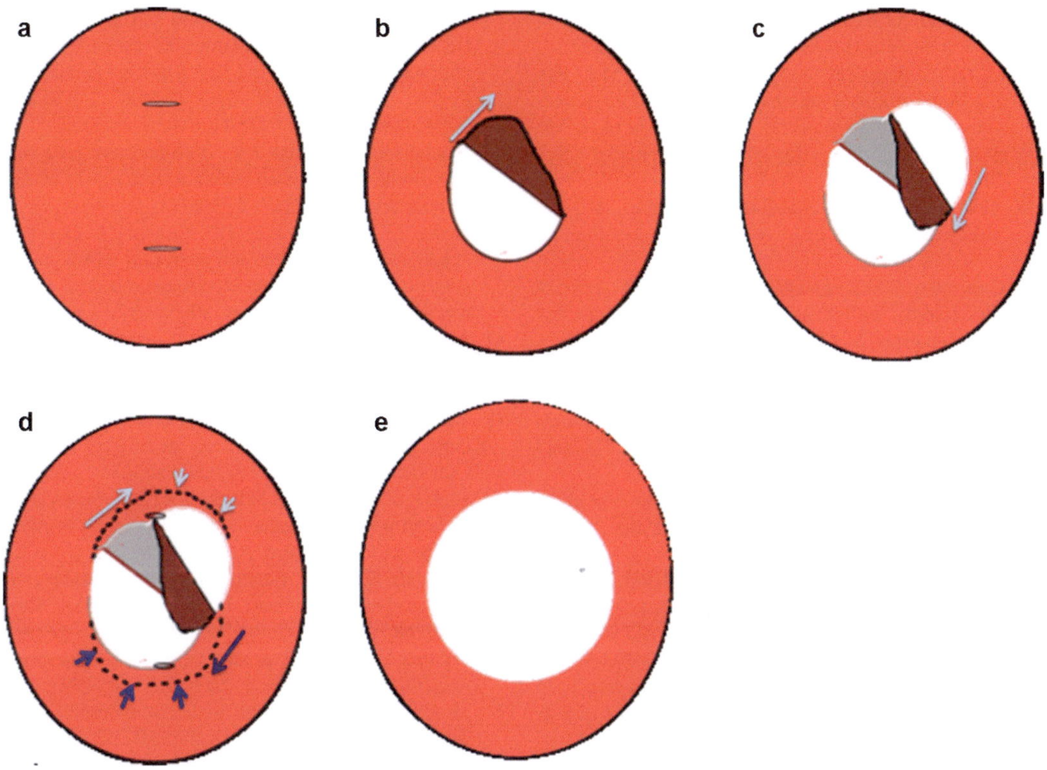

Fig. 6.6 In older children the capsule is less elastic and after the two initial stabs are made (**a**) and the proximal tear initiated, the tear may be found to be too narrow. Under these circumstances the initial flap is pushed slightly to the left (**b**; *blue arrow* shows direction of force to create flap, *maroon*) and then the distal flap and tear pulled slightly to the right (**c**; - initial flap is now shown *grey,* and distal flap is *maroon*. The *blue arrow* shows direction of pull to create maroon flap). In this way the initial flap can be taken around to include the original distal stab (**d** *light blue arrows*) and the distal flap can be pulled back to also include the original proximal stab (*royal blue arrows*), thus completing the rhexis (**e**)

stances authors have described using endo-illumination within the anterior chamber either with self-retaining chandelier light [21] or a straight endo-illuminator. The microscope lights need to be turned off, as do the room lights and then the view of the lens is remarkably good.

In such circumstances if an endoscope is available [22], this can also be used but in this author's experience using the endoilluminator is actually enough.

Recently there has also been a report of cataract surgery in cases of kerato-lenticualr adhesion (Peters anomaly type 2) and a technique to create anterior capsular opening, decompress the lens and then use a vitrectorhexis technique to avoid tearing the adherent capsule off the endothelium to prevent further opacification [23].

References

1. Langwińska-Wośko E, Broniek-Kowalik K, Szulborski K. The impact of capsulorhexis diameter, localization and shape on posterior capsule opacification. Med Sci Monit. 2011;17(10):CR577–82.
2. Trivedi RH, Wilson Jr ME, Bartholomew LR. Extensibility and scanning electron microscopy evaluation of 5 pediatric anterior capsulotomy techniques in a porcine model. J Cataract Refract Surg. 2006;32(7):1206–13.
3. Andreo LK, Wilson ME, Apple DJ. Elastic properties and scanning electron microscopic appearance of manual continuous curvilinear capsulorhexis and vitrectorhexis in an animal model of pediatric cataract. J Cataract Refract Surg. 1999;25(4):534–9.
4. Wilson Jr ME, Trivedi RH, Bartholomew LR, Pershing S. Comparison of anterior vitrectorhexis and continuous curvilinear capsulorhexis in pediatric cat-

aract and intraocular lens implantation surgery: a 10-year analysis. J AAPOS. 2007;11(5):443–6.
5. Li SY, Zhang ZP, Ji SJ, Liu HY, Si MY, Fan KS. Application of minimally invasive 23G vitrectomy via corneal approach for the treatment of pediatric cataract. Eur Rev Med Pharmacol Sci. 2014;18(17):2413–8.
6. Kloti R. Bipolar-Nassfeld-Diathermie in der Mikrochirugie. Klin Monatsbl Augenheilkd. 1984;442:184.6.
7. Gassmann F, Schimmelpfennig B, Kloti R. Anterior capsulotomy by means of bipolar radio-frequency endodiathermy. J Cataract Refract Surg. 1988;14:673.
8. Comer RM, Abdulla N, O'Keefe M. Radiofrequency diathermy capsulorhexis of the anterior and posterior capsules in pediatric cataract surgery: preliminary results. J Cataract Refract Surg. 1997;23 Suppl 1:641–4.
9. Mohammadpour M, Erfanian R, Karimi N. Capsulorhexis: pearls and pitfalls. Saudi J Ophthalmol. 2012;26(1):33–40.
10. Bartholomew LR, Wilson Jr ME, Trivedi RH. Pediatric anterior capsulotomy preferences of cataract surgeons worldwide: comparison of 1993, 2001, and 2003 surveys. J Cataract Refract Surg. 2007;33(5):893–900.
11. Wilson Jr ME. Anterior lens capsule management in pediatric cataract surgery. Trans Am Ophthalmol Soc. 2004;102:391–422.
12. Dick HB, Aliyeva SE, Hengerer F. Effect of trypan blue on the elasticity of the human anterior lens capsule. J Cataract Refract Surg. 2008;34(8):1367–73.
13. Tassignon MJ, Taal M, Ni Dhubhghaill SS. On devices for creating a continuous curvilinear capsulorhexis. J Cataract Refract Surg. 2014;40(10):1754–5.
14. Tassignon MJ, Gobin L, Mathysen D, Van Looveren J, De Groot V. Clinical outcomes of cataract surgery after bag-in-the-lens intraocular lens implantation following ISO standard 11979–7:2006. J Cataract Refract Surg. 2011;37(12):2120–9.
15. Nischal KK, Nischal KK. Two-incision push-pull capsulorhexis for pediatric cataract surgery. J Cataract Refract Surg. 2002;28(4):593–5.
16. Hamada S, Low S, Walters BC, Nischal KK. Five-year experience of the 2-incision push-pull technique for anterior and posterior capsulorrhexis in pediatric cataract surgery. Ophthalmology. 2006;113(8):1309–14.
17. Kesarwani SS, Sahu SK. Push-pull technique of capsulorhexis for fibrous plaques on anterior capsules in pediatric cataract surgery. J AAPOS. 2011;15(5):493–4.
18. Naranjo-Tackman R. How a femtosecond laser increases safety and precision in cataract surgery? Curr Opin Ophthalmol. 2011;22(1):53–7.
19. Dick HB, Schelenz D, Schultz T. Femtosecond laser-assisted pediatric cataract surgery: Bochum formula. J Cataract Refract Surg. 2015;41(4):821–6.
20. Dick HB, Schultz T. Femtosecond laser-assisted cataract surgery in infants. J Cataract Refract Surg. 2013;39(5):665–8.
21. Oshima Y, Shima C, Maeda N, Tano Y. Chandelier retroillumination-assisted torsional oscillation for cataract surgery in patients with severe corneal opacity. J Cataract Refract Surg. 2007;33(12):2018–22.
22. Moore JE, Herath GD, Sharma A. Continuous curvilinear capsulorhexis with use of an endoscope. J Cataract Refract Surg. 2004;30(5):960–3.
23. Medsinge A, Nischal KK. Cataract surgery in children with congenital keratolenticular adhesion (peters anomaly type 2). J AAPOS. 2015;19(1):24–8.

Lensectomy and Anterior Vitrectomy

7

M. Edward Wilson, Katherine S. Wood, and Rupal H. Trivedi

7.1 Introduction

Lensectomy is the term most commonly used to describe removal of the lens in an infant eye using mechanized irrigation/aspiration and cutting instrumentation when an intraocular lens (IOL) is not being implanted at the primary surgery. Lensectomy has evolved in the last few decades. The original automated, mechanical lensectomy/vitrectomy technique was designed to prevent secondary visual axis opacification (VAO), by removing as much of the lens capsule as possible. While this was largely accomplished, if the patient required an IOL in the future, the pediatric surgeon's only options were to implant the IOL in the anterior chamber or to fixate the IOL in the sulcus either with sutures or scleral tunnels, as there was often inadequate capsule support for a lens in its anatomical location. Lensectomy and anterior vitrectomy as we know it evolved in an effort to preserve enough anatomy for future secondary IOL implantation, while preventing opacification as a secondary aim.

Herein we describe the technique of lensectomy and anterior vitrectomy when an IOL is not being implanted during the primary procedure. A lensectomy, as we will describe it, includes anterior central capsulorhexis/capsulectomy, lens aspiration, posterior central capsulorhexis/capsulectomy, and mechanized anterior vitrectomy. In infants, the anterior capsule and posterior capsule openings are usually matched in size and shape to facilitate, in the absence of an IOL, a sealed capsular bag remnant, trapping any re-proliferated cortex that may accumulate in the months following surgery when any residual young lens epithelial cells are still in their active growth mode.

7.2 Advantages and Disadvantages of Lensectomy Without IOL Implantation

A lensectomy and vitrectomy without immediate IOL implantation is common for infants. In many ways it is more favorable to not implant an IOL in this age group. These advantages include:

1. A less invasive procedure: Without IOL implantation the incisions can be smaller—only two 23 or 25 gauge corneal stab wounds are required. Additionally, the extra inflammation associated with IOL implantation can be avoided, and without the larger IOL incision a patch and a shield are not necessary.

M.E. Wilson, MD (✉) • K.S. Wood, MS-II
R.H. Trivedi, MD, MSCR
Department of Ophthalmology, Storm Eye Institute, Medical University of South Carolina, 167 Ashley Avenue, MSC 676, Charleston, SC 29425-6760, USA
e-mail: wilsonme@musc.edu

I.C. Lloyd, S.R. Lambert (eds.), *Congenital Cataract*, DOI 10.1007/978-3-319-27848-3_7

An extended-wear silicone contact lens can be inserted at the end of the surgical procedure and left in place for the first postoperative month. This is a psychological boost for the parents, who appreciate that their child can "start seeing" right away. Postoperative drops can be started right away as well.

2. Decreased risk of VAO: Without an IOL, the anterior and posterior capsular remnants fuse more readily, and a Soemmerring ring is less likely to obscure the visual axis. An IOL prevents the anterior and posterior capsule edges from fusing and may force cortex to escape the Soemmerring ring, increasing the likelihood of VAO.
3. More precise vision correction. Aphakic contact lenses can be adjusted as the eye grows, allowing for precise visual correction. Parents often prefer contact lenses because they are more manageable than glasses for most infants. Later in childhood, glasses can be worn more easily.

The disadvantage of leaving an infant aphakic and correcting vision using contact lenses is twofold. If the lens is lost or if caregivers stop using the contact lens, significant periods of uncorrected aphakic vision can result. This may worsen amblyopia. Contact lenses are expensive and although they are medically necessary, insurance plans or government payers may not cover them. Another disadvantage is that corneal ulcers may develop from wearing contact lenses long-term.

The Infant Aphakia Treatment Study (IATS), a randomized clinical trial comparing primary IOL implantation to primary aphakia corrected with a contact lens, found no significant difference between the median visual acuity of operated eyes in children who underwent primary IOL implantation and those left aphakic.[1] However, there were significantly more adverse events and additional intraoperative procedures in the IOL group. When operating on an infant younger than 7 months of age with a unilateral cataract, IATS investigators recommended leaving the eye aphakic. These infants are likely to receive secondary IOL implantation and thus it is important to leave enough capsular support at the time of cataract surgery for future in-the-bag or sulcus fixation of an IOL.

7.3 Intraoperative Considerations

7.3.1 Intraoperative Mydriasis

Epinephrine(1:500,000 concentration) should be mixed with balanced salt solution (BSS; Alcon Laboratories, Fort Worth, Tx) to avoid intraoperative miosis and pediatric intraoperative floppy iris syndrome (PIFIS). Non-preserved epinephrine should be used even though it is considered an off-label use. We reported an infant with bilateral cataracts in which epinephrine was added to the irrigation fluid for one eye, but was inadvertently omitted from the fellow eye. In the eye that did not receive epinephrine, PIFIS was observed, despite the fact that both pupils dilated well preoperatively. [2]. Recently, a phenylephrine/ketorolac mixture (Omidria, Omeros, Seattle, WA) has been developed for maintaining mydriasis during cataract surgery. It is mixed into the BSS irrigation much like epinephrine but it is made specifically for ophthalmic surgery. The US FDA approved Omidria for use in adults and testing in infants and children is ongoing. We look forward to these results. If the pupil has not dilated well before the start of the procedure, aspirate the most reachable areas of the cortex while you wait for the epinephrine in the irrigation fluid to further enlarge the pupil. If necessary, pupil enlargers (iris hooks or a pupil expanding ring) may be used to assure thorough cortical aspiration [2].

7.3.2 Automated Versus Manual Approach to Lens Substance Aspiration

Pediatric cataracts can be aspirated using either a manual or automated approach. When using the automated approach, a peristaltic or Venturi-pump machine is used. The irrigation/aspiration (I/A) mode is selected. The vitreous infusion suction cutter was developed by Machemer et al. [3, 4] in 1970, and was developed primarily for the removal of vitreous and vitreous membranes. Pediatric cataracts can be aspirated with the vitrector handpiece in the cutter-off position. The advantage of using the vitrector handpiece (rather than a bimanual aspiration handpiece) is that the surgeon can perform multiple maneuvers (some with the cutter on and some with the cutter off) without removing the instrument from the eye, which decreases surgical trauma. These include anterior vitrectorhexis/capsulectomy, I/A, posterior vitrectorhexis/capsulectomy, and vitrectomy. We currently use the Constellation (Alcon surgical), a Venturi-pump driven machine designed primarily for adult vitrectomy procedures. We recommend that each surgeon refer to the instruction manual of the machine being used to learn about specific features unique to it.

7.3.3 Bimanual Approach

The lens substance can be aspirated using either a single port or a bimanual approach. While it is possible to use only one port, it can be difficult to complete the full aspiration and especially to remove the sub-incisional cortex with only one opening [5]. The bimanual approach was designed to make cortical removal easier. As opposed to the single port approach, which uses a single instrument that both irrigates and aspirates, the bimanual approach uses two side-port incisions, one for the irrigation system and one for the aspiration system. Each of these has a separate cannula. A J-shaped cannula is useful because it allows for easier removal of sub-incisional cortex [6]. To maintain the anterior chamber (AC), the irrigation system must have flow resistance lower than that of the aspiration system. This can be achieved using cannulas with shorter lengths and larger lumen diameters [7]. A bimanual approach is especially advantageous for the pediatric eye due to its reduced scleral rigidity. Bimanual irrigation/aspiration (I/A) allows for better control of the AC and decreased fluctuation in AC volume. This is important because AC shallowing can cause iris "bounce," which increases inflammation. Having a tight fit of the instruments into the paracenteses also helps to maintain chamber stability.

7.3.4 Limbal Versus Pars Plicata Approach

There are two main approaches used to perform lensectomy: the limbal/corneal, and the pars plana/pars plicata [8–15].

7.3.5 Limbal/Corneal Approach

Advantages of the limbal/corneal approach include familiarity to the anterior segment surgeon, that the conjunctiva is not disturbed and an adequate capsular rim is more likely to be maintained for secondary IOL implantation later in life. Disadvantages of this approach include a greater risk for iris manipulation or trauma due to the presence of the vitrector in the anterior chamber. To avoid the risk of iris damage, the vitrector's cutting port should always be angled away from the iris. If it is not, a sudden shallowing of the AC may result in the iris coming into contact with the vitrector port while it is in cutting mode and being damaged.

Under general anesthesia, two corneal stab incisions are made, usually at the 10 and 2 o'clock positions (Fig 7.1). The incisions should be made at the terminal end of the limbal blood vessels as they approach the cornea. If they are too far from the cornea, ballooning of the conjunctiva may occur due to fluid that tracks back into the subconjunctival space during lensectomy. As previously, one incision is for the irrigation cannula, which is connected to a bottle of BSS, and one is for the aspiration/cutting handpiece. The incisions are made with a side-port knife or a small MVR blade. Take care to match the size of the incisions as closely as possible with the gauge of the instruments to ensure minimal fluid leakage and AC stability. As the knife is inserted it is aimed posteriorly, but is flattened out into the iris plane after its tip enters the AC. This will produce a tunnelled incision approximately 1 mm long. It is important to keep in mind that the same maneuver

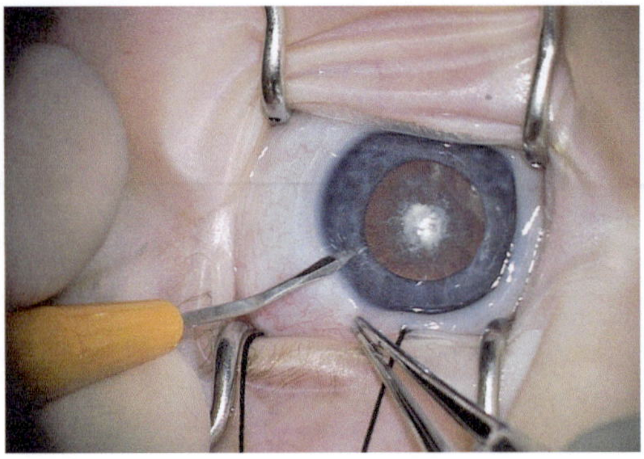

Fig. 7.1 Side-port incision in 3-month old child with bilateral nuclear cataract

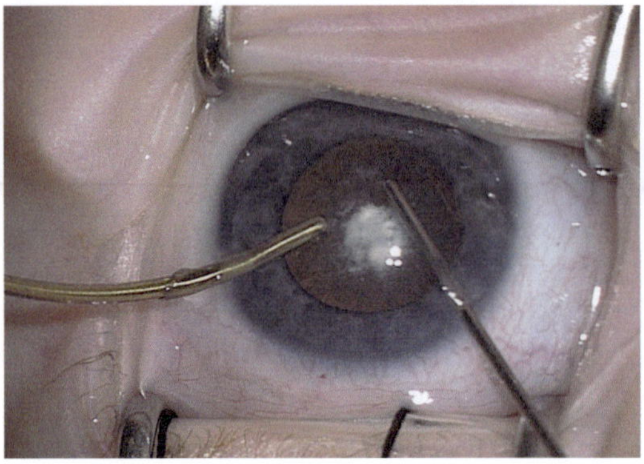

Fig. 7.2 Irrigation cannula and vitrector performing vitrectorrhexis

will produce a longer tunneled incision than expected in infant eyes due to their low tissue rigidity. With a longer incision, the anterior chamber will be entered closer to the visual axis than intended and will make maneuvering more difficult due to an "oar-locking" phenomenon. When removing the knife, remove it precisely along its path of entry. Failure to do so will result in "side-slicing" and thus leakage around the instruments and greater likelihood of AC instability. The non-dominant side incision should be made first (the left-hand incision for a right-handed surgeon). When the non-dominant incision is made first the irrigation cannula can be placed into the incision to keep the AC at a constant volume and allow the surgeon to make the second incision. Otherwise, an ophthalmic viscosurgical device might have to be placed, which is not otherwise necessary when an IOL is not being placed.

Our preferred infusion instruments are 23-gauge blunt-tip, angled, beveled irrigating cannula or a 25-gauge anterior chamber maintainer (Lewicky, Bausch & Lomb). For the irrigation supply we highly recommend a Venturi-pump positive-pressure irrigation system. The active pump can be set to the desired fluid delivery rather than adjusting a gravity-fed bottle-height. Anterior chamber stability for soft infant eyes is much better with the Venturi-pump system. The irrigation should be turned on and set to the *irrigation continuous* mode before entering the eye. We prefer an initial setting of 50 for the fluid flow on the Constellation machine. This is adjusted up or down depending on how much fluid leaks out around the instruments and how much lens cortex and nucleus is aspirated from the eye.

A 23 or 25-gauge vitrectomy handpiece (Constellation, Alcon) is often used for aspiration and cutting. We now prefer the 25-gauge size because it has demonstrated efficiency and effectiveness even when we have used it to remove dense fibrotic membranes and gummy cortex. The aspiration handpiece that matches the bimanual irrigation cannula is also placed on the surgical table for use during cortex aspiration, if needed. However, using the vitrector handpiece for both the cutting steps and the aspiration steps reduces the need to enter and exit the eye multiple times. Another consideration is that the instruments be equal or nearly equal in size. At present, bimanual I/A handpieces are not available smaller than 23-gauge. Therefore, we use a 23-gauge irrigation cannula and a 25-gauge vitrector (Fig 7.2). As mentioned previously, switching hands and instruments is a useful strategy for aspirating subincisional lens material. An alternative to switching hands is to use the irrigation cannula to hydrodissect the stubborn cortex and push it to the pupillary space, so that it can be more easily aspirated. For surgeons who prefer to use an AC maintainer, the 25-gauge Lewicky (Bausch and Lomb) instrument is now available along with the larger 23-gauge of the same name. This is a matter of surgeon preference.

The anterior chamber is entered first with the irrigating cannula in the surgeon's non-dominant

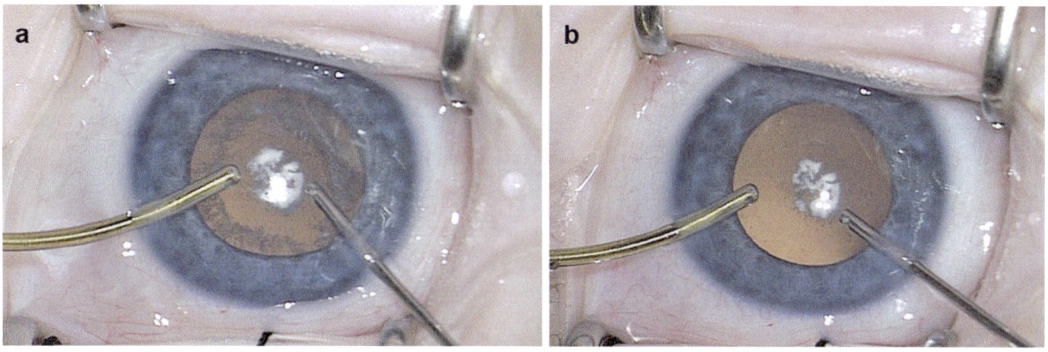

Fig. 7.3 (**a**, **b**) Bimanual aspiration of the lens cortex and nucleus. Note posterior capsule plaque

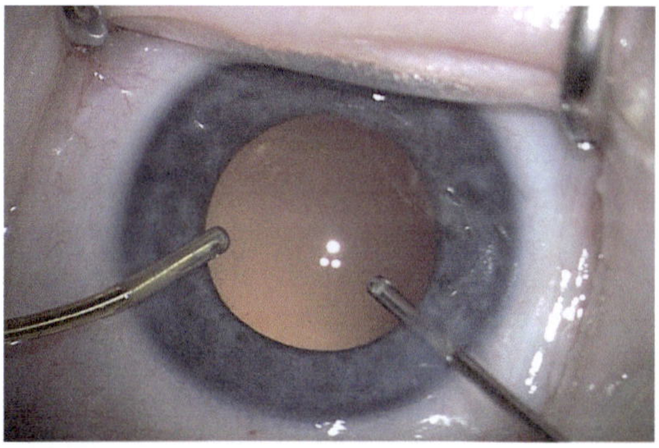

Fig. 7.4 Posterior capsulectomy and vitrectomy

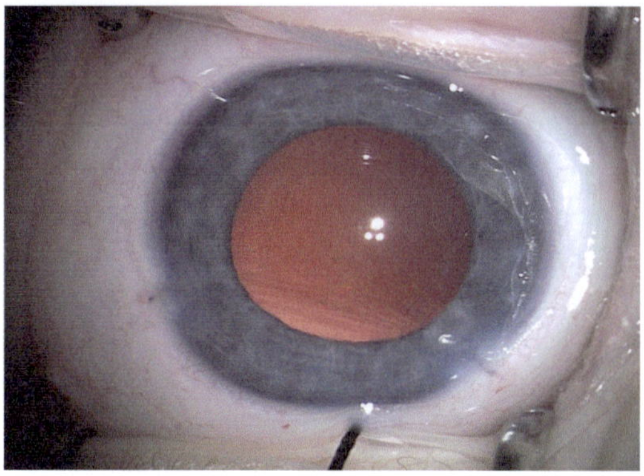

Fig. 7.5 10-0 Vicryl suture to close both the incisions

hand. The beveled tip is inserted into the incision along the plane of the incision, using slight twirling motions if necessary. The vitrector is inserted similarly. Twirling motions facilitate entry once again. Resist the temptation to enlarge the incision.

The anterior capsulorhexis is made first. We recommend using a vitrectorhexis technique unless a primary IOL is being inserted. A manual tear capsulorhexis is more suited for IOL insertion but the vitrectorhexis works well for the lensectomy and vitrectomy technique we are describing here. A Venturi-pump driven vitrector cuts anterior capsule more easily than a vitrector handpiece attached to a peristaltic-pump machine. We now use the 25-gauge vitrector set at 7500 cuts per minute. The cutting port is placed in the eye facing directly posterior. The aspiration foot petal is depressed until there is enough aspiration to bring the capsule into the cutter. The vitrector cutter is used to create a round 4.5 mm central vitrectorhexis.

The vitrector is then taken off of the cutting mode so that it functions as an aspiration-only instrument. This is done using the foot petal and without removing the instruments from the eye. Bimanual aspiration of lens cortex and nucleus is accomplished (Fig 7.3a, b). The vitrectomy cutter can then be turned back on, using the foot petal, and a matching posterior vitrectorhexis is created (Fig 7.4). We recommend a generous central anterior vitrectomy, aiming to remove 1/3rd of the vitreous volume.

The paracentesis incisions are most often closed with a single interrupted 10-0 Vicryl suture each (Fig 7.5). A drop of 5 % povidone-iodine along with atropine and steroid/antibiotic drops is placed on the eye at the end of surgery. An appropriate Silsoft aphakic contact lens placed on the eye as well (Fig 7.6). The child is then awakened and recovered.

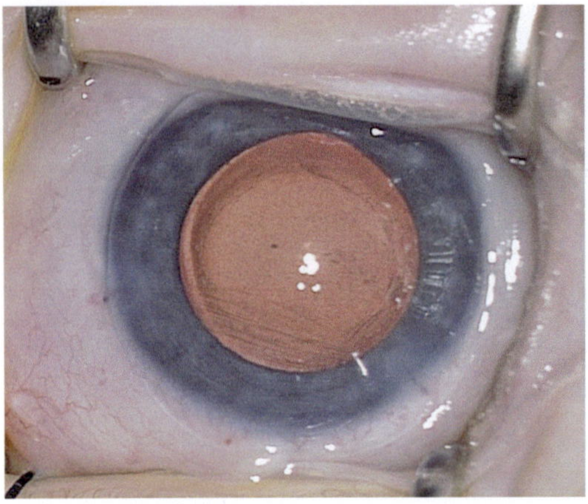

Fig. 7.6 Silsoft contact lens (26 D, 7.5 mm base curve) inserted immediately at the end of the surgery

7.4 Pars Plana Approach

When an IOL is being implanted, many surgeons prefer a pars plana/plicata approach for the central posterior capsulectomy. However, when an IOL is not being implanted at the time of cataract surgery, this approach is not commonly used unless vitreoretinal pathology is also being addressed during the surgery. Pediatric retina surgeons favor this approach, but pediatric anterior segment surgeons are more likely to favor a limbal/corneal approach. The pars plana approach is advantageous because it minimizes the risk of trauma to the iris and cornea, due to its inherent lack of maneuvering within the anterior chamber. The disadvantage is that there is an increased likelihood of removing too much capsule, so that a sulcus-fixated or capsular-fixated secondary IOL cannot be supported.

The pars plana/pars plicata lensectomy technique utilizes the same vitrectomy cutting handpiece described above. To begin, two incisions are made in the conjunctiva to expose the sclera at the level of the pars plana/plicata: one at the 10 o'clock position and one at the 2 o'clock position. Next, two scleral perforations are made using a microvitreoretinal (MVR) knife or a Stiletto knife (DORC, the Netherlands) to match the gauge of the instruments used for the rest of the procedure (20, 23, 25, 27 gauge). The perforations are also made at the level of the pars plana/plicata, one for the infusion cannula and one for the vitrectomy probe. A guideline for stab incision placements is 2 mm posterior to the limbus for infants. When completing a lensectomy and anterior vitrectomy via this approach, leave a peripheral rim of capsular bag, with anterior, equatorial, and posterior capsule. The capsular remnants are important for secondary IOL implantation later on, as they create a shelf for a posterior chamber implant to rest on. The pars plana/plicata scleral incisions are usually closed using 8-0, 9-0, or 10-0 synthetic absorbable suture. Sutureless pars plana sclerotomies in children have been reported, however, suturing these wounds in children is recommended [16]. The conjunctiva overlying the incisions may be closed as well.

7.5 Contact Lens Selection

Following the lensectomy, the patient's aphakia must be managed using either aphakic glasses or contact lenses. Glasses can be heavy and burdensome for infant patients to wear, so contact lenses are often chosen, especially for unilateral aphakia. There are two main choices: rigid gas permeable lenses and silicone elastomeric lenses. Most surgeons place a contact lens on an aphakic infant's eye within a week after surgery. A trial lens is placed in the office during one of the postoperative visits and an over-refraction is done to decide on the exact lens to be ordered for that infant. We prefer silicone, extended wear contact lenses (SilSoft, Bausch and Lomb, Rochester, NY) for infants and wanted a way to select the appropriate contact lens at the conclusion of the surgery. Poor refractive outcome data followed the practice of using a +32 D power for all infants [17, 18]. Trivedi et al. demonstrated that preoperative biometry, specifically axial length (AL), could be used to calculate contact lens power [17, 18]. We have also now created a lens constant for the Silsoft lens that can be used with modern IOL formulas to estimate the power for distance. Infants should have appropriate overcorrection (+2 D) added to provide near-point correction. We have found that a 7.5-base curve is appropriate in small infants, so we dispense a lens of that base curve at the calculated power (the lens comes in +20 to +32 power in 3 diopter steps). Axial length alone can be used as well. We recommend a +32-D CL when the preoperative AL is less than 17 mm, a

+29-D Cl when the preoperative AL is between 17 and 18.5 mm, a +26-D CL when the preoperative AL is 18.5–19.5 D, a +23-D CL when the preoperative AL is between 19.5 and 20 mm (21 mm), and a +20-D CL for an AL of 20–21 mm (20 D for >21 mm) [17].

7.6 Summary

The lensectomy procedure is the least traumatic method of removing a congenital cataract in infancy. When done properly, it requires only one entry into the eye, allowing for a fast and simple surgery. Anterior chamber stability and the absence of iris manipulation lead to low levels of post-operative inflammation. The central anterior and posterior capsule is removed but only to about 4.5 mm in diameter, allowing for a secondary IOL placement a few years later. Improvements in instrumentation design and pump efficiency have resulted in smaller gauge tools with minimal loss of effectiveness or efficiency. In the future, even smaller instruments will be used. Placing a contact lens at the end of the surgery allows the visual rehabilitation to begin immediately. This also minimizes the delay in getting the postoperative topical medications started. For us, this has eliminated the need for sub-conjunctival injections. After a properly performed lensectomy, secondary in-the-bag IOL implantation can usually be done safely and easily when the child is a few years older.

References

1. Infant Aphakia Treatment Study G, Lambert SR, Lynn MJ, Hartmann EE, DuBois L, Drews-Botsch C, Freedman SF, Plager DA, Buckley EG, Wilson ME. Comparison of contact lens and intraocular lens correction of monocular aphakia during infancy: a randomized clinical trial of HOTV optotype acuity at age 4.5 years and clinical findings at age 5 years. JAMA Ophthalmol. 2014;132(6):676–82. doi:10.1001/jamaophthalmol.2014.531.
2. Wilson Jr ME, Trivedi RH, Mistr S. Pediatric intraoperative floppy-iris syndrome. J Cataract Refract Surg. 2007;33(7):1325–7. doi:10.1016/j.jcrs.2007.03.025.
3. Machemer R, Buettner H, Norton EW, Parel JM. Vitrectomy: a pars plana approach. Trans Am Acad Ophthalmol Otolaryngol. 1971;75(4):813–20.
4. Machemer R, Parel JM, Norton EW. Vitrectomy: a pars plana approach. Technical improvements and further results. Trans Am Acad Ophthalmol Otolaryngol. 1972;76(2):462–6.
5. Brauweiler P. Bimanual irrigation/aspiration. J Cataract Refract Surg. 1996;22(8):1013–6.
6. Dewey SH. Cortical removal simplified by J-cannula irrigation. J Cataract Refract Surg. 2002;28(1):11–4. S0886335001011683 [pii].
7. Jeng BH, Huang D. Anterior chamber stability during bimanual irrigation and aspiration. Theoretical and experimental analysis. J Cataract Refract Surg. 2001;27(10):1670–8. S0886-3350(01)00860-4 [pii].
8. Pandey SK, Wilson ME, Trivedi RH, Izak AM, Macky TA, Werner L, Apple DJ. Pediatric cataract surgery and intraocular lens implantation: current techniques, complications, and management. Int Ophthalmol Clin. 2001;41(3):175–96.
9. Ram J, Pandey SK. Infantile cataract surgery: current techniques, complications and their management. In: Dutta LC, editor. Modern ophthalmology. New Delhi: Jaypee Brothers Medical Publications(P) Ltd; 2000. p. 378–84.
10. Wilson ME, Pandey SK, Thakur J. Pediatric cataract surgery in the developing world. Br J Ophthalmol. 2003;87:14–9.
11. Basti S, Ravishankar U, Gupta S. Results of a prospective evaluation of three methods of management of pediatric cataracts. Ophthalmology. 1996;103(5):713–20.
12. Parks MM. Posterior lens capsulectomy during primary cataract surgery in children. Ophthalmology. 1983;90(4):344–5.
13. Taylor D. Choice of surgical technique in the management of congenital cataract. Trans Ophthalmol Soc U K. 1981;101(1):114–7.
14. Meier P, Sterker I, Wiedemann P. Pars plana lentectomy for treatment of congenital cataract. Graefes Arch Clin Exp Ophthalmol. 2001;239:649–55.
15. Ahmadieh H, Javadi MA, Ahmady M, et al. Primary capsulectomy, anterior vitrectomy, lensectomy, and posterior chamber lens implantation in children: limbal versus pars plana. J Cataract Refract Surg. 1999; 25:768–75.
16. Lam DS, Chua JK, Leung AT, Fan DS, Ng JS, Rao SK. Sutureless pars plana anterior vitrectomy through self-sealing sclerotomies in children. Arch Ophthalmol. 2000;118(6):850–1.
17. Trivedi RH, Wilson ME. Selection of an initial contact lens power for infantile cataract surgery without primary intraocular lens implantation. Ophthalmology. 2013;120(10):1973–6. doi:10.1016/j.ophtha.2013.03.013.
18. Trivedi RH, Lambert SR, Lynn MJ, Wilson ME, Infant Aphakia Treatment Study G. The role of preoperative biometry in selecting initial contact lens power in the Infant Aphakia Treatment Study. J AAPOS Off Publ Am Assoc Pediatr Ophthalmol Strabismus Am Assoc Pediatr Ophthalmol Strabismus. 2014; 18(3):251–4. doi:10.1016/j.jaapos.2014.01.012.

8 Selecting an Intraocular Lens Power

Deborah K. VanderVeen

Once the decision has been made to operate on a child with a congenital cataract, a choice must be made about the optimal mode for correction of aphakia. Options include contact lens correction of aphakia, aphakic spectacle correction, and primary intraocular lens (IOL) implantation. Factors that should be considered include the age of the patient, whether the cataract is unilateral or bilateral, and whether the eye, the child, and the family are good candidates with regard to each mode of correction. Eyes with microcornea (<9 mm), microphthalmia, or pre-existing conditions such as glaucoma or uveitis are not good candidates for IOL implantation. The ability of a child or family to tolerate contact lenses or spectacles should be considered, and while infants with bilateral cataracts tend to do well with all options, interocular competition makes rehabilitation challenging in unilateral cases. Often a combination of refractive strategies is employed, as infants undergoing very early surgery may have initial correction of aphakia via contact lenses or aphakic spectacles with later secondary IOL implantation, and older infants and children typically do well with primary IOL implantation.

Once the decision has been made to place an IOL, the main considerations are the optimal power for the child at the time of surgery, the degree of ocular growth and myopic shift expected with regard to the final refractive status, and factors affecting biometry and IOL calculation.

8.1 Globe Size and Ocular Growth

The infant eye has a larger anterior to posterior segment ratio, steeper corneal curvature, a less deep anterior chamber, relatively thick lens, less scleral rigidity, and very short axial length compared with the adult eye. An eye with congenital cataract may have other anatomic abnormalities as well, such as microcornea, anterior segment dysgenesis, or persistent fetal vasculature, all of which may impact accuracy of biometry measures or, ultimately, the ability to implant an IOL in the capsular bag.

Gordon and Donzis described growth characteristics of non-cataractous eyes in a cross-sectional study investigating refractive development in a population of patients with ages ranging from 30 weeks gestational age (premature) up to 36 years [1]. While very steep keratometry measures were found in young infants, the corneal curvature was found to approximate typical adult measures by 6 months of age. Axial growth occurs in a triphasic pattern, with rapid elongation in the early months up to 2 years of age, then a slower rate of elongation between 2 and 6 years, and then an estimated 1 mm of elongation

D.K. VanderVeen, MD
Department of Ophthalmology, Boston Children's Hospital, Harvard Medical School, 300 Longwood Avenue, Fegan 404, Boston, MA 02115, USA
e-mail: Deborah.vanderveen@childrens.harvard.edu

I.C. Lloyd, S.R. Lambert (eds.), *Congenital Cataract*, DOI 10.1007/978-3-319-27848-3_8

in the years leading into adulthood. Thus, by 2 years of age, a typical pediatric eye has reached approximately 90 % of the predicted adult axial length. The natural lens power decreases in a normal eye during ocular growth, counterbalancing the myopic shift that would be seen on the basis of axial elongation alone.

8.2 Globe Size and Ocular Growth in Eyes with Infantile Cataract

Wide variations may be found in keratometry and axial length measures for eyes with infantile cataract [2, 3].

8.2.1 Infant Aphakia Treatment Study

The Infant Aphakia Treatment Study group compared outcomes of infants with unilateral congenital cataract, operated on between 28 days to <7 months, who were randomized to receive either contact lens correction of aphakia or primary IOL implantation [4]. Eyes with microcornea (<9 mm) and persistent fetal vasculature (PFV) were excluded. Baseline characteristics of the eyes with cataract as well as the normal fellow eyes were reported [5]. The eyes with cataract, compared with the normal fellow eyes, had steeper baseline keratometry readings (46.4 ± 2.7 diopters vs. 45.5 ± 1.8 diopters), smaller corneal diameters (10.5 ± 0.7 mm vs. 10.8 ± 0.6 mm), and shorter axial lengths (18.0 ± 1.3 mm vs. 18.6 ± 0.9 mm). Eyes with congenital cataract had a mean estimated axial length of 17.2 mm at 1 month of age and 19.9 mm at 6 months of age, which represents a mean growth rate of 0.5 mm per month during that span.

The Infant Aphakia Treatment Study cohort also provided information about ocular growth rates during the first year of life [5]. By 1 year of age, the ocular growth rates in operated eyes, while not age dependent, were greater in the eyes having primary IOL implantation (0.24 mm per month) compared to the eyes who had contact lens correction of aphakia (0.17 mm per month). The normal fellow eyes showed an age-dependent ocular axial growth rate, with an estimated mean change of 0.28 mm per month at 1 month of age compared with 0.14 mm per month at 6 months of age. Thus, the mean axial length at 1 year of age was 19.0 mm for aphakic eyes compared with 19.5 mm for pseudophakic eyes operated on at 1 month of age, and 20.6 mm for aphakic and 21.1 mm for pseudophakic eyes operated on at 6 months of age. The normal fellow eyes showed a mean axial length of 20.7 ± 0.6 mm at 1 year of age. By 5 years [6], the eyes that had primary IOL implantation showed a median refractive error of −2.25 diopters, however a wide range was noted (+5.00 to −19.00 diopters).

8.2.2 Axial Elongation Rates

Early ocular growth has been studied in several other cohorts that included unilateral and bilateral congenital cataract patients operated on at wider range of ages. All studies show higher degrees of mean axial elongation and myopic shift in children under 2 years of age, with the greatest change in the first 6 months after surgery [7]. Vasavada and colleagues [8] prospectively studied a large group of children, and at a mean follow up of almost 5 years found a higher rate of axial growth in children operated on at under 1 year of age (4.04 mm, 23.5 %) compared with those operated on between 1 and 3 years of age (1.07 mm, 4.8 %) or those operated on between 4 and 10 years of age (0.97 mm, 4.3 %). Unilateral cases operated in the first year showed a significantly greater rate of axial elongation compared with the fellow normal eye, and while there was also a higher rate compared with bilateral cases, this did not reach statistical significance. In other reports [2, 7, 9–12], axial elongation rates after surgery for unilateral or bilateral congenital and developmental cataracts have been found to be similar to normative data for eye growth or similar to the normal fellow eye. None of these studies specifically analyzed the role of amblyopia on axial elongation rates.

8.2.3 Myopic Shift

Refractions to assess myopic shift after surgery in infants and young children show some variability based on age at surgery and length of follow up, however, all reports for children operated on in infancy or less than 2 years of age showed a mean myopic shift of about six diopters (Table 8.1). The rate of refractive growth in pseudophakic eyes has been shown to be less than that of aphakic eyes [13, 14], but the effective myopic shift is greater because of the optical effect of the effective IOL position, moving further from the retina, in a growing eye.

Even children undergoing later surgery have some myopic shift, which is not unexpected with continued axial growth. A mean change of -0.99 ± 0.22 diopters over a mean follow up of 3.2 years was found in a series of children who underwent primary IOL implantation between 3 and 9 years of age [23]. For older children with unilateral cataract aged 5–15 years, similar changes in axial length, keratometry, and myopic shift were seen between the operated eye and the normal fellow eye [24]. Finally, myopic shift may continue after the tenth birthday, as one cohort showed a mean shift in refraction per year of -0.30 ± 0.38 diopters (mean shift to last follow up of -1.13 ± 1.36 diopters) in the second decade of life.

8.2.4 Other Conditions Affecting Axial Elongation and Myopic Shift

Glaucoma is not infrequent in children undergoing early cataract surgery, with long-term rates of up to approximately 30 % [6, 25]. Elevated intraocular pressure in infantile eyes commonly results in anatomic changes that may affect corneal curvature or result in increased axial elongation and myopic shift; many studies of ocular growth thus exclude eyes with recognized ocular hypertension or glaucoma.

Finally, some studies have demonstrated associations between axial elongation and deprivation amblyopia or vision. In patients with unilateral cataract, a smaller preoperative interocular axial length difference at surgery (suggesting less stimulus deprivation induced axial elongation) may be predictive of good post-operative visual acuity [26]. A correlation between higher rates of refractive growth and poor final visual acuity, particularly for unilateral cases, has been demonstrated in children with cataract surgery before 1 year of age [27]. Finally, for children undergoing unilateral cataract surgery between 2 and 6 years of age, no difference in final visual acuity or myopic shift was found by aiming for emmetropia vs. leaving residual hyperopia (≥2 diopters) [27].

8.3 Biometry in Young Children

Limited cooperation and density of the cataract in young infants and children usually prevent optical coherence measurements of keratometry and axial length. Ultrasound biometry is typically performed with the child under general anesthesia, at the time of cataract surgery, so portable equipment for keratometry and axial length measures must be available. While contact and immersion ultrasound technique for axial length measurements often give similar accuracy with regard to expected post-operative refraction [28, 29], when there is a significant discrepancy, immersion ultrasound is more predictable [30].

8.4 Predictability of IOL Calculation Formulas in the Pediatric Population and Prediction Error

Understanding typical performance of IOL calculation formulas in the pediatric population is helpful. Prediction error, which represents the difference between the predicted and actual post-operative refraction (obtained within a few weeks after surgery), is used to compare accuracy of formulas and early refractive outcomes. Commonly available formulas include the Sanders-Retzlaff-Kraff (SRK) II regression formula, the SRK Theoretic (SRK/T), Holladay 1, Hoffer Q, and Haigis formulas. While IOL calculation formulas are highly predictable within the range of typical keratometry and axial length measures found in older children and

Table 8.1 Myopic shift after cataract surgery in pseudophakic infantile eyes

Study	Age at surgery (mean)	Number of eyes	Mean follow-up	Myopic shift, diopters (D)	Comments
Dahan and Drusedau (1997) [15]	<18 months (9.36±6.12 months) *Subset of 156 eyes of 99 children up to 8 years of age*	68	6.93±3.42 years	−6.39±3.68 D	Greater myopic shift in younger age groups
Griener et al. (1999) [9]	2–4 months	11 All unilateral	5.6 years	−6.12 D (range −3.75 to −12.75 D)	
Lambert et al. (1999) [16]	<6 months (10±6 weeks)	11 All unilateral	1 year	−5.49 D (range 2–14 D)	Two patients with glaucoma had greatest rate of myopic shift
McClatchey et al. (2000) [13]	<6 months (0.30 year) 6–12 months (0.60 year) *Subsets of 100 pseudophakic eyes of 83 patients up to 10 years of age*	22 14 unilateral 22 12 unilateral	8 years 7.76 years	−6.68 D −7.82 D	Greater in unilateral cases <6 months and with less good final vision; for >6 months, unilateral shift less than bilateral cases
O'Keefe et al. (2001) [17]	<12 months (4 months)	27 13 unilateral	3.42 years	−6.0 D	Most shift occurred in first 24 months
Crouch et al. (2002) [18]	1–2 years *Subset of 52 eyes of 42 patients aged up to 18 years*	10	6.35 years	−5.96 D (range −3.06 to −8.87)	Greatest rate of growth occurred between 1 and 3 years, with more linear trend later
Fan et al. (2006) [7]	<1 year (6.7±3.9 month)	34 6 unilateral	3 years	−7.11±3.17 D (range −47 to −10.69 D)	Greatest change 6 months after surgery
Gouws et al. (2006) [19]	<1 year (15 weeks)	28 8 unilateral	7.92 years	At 36 months after surgery: −3.44 D (range +2.00 to −15.00 D)	Greater mean shift for unilateral cases (−5.53 vs. −2.77 D)
Ashworth et al. (2007) [20]	<1 year (18.9±16.2 weeks)	33 17 unilateral	3.70±2.55 years	At 1 year after surgery: −5.43±3.7 D	Greater shift in the first year after surgery and for those operated <10 weeks of age (−6.26±2.91)
Astle et al. (2007) [21]	<24 months	34 eyes 18 unilateral	2.94 years	−5.43 D (range −11.88 to +.50)	Subset of infants <12 months, similar rate of −5.33 D
Hoevenaars et al. (2011) [22]	<1 year *Subset of 70 eyes of 46 patient aged up to 18 years*	10 6 unilateral	3 years	−5.26 (range 0 to −8.13 D)	Greater shift in unilateral cases

adults, the wide range of keratometry and axial length combinations found in infantile eyes as well as the anatomic variances that may alter effective lens position can impact the ability of a formula to perform optimally [31, 32]. While some studies comparing formula performance have found that the SRK II formula works at least as well as theoretic formulas for pediatric eyes [29, 33–36], others found that theoretic formulas perform significantly better [37, 38]. Formulas specifically designed for shorter eyes seem to perform inconsistently in infantile eyes, so there is no clear evidence that they are superior [38, 39].

Overall, prediction error using any of the formulas is higher in pediatric cohorts compared with that in adult studies, with mean absolute prediction errors typically ranging from 0.7 to 1.5 diopters. [29, 30, 34, 35, 37, 40]. Higher prediction error has been associated with steep keratometry measures [22, 29], younger age at surgery [29], and short axial length [37, 39, 40]. Errors in axial length measurement can result in large prediction errors in pediatric eyes using all formulas [41]. Two large series involving children under 2 years of age have shown that SRK II formula may be the least variable [34] and that predictability is not influenced by axial length [36]. The SRK/T formula was used for infant eyes with reasonable mean prediction error (1.63 diopters), but a wide range in error was noted [20]. The Infant Aphakia Treatment Study utilized the Holladay 1 formula, with a mean prediction error of 1.7 ± 1.3 diopters (median, 1.2 diopters) [3], but comparison of mean and median prediction error for various formulas showed that the SRK/T and T2 formulas would have performed equally well or better [38, 42]. An association of higher prediction error with shorter axial length <18.0 mm at surgery was found in these infantile eyes. In another cohort of eyes with axial length <20 mm, SRK II performed the best, with a mean absolute prediction error of 1.84 ± 3.55 diopters [43].

8.5 IOL Power Selection Strategies

Given that ocular growth and myopic shift is expected for every infant eye that has IOL implantation, various strategies have been proposed for finding a target refraction in the early postoperative period that will provide reasonable amount of correction early, not induce significant anisometropia in the short or long term for unilateral cases, and not result in significant refractive error after eye growth is complete.

Several guidelines for IOL power selection have been published (Table 8.2). The majority recommend selection of a desired postoperative refraction based on age at surgery; more recent publications tend to recommend more residual hyperopia. Others recommend reducing the IOL power by a percentage of the IOL predicted to result in emmetropia, or by axial length at the time of surgery. All of these strategies will leave an infant eye significantly hyperopic immediately after the surgery, in anticipation of at least six diopters of myopic shift in the early years and a predicted refractive result of low to moderate myopia by adulthood. In addition to these general guidelines, Hoevenaars and colleagues advocated for residual hyperopia of as much as 7–8 diopters when operating at 3 months of age, with slightly higher amounts for unilateral cases. The Infant Aphakia Treatment Study aimed for postoperative hyperopia of +8.0 diopters for children operated on at 4–6 weeks of age and +6.0 diopters for children over 6 weeks of age [4].

Another tool that is useful when selecting an IOL power is McClatchey's Pediatric IOL Calculator [46]. McClatchey and Parks [47] studied aphakic refractions from a large series of patients operated on before age 10 years with at least 7 years follow up to calculate the range of final refractions for those eyes if primary IOL implantation had occurred instead, aiming for emmetropia at the time of surgery. These calculations predicted a median pseudophakic refraction at last follow of −6.6 diopters with a variance (−36.3 to +2.9 diopters), especially for children operated on in the first 2 years of life. From this data, McClatchey developed the program to predict the range of possible final refractive outcomes and standard deviation for an eye based on baseline biometry measures, age at surgery, and IOL implanted. Others have also used the program to confirm early predictability compared with standard IOL calculation formulas [43].

Table 8.2 Post-operative target refraction tables for residual hyperopia in young children

Age at surgery (years)	Dahan 1997 [15] % undercorrection[a]	Enyedi 1998 [44]	Crouch 2002 [18]	Plager 2002 [45]
<1	20 %			
1	20 %	+6	+4.0 D	
2	10 %	+5	+3.5 D	
3	10 %	+4	+2.5 D	+5
4	10 %	+3	+2.5 D	+4
5	10 %	+2	+2.0 D	+3
6	10 %	+1	+2.0 D	+2.25
7	10 %	Plano[b]	+1.0 D	+1.5
8	10 %		+1.0 D	+1.0
10	Plano[b]		Plano[b]	+.5[b] + 0.5%

D diopters

[a]Meaning, use 80 % or 90 % of IOL power needed by biometry based calculations for emmetropia. Alternatively, Dahan and colleagues suggested IOL power selection based on axial length in mm (IOL power): 17 mm (28 D), 18 mm (27 D), 19 mm (26 D), 20 mm (24 D), 21 mm (22 D)

[b]Emmetropia or slight myopia after this age

8.6 Special Circumstances

8.6.1 Secondary IOL Implantation

Many infants will not have primary IOL implantation but will have contact lens or spectacle correction of aphakia initially, with a secondary procedure for IOL implantation later [48]. Techniques and outcomes for secondary IOL surgery have been described [49–52] and are reviewed in Chap. 10.

Similar strategies for IOL power selection apply for secondary IOL implantation surgery. However, since the child will be older, more will be known about the visual potential of the operative eye, presence and depth of amblyopia, and refractive status and vision of the fellow eye, and these factors may influence the targeted post-operative refraction. Calculations should consider difference in the effective lens position if IOL implantation occurs within the capsular bag or in the ciliary sulcus. Refractive outcomes and predictability of IOL calculation formulas are similar to those in primary IOL implantation, with mean absolute prediction error ranging from 0.9 ± 0.9 diopters to 2.15 ± 1.68 diopters [52–55]. Higher prediction error has been seen with both lower age at surgery [54] and shorter axial length [52].

Alternative strategies to calculate IOL power for secondary IOL surgery from aphakic refractions have been proposed [56, 57], however, these are estimation methods and not as accurate as biometry-based IOL calculation formulas [55].

8.6.2 Piggyback IOLs

Another technique that has been used to correct high degrees of hyperopia in infancy is the piggyback technique, in which a permanent IOL is placed in the capsular bag and a second IOL is placed in the ciliary sulcus [58]. This is also known as temporary polypseudophakia [59], since the intent is to remove the anterior IOL once ocular growth results in too much myopia. The initial target refraction is emmetropia, with optimally 20 % of the total IOL power represented by the anterior IOL. The Pediatric Piggyback IOL Calculator is an Excel-based spreadsheet that can estimate the range of refractions over time when a piggyback lens is used and help the surgeon estimate the timing and refractive effects of removing the anterior IOL [60].

8.7 Summary

- Baseline eye characteristics, laterality, patient age, risk of early glaucoma, and a long-term visual rehabilitation plan should be carefully considered before IOL placement and when selecting an IOL power for an individual child.

- Significant axial elongation and myopic shift will occur, with typically at least six diopters for pseudophakic eyes operated on in infancy, and a wide range of final refractive outcomes may be seen. The greatest myopic shift occurs in the first 6 months after surgery and by 2 years of age, with continued but slower and more linear changes after that.
- Biometry is more challenging and larger prediction errors are seen when targeting a desired post-operative refraction in infantile eyes.
- SRK/T and Holladay formulas, since some studies have found that the SRK II formula is less accurate.

References

1. Gordon RA, Donzis PB. Refractive development of the human eye. Arch Ophthalmol. 1985;103(6):785–9.
2. Flitcroft DI, Knight-Nanan D, Bowell R, Lanigan B, O'Keefe M. Intraocular lenses in children: changes in axial length, corneal curvature, and refraction. Br J Ophthalmol. 1999;83(3):265–9.
3. VanderVeen DK, Nizam A, Lynn MJ, Bothun ED, McClatchey SK, Weakley DR, DuBois LG, Lambert SR, Infant Aphakia Treatment Study Group. Predictability of intraocular lens calculation and early refractive status: the Infant Aphakia Treatment Study. Arch Ophthalmol. 2012;130(3):293–9. doi:10.1001/archophthalmol.2011.358.
4. The Infant Aphakia Treatment Study Group. Design and clinical measures at enrollment. Arch Ophthalmol. 2010;128(1):21–7.
5. Lambert SR, Lynn MJ, DuBois LG, Cotsonis GA, Hartmann EE, Wilson ME, Infant Aphakia Treatment Study Group. Axial elongation following cataract surgery during the first year of life in the Infant Aphakia Treatment Study. Invest Ophthalmol Vis Sci. 2012; 53(12)):7539–45. doi:10.1167/iovs.12-10285.
6. Lambert SR, Lynn MJ, Hartmann EE, DuBois L, Drews-Botsch C, Freedman SF, Plager DA, Buckley EG, Wilson ME, Group IATS. Comparison of contact lens and intraocular lens correction of monocular aphakia during infancy: a randomized clinical trial of HOTV optotype acuity at age 4.5 years and clinical findings at age 5 years. JAMA Ophthalmol. 2014;132(6):676–82. doi:10.1001/jamaophthalmol.2014.531.
7. Fan DS, Rao SK, Yu CB, Wong CY, Lam DS. Changes in refraction and ocular dimensions after cataract surgery and primary intraocular lens implantation in infants. J Cataract Refract Surg. 2006;32((7):1104–8.
8. Vasavada AR, Raj SM, Nihalani B. Rate of axial growth after congenital cataract surgery. Am J Ophthalmol. 2004;138(6):915–24. doi:10.1016/j.ajo.2004.06.068.
9. Griener ED, Dahan E, Lambert SR. Effect of age at time of cataract surgery on subsequent axial length growth in infant eyes. Cataract Refract Surg. 1999;25 (9):1209–13.
10. Hutchinson AK, Wilson ME, Saunders RA. Outcomes and ocular growth rates after intraocular lens implantation in the first 2 years of life. J Cataract Refract Surg. 1998;24(6):846–52.
11. Hussin HM, Markham R. Changes in axial length growth after congenital cataract surgery and intraocular lens implantation in children younger than 5 years. J Cataract Refract Surg. 2009;35(7):1223–8. doi:10.1016/j.jcrs.2009.03.015.
12. Sminia ML, de Faber JT, Doelwijt DJ, Wubbels RJ, Tjon-Fo-Sang M. Axial eye length growth and final refractive outcome after unilateral paediatric cataract surgery. Br J Ophthalmol. 2010;94(5):547–50. doi:10.1136/bjo.2009.160192.
13. McClatchey SK, Dahan E, Maselli E, Gimbel HV, Wilson ME, Lambert SR, Buckley EG, Freedman SF, Plager DA, Parks MM. A comparison of the rate of refractive growth in pediatric aphakic and pseudophakic eyes. Ophthalmology. 2000;107(1):118–22.
14. Superstein R, Archer SM, Del Monte MA. Minimal myopic shift in pseudophakic versus aphakic pediatric cataract patients. J AAPOS. 2002;6:271–6.
15. Dahan E, Drusedau MU. Choice of lens and dioptric power in pediatric pseudophakia. J Cataract Refract Surg. 1997;23 Suppl 1:618–23.
16. Lambert SR, Buckley EG, Plager DA, Medow NB, Wilson ME. Unilateral intraocular lens implantation during the first six months of life. J AAPOS. 1999; 3(6):344–9.
17. O'Keefe M, Fenton S, Lanigan B. Visual outcomes and complications of posterior chamber intraocular lens implantation in the first year of life. J Cataract Refract Surg. 2001;27(12):2006–11.
18. Crouch ER, Pressman SH. Prospective analysis of pediatric pseudophakia: myopic shift and postoperative outcomes. J AAPOS. 2002;6(5):277–82.
19. Gouws P, Hussin HM, Markham RH. Long term results of primary posterior chamber intraocular lens implantation for congenital cataract in the first year of life. Br J Ophthalmol. 2006;90(8):975–8. doi:10.1136/bjo.2006.094656.
20. Ashworth JL, Maino AP, Biswas S, Lloyd IC. Refractive outcomes after primary intraocular lens implantation in infants. Br J Ophthalmol. 2007;91(5):596–9. doi:10.1136/bjo.2006.108571.
21. Astle WF, Ingram AD, Isaza GM, Echeverri P. Paediatric pseudophakia: analysis of intraocular lens power and myopic shift. Clin Experiment Ophthalmol. 2007;35(3):244–51. doi:10.1111/j.1442-9071.2006.01446.x.
22. Hoevenaars NE, Polling JR, Wolfs RC. Prediction error and myopic shift after intraocular lens

implantation in paediatric cataract patients. Br J Ophthalmol. 2011;95(8):1082–5. doi:10.1136/bjo.2010.183566.
23. Hutchinson AK, Drews-Botsch C, Lambert SR. Myopic shift after intraocular lens implantation during childhood. Ophthalmology. 1997;104(11):1752–7.
24. Inatomi M, Kora Y, Kinohira Y, Yaguchi S. Long-term follow-up of eye growth in pediatric patients after unilateral cataract surgery with intraocular lens implantation. J AAPOS. 2004;8(1):50–5. doi:10.1016/S1091853103002544.
25. Chen TC, Walton DS, Bhatia LS. Aphakic glaucoma after congenital cataract surgery. Arch Ophthalmol. 2004;122(12):1819–25. doi:10.1001/archopht.122.12.1819.
26. Gochnauer AC, Trivedi RH, Hill EG, Wilson ME. Interocular axial length difference as a predictor of postoperative visual acuity after unilateral pediatric cataract extraction with primary IOL implantation. J AAPOS. 2010;14(1):20–4. doi:10.1016/j.jaapos.2009.10.015.
27. Lambert SR, Archer SM, Wilson ME, Trivedi RH, del Monte MA, Lynn M. Long-term outcomes of undercorrection versus full correction after unilateral intraocular lens implantation in children. Am J Ophthalmol. 2012;153(4):602–608, 608.e601. doi:10.1016/j.ajo.2011.08.046.
28. Ben-Zion I, Neely DE, Plager DA, Ofner S, Sprunger DT, Roberts GJ. Accuracy of IOL calculations in children: a comparison of immersion versus contact A-scan biometery. J AAPOS. 2008;12(5):440–4. doi:10.1016/j.jaapos.2008.03.016.
29. Moore DB, Ben Zion I, Neely DE, Plager DA, Ofner S, Sprunger DT, Roberts GJ. Accuracy of biometry in pediatric cataract extraction with primary intraocular lens implantation. J Cataract Refract Surg. 2008;34(11):1940–7. doi:10.1016/j.jcrs.2008.07.019.
30. Trivedi RH, Wilson ME. Prediction error after pediatric cataract surgery with intraocular lens implantation: contact versus immersion A-scan biometry. J Cataract Refract Surg. 2011;37(3):501–5. doi:10.1016/j.jcrs.2010.09.023.
31. Mezer E, Rootman DS, Abdolell M, Levin AV. Early postoperative refractive outcomes of pediatric intraocular lens implantation. J Cataract Refract Surg. 2004;30(3):603–10. doi:10.1016/j.jcrs.2003.07.002.
32. Eibschitz-Tsimhoni M, Tsimhoni O, Archer SM, Del Monte MA. Discrepancies between intraocular lens implant power prediction formulas in pediatric patients. Ophthalmology. 2007;114(2):383–6. doi:10.1016/j.ophtha.2006.06.063.
33. Narvaez J, Zimmerman G, Stulting RD, Chang DH. Accuracy of intraocular lens power prediction using the Hoffer Q, Holladay 1, Holladay 2, and SRK/T formulas. J Cataract Refract Surg. 2006;32(12):2050–3. doi:10.1016/j.jcrs.2006.09.009.
34. Neely DE, Plager DA, Borger SM, Golub RL. Accuracy of intraocular lens calculations in infants and children undergoing cataract surgery. J AAPOS. 2005;9(2):160–5. doi:10.1016/j.jaapos.2004.12.010.
35. Andreo LK, Wilson ME, Saunders RA. Predictive value of regression and theoretical IOL formulas in pediatric intraocular lens implantation. J Pediatr Ophthalmol Strabismus. 1997;34(4):240–3.
36. Kekunnaya R, Gupta A, Sachdeva V, Rao HL, Vaddavalli PK, Om Prakash V. Accuracy of intraocular lens power calculation formulae in children less than two years. Am J Ophthalmol. 2012;154(1):13–19.e12. doi:10.1016/j.ajo.2011.11.031.
37. Nihalani BR, VanderVeen DK. Comparison of intraocular lens power calculation formulae in pediatric eyes. Ophthalmology. 2010;117(8):1493–9. doi:10.1016/j.ophtha.2009.12.031.
38. VanderVeen DK, Trivedi RH, Nizam A, Lynn MJ, Lambert SR, Infant Aphakia Treatment Study Group. Predictability of intraocular lens power calculation formulae in infantile eyes with unilateral congenital cataract: results from the Infant Aphakia Treatment Study. Am J Ophthalmol. 2013;156(6):1252–1260.e1252. doi:10.1016/j.ajo.2013.07.014.
39. Trivedi RH, Wilson ME, Reardon W. Accuracy of the Holladay 2 intraocular lens formula for pediatric eyes in the absence of preoperative refraction. J Cataract Refract Surg. 2011;37(7):1239–43. doi:10.1016/j.jcrs.2011.01.021.
40. Tromans C, Haigh PM, Biswas S, Lloyd IC. Accuracy of intraocular lens power calculation in paediatric cataract surgery. Br J Ophthalmol. 2001;85(8):939–41.
41. Eibschitz-Tsimhoni M, Tsimhoni O, Archer SM, Del Monte MA. Effect of axial length and keratometry measurement error on intraocular lens implant power prediction formulas in pediatric patients. J AAPOS. 2008;12(2):173–6. doi:10.1016/j.jaapos.2007.10.012.
42. VanderVeen DK, Trivedi RH, Nizam A, Lynn MJ, Lambert SR, for the Infant Aphakia Treatment Study Group. Response to letter to the editor re: predictability of intraocular lens power calculation formulae in infantile eyes with unilateral congenital cataract: results from the Infant Aphakia Treatment Study. Am J Ophthalmol. 2014;157:1333.
43. Joshi P, Mehta R, Ganesh S. Accuracy of intraocular lens power calculation in pediatric cataracts with less than a 20 mm axial length of the eye. Nepal J Ophthalmol. 2014;6(11):56–64. doi:10.3126/nepjoph.v6i1.10773.
44. Enyedi l B, Peterseim MW, Freedman SF, Buckley EG. Refractive changes after pediatric intraocular lens implantation. Am J Ophthalmol. 1998;126(6):772–81.
45. Plager DA, Kipfer H, Sprunger DT, Sondhi N, Neely DE. Refractive change in pediatric pseudophakia: a 6-year follow-up. J Cataract Refract Surg. 2002;28(5):810–5.
46. McClatchey SK. Intraocular lens calculator for childhood cataract. J Cataract Refract Surg. 1998;24(8):1125–9.
47. McClatchey SK, Parks MM. Theoretic refractive changes after lens implantation in childhood. Ophthalmology. 1997;104(11):1744–51.
48. Kim DH, Kim JH, Kim SJ, Yu YS. Long-term results of bilateral congenital cataract treated with early cataract surgery, aphakic glasses and secondary IOL

implantation. Acta Ophthalmol. 2012;90(3):231–6. doi:10.1111/j.1755-3768.2010.01872.x.
49. Wilson ME, Englert JA, Greenwald MJ. In-the-bag secondary intraocular lens implantation in children. J AAPOS. 1999;3(6):350–5.
50. Wilson ME, Hafez GA, Trivedi RH. Secondary in-the-bag intraocular lens implantation in children who have been aphakic since early infancy. J AAPOS. 2011;15(2):162–6. doi:10.1016/j.jaapos.2010.12.008.
51. Buckley EG. Scleral fixated (sutured) posterior chamber intraocular lens implantation in children. J AAPOS. 1999;3(5):289–94.
52. Nihalani BR, VanderVeen DK. Secondary intraocular lens implantation after pediatric aphakia. J AAPOS. 2011;15(5):435–40. doi:10.1016/j.jaapos.2011.05.019.
53. Moore DB, Ben Zion I, Neely DE, Roberts GJ, Sprunger DT, Plager DA. Refractive outcomes with secondary intraocular lens implantation in children. J AAPOS. 2009;13(6):551–4. doi:10.1016/j.jaapos.2009.09.012.
54. Shenoy BH, Mittal V, Gupta A, Sachdeva V, Kekunnaya R. Refractive outcomes and prediction error following secondary intraocular lens implantation in children: a decade-long analysis. Br J Ophthalmol. 2013;97(12):1516–9. doi:10.1136/bjophthalmol-2012-302775.
55. Abdel-Hafez G. Comparison of aphakic refraction formulas for secondary in-the-bag intraocular lens power estimation in children. J AAPOS. 2011;15(5):432–4. doi:10.1016/j.jaapos.2011.05.021.
56. Hug T. Use of the aphakic refraction in intraocular lens (IOL) power calculations for secondary IOLs in pediatric patients. J Pediatr Ophthalmol Strabismus. 2004;41(4):209–11.
57. Khan AO, AlGaeed A. Paediatric secondary intraocular lens estimation from the aphakic refraction alone: comparison with a standard biometric technique. Br J Ophthalmol. 2006;90(12):1458–60. doi:10.1136/bjo.2006.100834.
58. Gayton JL, Sanders VN. Implanting two posterior chamber intraocular lenses in a case of microphthalmos. J Cataract Refract Surg. 1993;19(6):776–7.
59. Wilson ME, Peterseim MW, Englert JA, Lall-Trail JK, Elliott LA. Pseudophakia and polypseudophakia in the first year of life. J AAPOS. 2001;5(4):238–45. doi:10.1067/mpa.2001.116867.
60. Boisvert C, Beverly DT, McClatchey SK. Theoretical strategy for choosing piggyback intraocular lens powers in young children. J AAPOS. 2009;13(6):555–7. doi:10.1016/j.jaapos.2009.10.001.

9 Intraocular Lens Implantation in the Capsular Bag and Posterior Capsulotomy Techniques

Jane L. Ashworth and Ian Christopher Lloyd

The techniques used for IOL implantation and management of the posterior capsule are crucial factors in maintaining postoperative clarity of the visual axis and thus achieving an optimal visual outcome following paediatric cataract surgery. Visual axis re-opacification (VAO) is the most common postoperative complication following IOL implantation in children and occurs universally in infants and very frequently in young children if the posterior capsule remains intact at surgery [1, 2].

IOL implantation within the capsular bag minimises the risk of postoperative complications such as lens dislocation and postoperative inflammation. Posterior capsulotomy and anterior vitrectomy performed at the time of surgery reduces the risk of visual axis re-opacification in young children undergoing cataract surgery. This chapter discusses the evidence for the safe use of an IOL in congenital cataract surgery, the type of IOL suitable for use in paediatric cataract surgery, implantation and IOL fixation techniques, when posterior capsulotomy and anterior vitrectomy are needed, and surgical technique options.

J.L. Ashworth, PhD, FRCOphth (✉)
Department of Paediatric Ophthalmology, Manchester Royal Eye Hospital, University of Manchester, Manchester, UK
e-mail: Jane.Ashworth@cmft.nhs.uk

I.C. Lloyd, MB, FRCS, FRCOphth
Department of Clinical and Academic Ophthalmology, Great Ormond Street Hospital for Children, London WC1N 7EH, UK

Paediatric Ophthalmology, Manchester Royal Eye Hospital, University of Manchester, Manchester, UK
e-mail: IanChristopher.Lloyd@gosh.nhs.uk

9.1 When to Implant an Intraocular Lens in Pediatric Cataract Surgery

IOL implantation is a safe and predictable procedure for older children and it is probably safe to say that most paediatric cataract surgeons now routinely carry out IOL implantation when performing cataract surgery in children over 2 years of age. However two recently published studies have provided evidence with regard to the efficacy and safety of IOL implantation in younger children. The Infant Aphakia Treatment Study (IATS) and IOLu2 study have both highlighted the greater frequency of peri- and postoperative complications associated with IOL implantation in very young children in comparison to those left aphakic [3–5]. IATS was a randomised controlled trial which demonstrated that IOL implantation in infants with unilateral pediatric cataract (undergoing surgery at 6 months of age or less) produced no significant difference in visual acuity outcome at 4.5 years in comparison with infants left aphakic and managed with contact lens refractive correction [6]. In addition, IATS found IOL implantation was associated with more frequent postoperative adverse events, particularly lens re-proliferation into the visual axis, pupillary membrane formation and

I.C. Lloyd, S.R. Lambert (eds.), *Congenital Cataract*, DOI 10.1007/978-3-319-27848-3_9

corectopia. The authors also reported a greater rate of re-operations in the IOL implanted infants (21 % in the contact lens group compared to 72 % in the IOL group). The IOLu2 study studied a large cohort of British and Irish children with unilateral and bilateral congenital cataracts who were all operated on under 2 years of age. It demonstrated a trend towards better visual outcome in children with bilateral IOL implantation at 1 year after surgery in comparison to those who had been left aphakic, but like IATS found a higher re-operation rate in the IOL group [5].

We believe the current evidence therefore suggests that IOL implantation should be undertaken with caution in infants with unilateral congenital cataract undergoing surgery at 6 months old or less (perhaps unless periods of uncorrected aphakia are deemed likely to occur). Discussion about appropriate surgical management with the parents/carers of infants with bilateral cataract should outline the current evidence relating to the use (or not) of IOLs in congenital cataract surgery. Any perceived marginal benefit to vision in bilateral cases must be balanced by the increased risk of post-operative complications which can necessitate further surgical procedures. This risk can lead to multiple general anaesthetics and possible adverse cognitive/neurodevelopmental effects on the vulnerable developing infant brain.

It should be noted that many eyes with congenital cataract are micro-ophthalmic or have co-existent significant anterior segment abnormalities. These anatomical factors, if significant, should preclude insertion of an IOL at the time of surgery.

9.2 Which Type of IOL to Use

IOLs made from hydrophobic acrylic are preferred by the majority of surgeons who carry out paediatric cataract surgery [7]. IATS surgeons used Acrysof SN60AT IOL (a 1 piece hydrophobic acrylic IOL, Alcon Laboratories, Fort Worth, Texas) implanted into the capsular bag, or Acrysof MA60AT 3 (a 3 piece hydrophobic acrylic IOL, Alcon Laboratories) implanted into the sulcus. The Acrysof MA30AT has a smaller optic size (5.5 mm compared to 6.0 mm) and is easier to fit into the smaller capsular bag of infants less than 1 year of age (Fig. 9.1). No difference in VAO rates was found in a study comparing 4 different hydrophobic acrylic IOLs (Acrysof MA60AC, SA60AT, SN60AT, SN60WF) commonly used in children undergoing cataract surgery at less than 12 months of age [8]. Other hydrophobic acrylic IOLs which can be considered for use in children include the Bausch and Lomb enVista and Hoya iSert IOLs. The Bausch and Lomb IOL is claimed to be free of the "glistenings" seen in the optic of some hydrophobic lenses. However in the author's experience these, when present, are rarely symptomatic.

The use of rigid PMMA IOLs has been shown to be associated with a higher risk of complications such as anterior capsular tears, iris prolapse, optic displacement anterior to the capsule, optic capture of the pupil and fibrinous uveitis. This is likely to be due to the larger wound size needed for their insertion [9], and the associated operative and post-operative complications (uveitis, pigment deposition, iridocorneal adhesions and posterior synechiae). However IOL type (PMMA or acrylic) does not appear to significantly influence the incidence of PCO following cataract surgery in children [9] but onset of significant PCO may

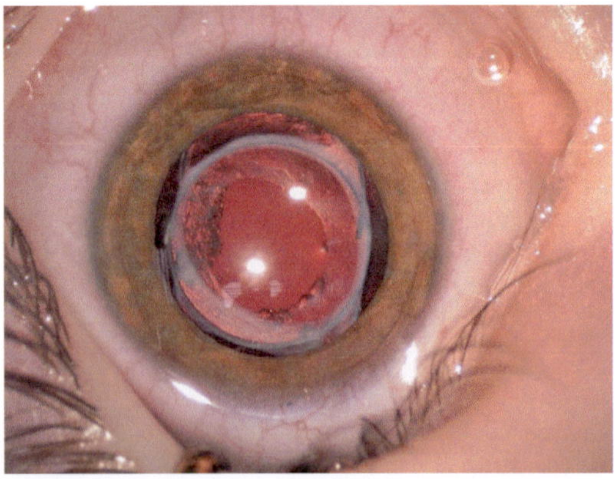

Fig. 9.1 Four year old with LEC migration approaching visual axis. Three piece MA30 acrylic IOL "in the bag" after anterior CCC, lensectomy, posterior CCC and anterior vitrectomy carried out in infancy

be inhibited for longer following acrylic IOL insertion [10–13].

9.3 Technique of IOL Insertion

The authors prefer corneal incisions (rather than limbal or scleral). A superior incision with a keratome is made at the start of the lensectomy procedure and temporarily sutured closed again once it has been used for access to perform a capsulorhexis with forceps under viscoelastic. This suture maintains the stability of the anterior chamber of the eye for the subsequent lensectomy. Two incisions with an MVR blade are made at 90° to this incision i.e. at 3 and 9 o'clock and are used for the vitrector and infusion cannula. The lensectomy is performed as outlined in Chap. 7 (Wilson). An alternative technique is to use vitrector forceps for capsulorhexis using one of the two MVR incisions. One of these can then be enlarged after the lensectomy to enable IOL implantation (rather than using 3 incisions). In either approach, the corneal wound utilised is enlarged to approximately 3.0 mm in length, prior to insertion of the IOL. The capsular bag is filled with viscoelastic in order to ensure that the anterior and posterior capsules are well separated and thus provide sufficient space within the capsular bag for IOL insertion. Single piece preloaded injectable IOLs (for example the Acrysof SN60AT) may be used even in the presence of a posterior capulotomy [14]. However they require careful insertion as the leading haptic can snag on a weak or defective posterior capsule causing further capsular trauma and lens luxation into the vitreous cavity. This should be guarded against in cases of posterior lenticonus (Fig. 9.2). The single-piece SA60 IOL is folded into an IOL introducer which has been primed with viscoelastic. The introducer is inserted through the enlarged corneal wound into the plane of the anterior capsule and the lens is injected into the capsular bag gently, taking care not to inject the lens through the posterior capsule or disrupt the capsular bag.

A 3-piece IOL (for example the Acrysof MA30AT or MA60AT) can be placed directly in a controlled manner within the capsular bag and so may be less technically challenging in the presence of a posterior capsulotomy in younger children. The 3 piece Acrysof MA60AT and MA30AT lenses are folded manually in forceps and inserted through the enlarged corneal wound. The leading haptic is inserted through the wound first and placed carefully in a flat plane into the equator of the capsular bag, taking care not to snag or disrupt the posterior capsulotomy. The optic follows through the corneal wound and is allowed to slowly unfold in the plane of the anterior capsule. The trailing haptic is then grasped with forceps and, via pronation of the surgeons wrist, rotated into the plane of the capsular bag, whilst the optic is depressed gently with a second instrument (such as a lens dialler) introduced through the paracentesis. This ensures that the trailing haptic follows the optic into position within the capsular bag once gently released and that any dialling of the lens is minimal or unnecessary.

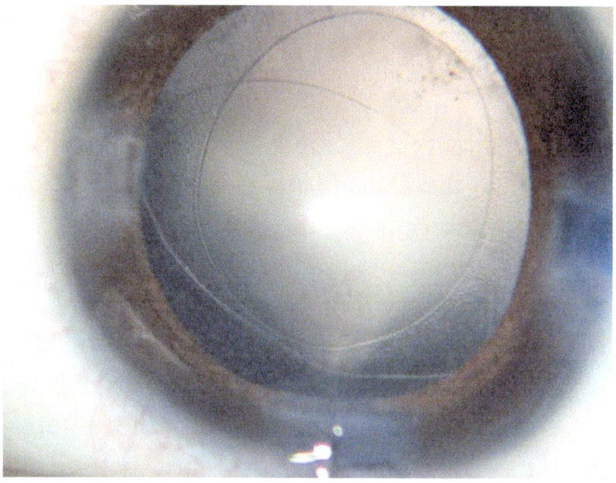

Fig. 9.2 Large oval posterior lenticonus defect apparent in eye of infant (prior to IOL insertion) after anterior circular capsulorhexis and lensectomy

9.4 IOL Position

There are several options open to the surgeon with regard to the position of the IOL in relation to the capsular bag.

The IOL can be positioned completely within the capsular bag between the anterior and posterior capsules (as in traditional adult extracapsular surgery) (Fig. 9.3). However in the presence of an abnormal, torn or unstable posterior capsule, optic "capture" can be achieved so that the lens haptics are placed anterior to the capsular bag, in the ciliary sulcus, with the optic of the IOL pushed posteriorly through an intact anterior capsulorhexis so that the optic is within the plane of the capsular bag. Other useful techniques to consider include placing the haptics in the sulcus but capturing the IOL through both the anterior and posterior capsulorhexes (optic behind the posterior capsule), or the haptics can be positioned within a capsular bag with posterior capture of the optic of the IOL through a stable posterior capsulorhexis (optic buttonholing) [1, 2, 15, 16]. Optic capture is performed in each of these techniques after initial positioning of the haptics (with adequate viscoelastic maintaining the anterior chamber). Gentle pressure is applied to the lens optic with a manipulator to push it through the capsular opening (Diagrams 9.1, 9.2, 9.3, and 9.4).

IOL implantation within the capsular bag produces a stable IOL with a reduced risk of postoperative inflammation compared to a sulcus fixated IOL. However IOL capture may provide stability and long-term centration of the IOL and prevents vitreous from extending anteriorly [15], and may reduce the incidence of and/or delay the onset of VAO [17, 18].

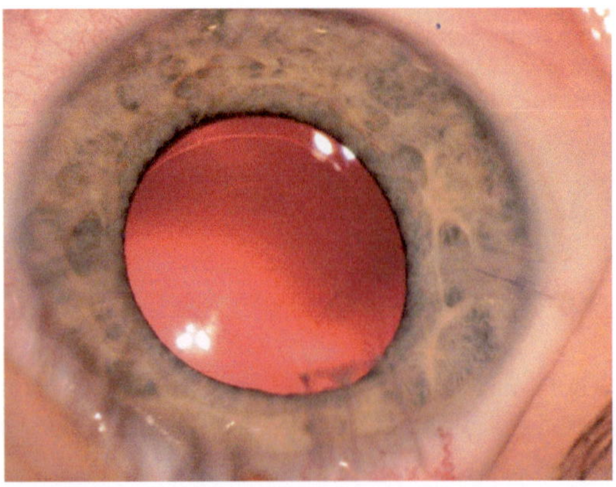

Fig. 9.3 Two year old with one piece SA60 acrylic IOL "in the bag" immediately after procedure - anterior CCC, lensectomy, posterior CCC and anterior vitrectomy

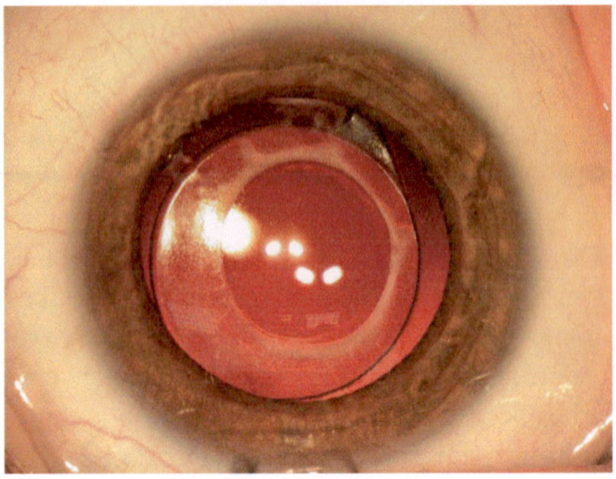

Fig. 9.4 Five year old with well centred one piece SA60 acrylic IOL "in the bag" 2 months after anterior CCC, lensectomy, posterior CCC and anterior vitrectomy

A technique, known as 'bag-in-the-lens' IOL implantation, has been used extensively in Europe [19]. Anterior and posterior capsulorhexes are performed of a similar size (5.0 mm) and, following IOL insertion, both leaves of the capsule are positioned into a groove between two flanges around the circumference of the IOL. This technique aims to eradicate lens epithelial cell (LEC) proliferation and migration by confining the LECs to the rim of capsular bag around the IOL.

9.5 When to Perform a Posterior Capsulotomy and Anterior Vitrectomy

Visual axis opacification (VAO) occurs rapidly and universally in young children when the posterior capsule is left intact, due to the greater tissue reactivity of younger lens epithelial cells (LEC) [1, 2]. Performance of a primary posterior capsulotomy (PCC) and anterior vitrectomy at the time of surgery reduces the incidence of, and delays the onset of, VAO [13, 16, 18, 20, 21] (Fig. 9.4). There remains uncertainty about the precise age up to which PCC and anterior vitrectomy is needed. It is undoubtedly also influenced by factors such as likely compliance with follow-up and access to a horizontally mounted Nd-YAG laser for capsulotomy. VAO is reported to be significantly higher in children aged 8 years and

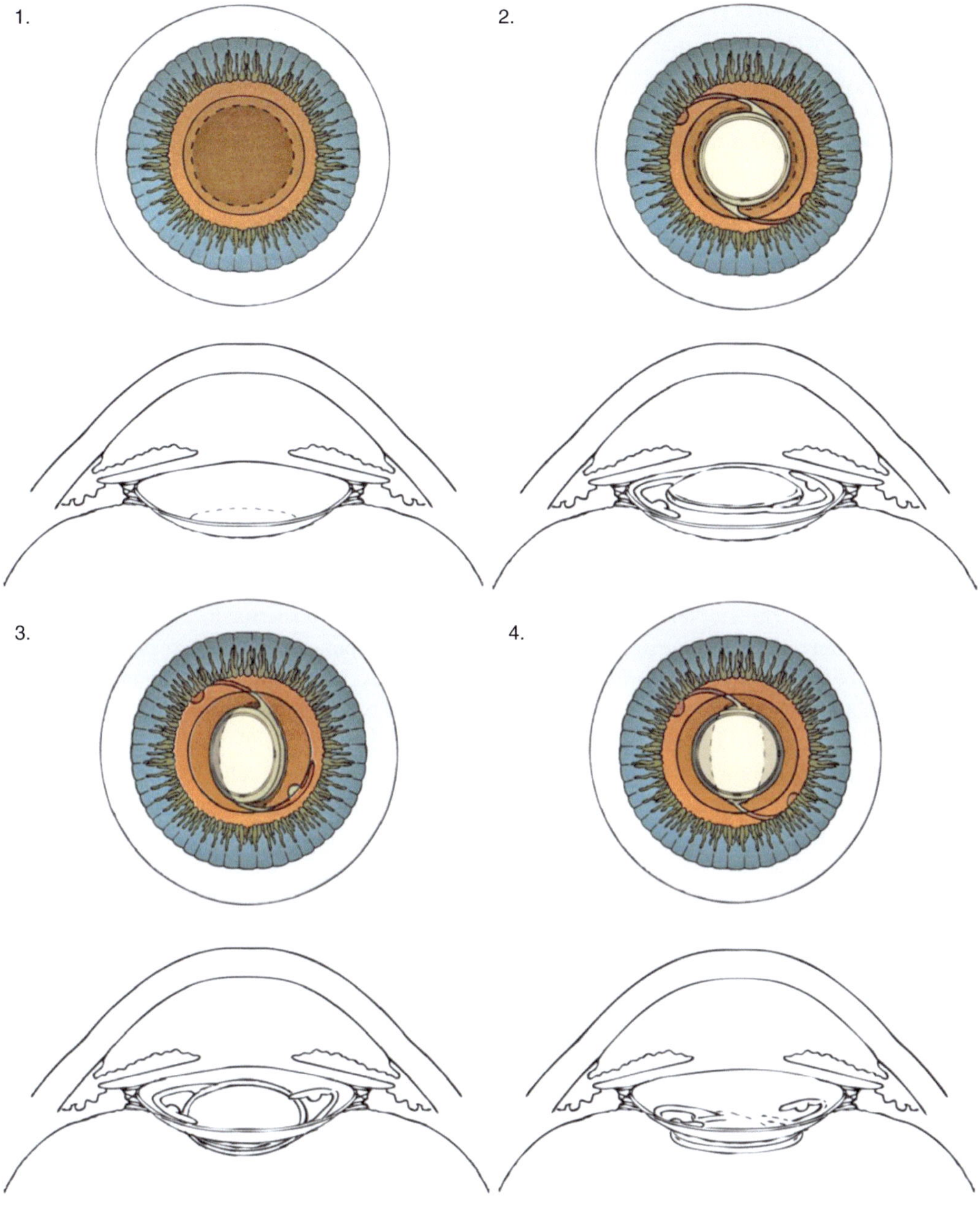

Diagrams 9.1, 9.2, 9.3, and 9.4 Sequence of images showing a three piece IOL converted from initial "in the bag" implantation to optic capture through a posterior CCC (Graphic by Dr C Kilduff)

younger at the time of surgery [22]. Other authors suggest that PPC is advisable when cataract surgery is carried out at less than 6 years old [23].

PCC alone is less effective in delaying or preventing VAO than PCC combined with anterior vitrectomy [18, 24], as the intact anterior hyaloid face may act as a scaffold for LEC migration and proliferation across the visual axis. PCC with posterior optic capture has been suggested as a technique to delay VAO in the absence of anterior vitrectomy [17], but it appears to be more effective in the prevention of VAO when combined with anterior vitrectomy [18]. Other studies have suggested that PCC and anterior vitrectomy are important steps in maintaining a clear visual axis after cataract surgery in patients younger than 7 years of age [25]. The authors perform PCC and anterior vitrectomy in all children of 5 years of age or younger.

9.6 Posterior Capsulotomy Techniques

Several techniques are available for performing posterior capsulotomy, and the one chosen will depend on the clinical features of each individual case, the surgeons experience and preference, and the equipment available. Frequently used techniques include a manual continuous curvilinear capsulorhexis (CCC), the 'two incision push pull' technique, and vitrectorhexis through a pars plana sclerostomy. The paediatric cataract surgeon should be comfortable performing PCC via a variety of techniques. This enables posterior capsulotomy to be carried out in a range of clinical situations, for example in the presence of a pre-existing posterior capsular defect or a posterior capsular plaque.

Posterior capsulotomy and anterior vitrectomy may be performed prior to insertion of the IOL (via manual CCC, 'two incision push pull' technique or vitrectorhexis followed by anterior vitrectomy). It can also follow IOL insertion (via vitrectorhexis from an anterior approach behind the IOL, via a pars plana incision with vitrectorhexis or via manual CCC followed by anterior vitrectomy. When PCC is carried out prior to IOL insertion, trypan blue 0.06% may be used to enable better visualisation of the posterior capsule if necessary [26]. This is instilled under viscoelastic and then the anterior chamber irrigated with balanced salt solution.

The posterior capsulotomy may be carried out with the vitrectomy cutter (vitrectorhexis) prior to insertion of the IOL, by insertion of the vitrector through a corneal paracentesis, and fashioning of a posterior capsular opening with the cutter under viscoelastic. The posterior capsulotomy should ideally be smaller than the size of the anterior capsulorhexis (approximately 4 mm), round and centrally placed so that the visual axis is cleared. This technique may be difficult in the presence of a posterior capsular plaque (for example in cases of persistent fetal vasculature) when intraocular forceps and/or scissors may be needed for removal of the central capsule. In cases of posterior lenticonus the posterior capsule is often very thin and friable and thus easily amenable to opening with this technique. If there is a pre-existing capsular defect, this can similarly be enlarged or trimmed as necessary with the cutter.

Some surgeons prefer to perform a manual posterior CCC; an initial opening is made in the posterior capsule using a needle following inflation of the capsular bag with viscoelastic, and then the capsulotomy is completed with forceps [27]. The CCC should be well centred and smaller than the anterior capsulorhexis. Excess injection of viscoelastic posterior to the capsule through the central puncture may increase the potential for the CCC to tear out to the equator.

The 'two-incision push-pull' capsulotomy technique has been well described [29–29] and is reported to provide a reliable method of making the posterior capsular opening; two parallel incision are made in the posterior capsule with a needle under viscoelastic, and these are then extended with forceps to create a central posterior capsulotomy opening. Hamada et al reported no incidents of inadvertent vitreous loss in 41 cases undergoing the two incision push pull technique for posterior capsulotomy [28]. This method can result in an oval rhexis and so a four-incision technique has been described in order to improve the configuration of the posterior capsulotomy (Mohammadpour JCRS) [30].

Pars plana capsulotomy and anterior vitrectomy can be performed after the IOL has been placed in the capsular bag [1, 31]. It is probably technically easier to implant the IOL before PCCC is made, and it may reduce the risk of vitreous strands coming forward during the remaining surgery. In this technique a sclerostomy incision is made at the pars plana/plicata superotemporally or superonasally. The position of this should be 2 mm posterior to the limbus in infants less than 12 months old, 2.5 mm posterior to the limbus in those 12–48 months, increasing to 3 mm from age 4 to 10 years and 3.5 mm after 10 years. An incision in the conjunctiva and tenons capsule is made with scissors, the sclera visualised and then an MVR blade used to make a sclerostomy. An infusion via the paracentesis in the anterior chamber is maintained and a vitrectomy cutter is passed through the sclerostomy behind the capsule and lens. The vitrector is used to create a central circular opening in the posterior capsule, as well as a limited anterior vitrectomy. The sclera incision is carefully checked and cleared of any vitreous. It is then sutured with 7.0 or 8.0 vicryl synthetic absorbable sutures. The overlying tenons layer and conjunctiva are also closed with vicryl sutures.

Manual posterior capsulorhexis can be performed with forceps following IOL placement through a pars plicata incision [1].

Other techniques described for carrying out posterior capsulorhexis include the use of radiofrequency diathermy [32] and Fugo blade assisted plasma ablation [33].

9.7 Anterior Vitrectomy Techniques

Anterior vitrectomy is carried out immediately following posterior capsulotomy, either before or after IOL insertion. Anterior vitrectomy can be performed under viscoelastic without anterior chamber infusion. This minimises the risk of vitreous hydration and extrusion of vitreous into the anterior chamber and possible wick formation. An anterior vitrectomy is carried out with the aim of removing approximately one third of the vitreous directly behind the posterior capsule. Intracameral preservative free triamcinolone acetonide can be used following the posterior capsulotomy to visualise the anterior vitreous face [34, 35], and can be used following vitrectomy and after IOL implantation to visualise and help in the eradication of any residual vitreous strands. The use of intracameral steroid raises the concern of subsequent secondary ocular hypertension or glaucoma. However a study of 43 eyes of children undergoing cataract surgery with the use of intraoperative triamcinolone revealed none had raised intraocular pressure at any point in 12 months follow-up [35].

9.8 Management of Posterior Capsular Abnormalities

Posterior capsular plaque occurs in 13 % of children up to 15 years old undergoing cataract surgery [36], and is often associated with persistent fetal vasculature. Smaller plaques can be removed by creating a manual PCC with forceps. However larger plaques may need removal via posterior vitrectorhexis. Occasionally intraocular scissors are required to remove thickened posterior capsular plaques. This can result in instability of the posterior capsulorhexis making it prone to tearing out. Caution must therefore be used on insertion of the IOL.

A rent in the PC may inadvertently arise during lensectomy, or a pre-existing capsular defect may become apparent (posterior lenticonus). In these situations, the posterior capsulotomy may need to be trimmed with the vitrector to ensure it is central and stable prior to IOL insertion. In this situation anterior vitrectomy should be carried out before IOL insertion, and consideration must be given as to the most stable position for the IOL in relation to the capsular bag; sulcus fixation of the IOL haptics with posterior capture of the optic is often the optimal approach.

9.9 Complications of IOL Insertion

Per-operative complications of IOL insertion include luxation of the IOL through the posterior capsule requiring IOL repositioning or even removal, disruption of the posterior capsule resulting in an unstable and over large posterior capsulotomy, and iris prolapse into the wound. Postoperative complications occurring following IOL insertion and PCCC include LEC reproliferation or pupillary membranes causing VAO, vitreous wicks, uveitis, corectopia, pigment deposition, posterior synechiae, and iridocorneal adhesions.

9.10 Summary

IOL implantation has transformed paediatric cataract surgery in the last 30 years particularly for children over the age of 2. Current evidence suggests that paediatric cataract surgeons should carry out IOL implantation in infants with some caution and only when clinically appropriate. Similarly age appropriate management of the posterior capsule and anterior vitreous is important to minimise visual axis opacification (VAO). It behoves the paediatric cataract surgeon to learn and be able to call on a variety of surgical techniques in order to achieve optimal visual results in all patients.

References

1. Vasavada AR, Praveen MR, Tassignon MJ, Shah SK, Vasavada VA, Van Looveren J, De Veuster I, Trivedi RH. Posterior capsule management in congenital cataract surgery. J Cataract Refract Surg. 2011;37(1):173–93.
2. Vasavada AR, Shah SK, Praveen MR, Vasavada VA, Trivedi RH, Karve SJ. Pars plicata posterior continuous curvilinear capsulorhexis. J Cataract Refract Surg. 2011;37(2):221–3.
3. Plager DA, Lynn MJ, Buckley EG, Wilson ME, Lambert SR. Complications, adverse events and additional intraocular surgery one year after cataract surgery in the Infant Aphakia Treatment Study. Ophthalmology. 2011;118(12):2330–4.
4. Plager DA, Lynn MJ, Buckley EG, Wilson ME, Lambert SR, Infant Aphakia Treatment Study Group. Complications in the first 5 years following cataract surgery in infants with and without intraocular lens implantation in the Infant Aphakia Treatment Study. Am J Ophthalmol. 2014;158(5):892–8.
5. Solebo AL, Russell-Eggitt I, Cumberland PM, Rahi JS, British Isles Congenital Cataract Interest Group. Risks and outcomes associated with primary intraocular lens implantation in children under 2 years of age: the IoLunder2 cohort study. Br J Ophthalmol. 2015;99(11):1471–6.
6. Infant Aphakia Treatment Study Group, Lambert SR, Lynn MJ, Hartmann EE, DuBois L, Drews-Botsch C, Freedman SF, Plager DA, Buckley EG, Wilson ME. Comparison of contact lens and intraocular lens correction of monocular aphakia during infancy: a randomized clinical trial of HOTV optotype acuity at age 4.5 years and clinical findings at age 5 years. JAMA Ophthalmol. 2014;132(6):676–82.
7. Medsinge A, Nischal KK. Pediatric cataract: challenges and future directions. Clin Ophthalmol. 2015;9:77–90.
8. Trivedi RH, Wilson ME, Vasavada AR, Shah SK, Vasavada V, Vasavada VA. Visual axis opacification after cataract surgery and hydrophobic acrylic intraocular lens implantation in the first year of life. J Cataract Refract Surg. 2011;37(1):83–7.
9. Rowe NA, Biswas S, Lloyd IC. Primary IOL implantation in children: a risk analysis of foldable acrylic v PMMA lenses. Br J Ophthalmol. 2004;88(4):481–5.
10. Küchle M, Lausen B, Gusek-Schneider GC. Results and complications of hydrophobic acrylic vs PMMA posterior chamber lenses in children under 17 years of age. Graefes Arch Clin Exp Ophthalmol. 2003;241(8):637–41.
11. Wilson Jr ME, Trivedi RH, Buckley EG, Granet DB, Lambert SR, Plager DA, Sinskey RM, Vasavada AR. ASCRS white paper. Hydrophobic acrylic intraocular lenses in children. J Cataract Refract Surg. 2007;33(11):1966–73.
12. Panahi-Bazaz MR, Zamani M, Abazar B. Hydrophilic Acrylic versus PMMA Intraocular Lens Implantation in Pediatric Cataract Surgery. J Ophthalmic Vis Res. 2009;4(4):201–7.
13. Ram J, Brar GS, Kaushik S, Gupta A, Gupta A. Role of posterior capsulotomy with vitrectomy and intraocular lens design and material in reducing posterior capsule opacification after pediatric cataract surgery. J Cataract Refract Surg. 2003;29(8):1579–84.
14. Trivedi RH, Wilson Jr ME. Single-piece acrylic intraocular lens implantation in children. J Cataract Refract Surg. 2003;29(9):1738–43.
15. Gimbel HV, DeBroff BM. Intraocular lens optic capture. J Cataract Refract Surg. 2004;30(1):200–6.
16. Dada T, Dada VK, Sharma N, Vajpayee RB. Primary posterior capsulorhexis with optic capture and intracameral heparin in paediatric cataract surgery. Clin Exp Ophthalmol. 2000;28(5):361–3.
17. Raina UK, Gupta V, Arora R, Mehta DK. Posterior continuous curvilinear capsulorhexis with and without optic capture of the posterior chamber intraocular lens in the absence of vitrectomy. J Pediatr Ophthalmol Strabismus. 2002;39(5):278–87.
18. Koch DD, Kohnen T. A retrospective comparison of techniques to prevent secondary cataract formation following posterior chamber intraocular lens implantation in infants and children. Trans Am Ophthalmol Soc. 1997;95:351–60.
19. Tassignon M, De Veuster I, Godts D, Kosec D, Van den Dooren K, Gobin L. Bag-in-the-lens intraocular lens implantation in the pediatric eye. J Cataract Refract Surg. 2007;33:611–7.
20. Guo S, Wagner RS, Caputo A. Management of the anterior and posterior lens capsules and vitreous in pediatric cataract surgery. J Pediatr Ophthalmol Strabismus. 2004;41(6):330–7.
21. Er H, Doganay S, Evereklioglu C, Erten A, Cumurcu T, Bayramlar H. Retrospective comparison of surgical techniques to prevent secondary opacification in pediatric cataracts. J Pediatr Ophthalmol Strabismus. 2000;37(5):294–8.

22. Vasavada AR, Trivedi RH, Nath VC. Visual axis opacification after AcrySof intraocular lens implantation in children. J Cataract Refract Surg. 2004;30(5): 1073–81.
23. Jensen AA, Basti S, Greenwald MJ, Mets MB. When may the posterior capsule be preserved in pediatric intraocular lens surgery? Ophthalmology. 2002;109(2):324–7.
24. Vasavada A, Desai J. Primary posterior capsulorhexis with and without anterior vitrectomy in congenital cataracts. J Cataract Refract Surg. 1997;23(1):645–51.
25. Kugelberg M, Zetterström C. Pediatric cataract surgery with or without anterior vitrectomy. J Cataract Refract Surg. 2002;28(10):1770–3.
26. Sharma N, Balasubramanya R, Dada VK, Vajpayee RB. Efficacy of trypan blue in posterior capsulorhexis with optic capture in pediatric cataracts. BMC Ophthalmol. 2006;6:12.
27. Dholakia SA, Praveen MR, Vasavada AR, Nihalani B. Completion rate of primary posterior continuous curvilinear capsulorhexis and vitreous disturbance during congenital cataract surgery. J AAPOS. 2006;10(4):351–6.
28. Hamada S, Low S, Walters BC, Nischal KK. Five-year experience of the 2-incision push-pull technique for anterior and posterior capsulorrhexis in pediatric cataract surgery. Ophthalmology. 2006;113(8):1309–14.
29. Nischal K. Two-incision push-pull capsularhexis for pedicatric cataract surgery. J Cataract Refract Surg. 2002;28(4):593–5.
30. Mohammadpour M. Four-incision capsularhexis in pediatric cataract surgery. J Cataract Refract Surg. 2007;33(7):1155–7.
31. Alexandrakis G, Peterseim MM, Wilson ME. Clinical outcomes of pars plana capsulotomy with anterior vitrectomy in pediatric cataract surgery. J AAPOS. 2002;6(3):163–7.
32. Comer RM, Abdulla N, O'Keefe M. Radiofrequency diathermy capsulorhexis of the anterior and posterior capsules in pediatric cataract surgery: preliminary results. J Cataract Refract Surg. 1997;23:641–4.
33. Sinha R, Bali SJ, Kumar C, Shekhar H, Sharma N, Titiyal JS, Vajpayee RB. Results of cataract surgery and plasma ablation posterior capsulotomy in anterior persistent hyperplastic primary vitreous. Middle East Afr J Ophthalmol. 2013;20(3):217–20.
34. Shah SK, Vasavada V, Praveen MR, Vasavada AR, Trivedi RH, Dixit NV. Triamcinolone-assisted vitrectomy in pediatric cataract surgery. J Cataract Refract Surg. 2009;35(2):230–2.
35. Praveen MR, Shah SK, Vasavada VA, Dixit NV, Vasavada AR, Garg VS, Trivedi RH. Triamcinolone-assisted vitrectomy in pediatric cataract surgery: intraoperative effectiveness and postoperative outcome. J AAPOS. 2010;14(4):340–4.
36. Praveen MR, Shah SK, Vasavada AR, Vasavada VA, Asnani PK, Anwar I, Trivedi RH. Incidence, management, and postoperative outcomes in pediatric eyes with coexisting posterior capsule plaque and cataract. J Cataract Refract Surg. 2010;36(12):2094–9.

10 Secondary IOLs in Children

Jan Tjeerd de Faber

Implantation of an intraocular lens has become the standard of care to correct the aphakic state that arises following the removal of cataract. Ideally, the IOL is placed within the capsular bag. This allows stable fixation at a position closest to the nodal point of the eye. However the use of IOLs in very young children remains controversial because of the reported increased complication rate in this group. Thus a clinical decision to leave the eyes aphakic is often made and the resultant aphakia and hypermetropic refractive error corrected with either contact lenses or spectacles. This enables the surgeon to carry out implantation of an IOL later in childhood or adult life when the refractive growth of the eye (emmetropisation) is finished or when contact lens intolerance occurs.

In these circumstances secondary implantation of an IOL is a good option. Several surgical approaches are possible.

A. In patients with adequate residual capsular support:
   - Placement of the IOL in the posterior chamber (ciliary sulcus) on top of remnants of the anterior and posterior lens capsule (Soemmerring's ring).
   - Placement of the IOL within the leaves of the surgically opened Soemmerring's ring (after removal of residual lens material).

B. In patients with little or no capsular support
   1. Scleral sutured or glued PC IOL.
   2. Iris sutured PC IOL
   3. Iris fixated Artisan IOL (posteriorly placed).
   4. Angle supported AC IOL
   5. Iris fixated Artisan AC IOL

In the presence of an intact and central (not subluxated) capsular bag and adequate zonular support, the most stable and physiological position for an IOL in children is within the bag. Most modern IOLs are designed for this location and have been shown to be highly biocompatible. However in some cases this is not possible, either because of anatomical abnormalities, due to the absence of capsular support in eyes after trauma or those with previously dislocated lenses (e.g. Marfan syndrome).

This chapter outlines the methods developed to enable intraocular lens implantation as a secondary procedure in aphakic paediatric eyes both with or without adequate capsular or zonular support. This includes anterior chamber angle and iris-fixated lenses, as well as posterior chamber iris-fixated lenses and scleral-sutured or glued lenses. Specific lenses and techniques are described, including possible complications [1–4].

J.T. de Faber, MD
Department of Pediatric Ophthalmology and Strabismus, The Rotterdam Eye Hospital, Rotterdam, The Netherlands
e-mail: defaber@telfort.nl

I.C. Lloyd, S.R. Lambert (eds.), *Congenital Cataract*, DOI 10.1007/978-3-319-27848-3_10

10.1 Secondary Implantation in the Presence of Capsular Support

An IOL can be placed in the ciliary sulcus when the remnants of the anterior and posterior capsule, the ring of Soemmerring, are strong enough to support it. The surgeon can choose to decrease the size and thickness of the Soemmerring's ring by opening it with a blade such as an MVR and by then removing the "doughnut" of lens material and after-cataract. This enables placement of an IOL between the residual anterior and posterior capsule leaves thus allowing secondary implantation in the capsular bag [5] (Fig. 10.1). When this is not possible, the IOL can be placed on top of Soemmerring's ring. However, the surgeon should be aware that increasing thickness of this ring during the first decades of life can push the optic and haptics anteriorly, causing shallowing of the anterior chamber. This in turn can lead to the formation of peripheral anterior synechiae (PAS) and secondary glaucoma.

Until the late 1990s rigid PMMA IOLs were the standard of care. The stiffness of the haptics in these IOLs prevented their forward movement. Currently most commonly used IOLs are made from flexible acrylic. When these are placed in the ciliary sulcus they are prone to anterior movement caused by the gradually increasing thickness of the Soemmerring's ring. I have seen this occur in several patients who presented some months after surgery with the IOL optic dislocated

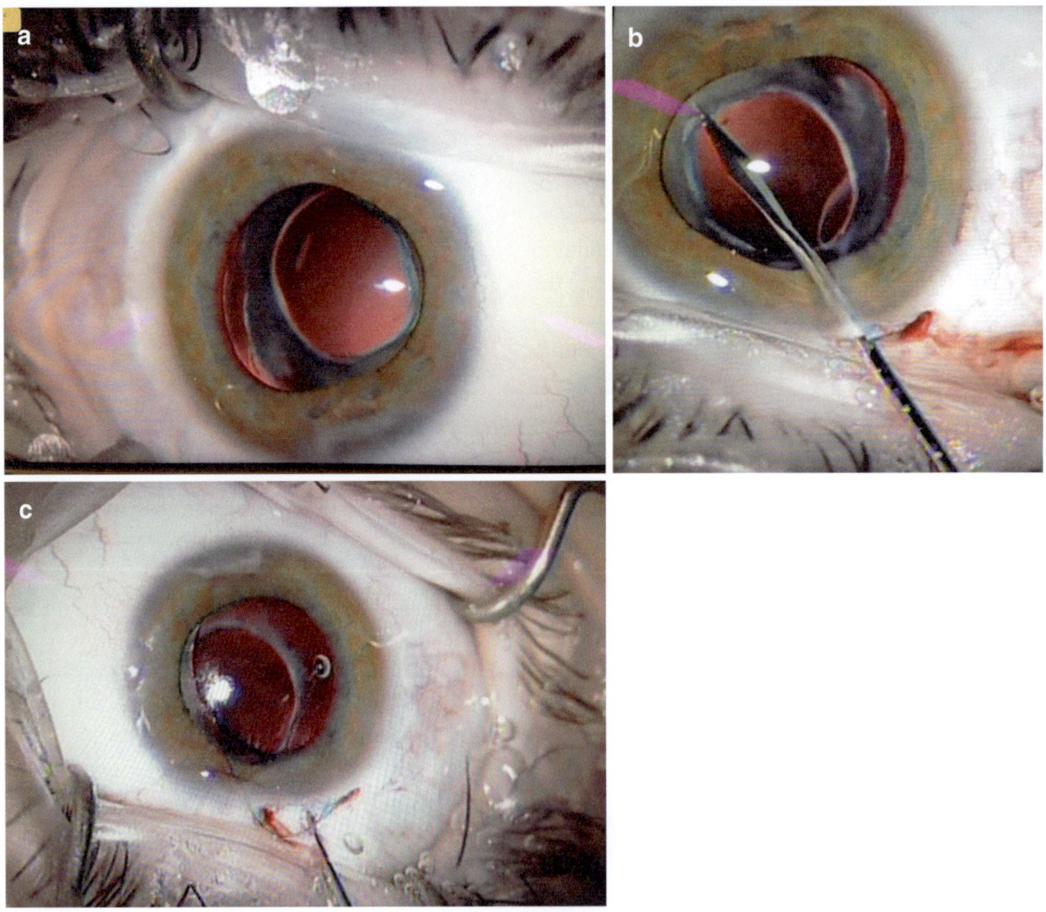

Fig. 10.1 (a–c) Opening a Soemmerring's ring and aspiration of the after cataract. Secondary IOL implanted in the sulcus. Note peripheral anterior synechiae at the 6 o'clock position

forwards into the AC. Examination reveals a distorted, stretched pupil due to entrapment of the optic of the IOL in the pupillary opening. Thus caution should be exercised in the use of this type of lens in the ciliary sulcus.

An alternative option is to open Soemmerring's ring and aspirate the lens remnants within it to recreate a capsular bag. These residual lens epithelial cells aggregate after the initial cataract surgery between the leaves of the anterior and posterior lens capsule. If the reformed capsular bag has enough residual posterior capsular support, a round edged IOL can be implanted into the bag. If the bag is structurally inadequate to support "in the bag" fixation, the IOL can be placed in the sulcus, which is now deeper because the thick Soemerring's ring has been removed or debulked.

10.2 Figures Showing IOLs in the Sulcus

IOL design has evolved over the last 20 years. Haptics (as well as optics) in many IOLs are now sharp edged (rather than round edged) in order to prevent migration of lens epithelial cells to the centre of the visual axis between the posterior capsule and the IOL itself. Serious problems have been reported after sharp edged IOLs had been placed inappropriately (or inadvertently) outside of the capsular bag. Never put a sharp edged IOL in the ciliary sulcus. It is likely to lead to serious complications including chafing of the posterior iris pigment epithelium, hyphaema, glaucoma, iris cysts, uveitis and even phthisis (Figs. 10.2, 10.3 and 10.4). An example is a 1 year old girl in whom an Acrysof SA60AT was unintentionally placed

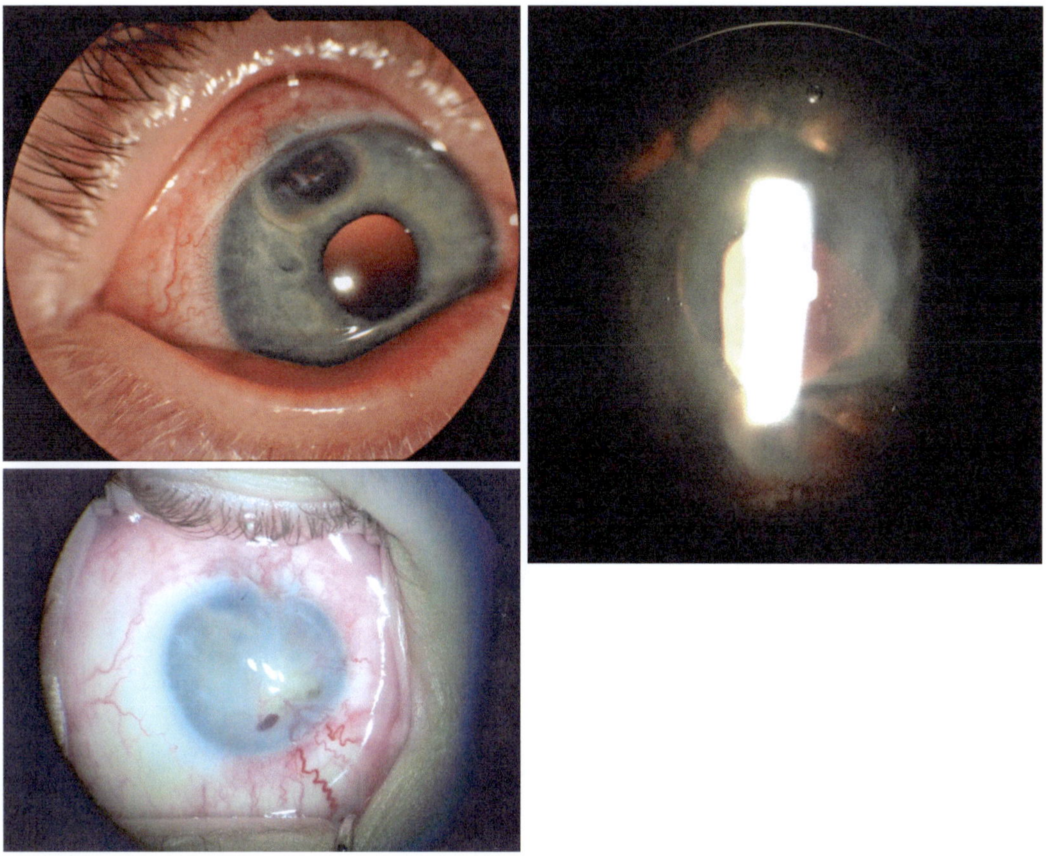

Figs. 10.2, 10.3 and 10.4 SA60AT IOL placed in the sulcus leading to iris cyst, iris chafing pigment dispersion, peripheral anterior synechiae, and glaucoma. After removal of the IOL the eye became blind and phthisical

in the sulcus, instead of in the capsular bag. She initially developed an iris cyst and later pigment dispersion, glaucoma and uveitis. The eye became blind at the age of 4 and then became phthisical. In the event of difficulties during the insertion of a sharp edged IOL into the bag, I would advise immediate removal of the IOL and substitute placement of a round edged 3-piece IOL (or alternatively a rigid PMMA IOL) in the ciliary sulcus with where possible, capture of the optic in the anterior capsulorhexis (Figs. 10.5 and 10.6).

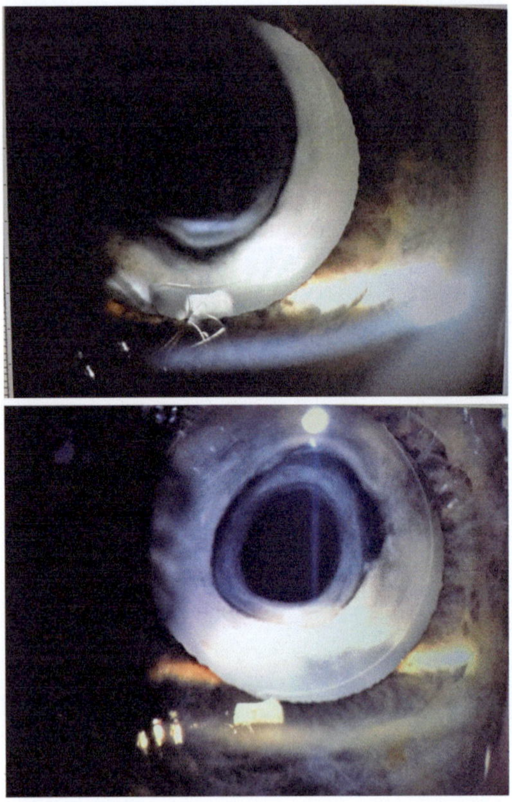

Figs. 10.5 and 10.6 PMMA IOL placed in the sulcus on top of the Soemmerring's ring

10.3 Artisan Iris Fixated AC IOL

When there is inadequate capsular support for placing an IOL in the ciliary sulcus, an option is the use of an Artisan iris fixated IOL in the AC.

The Artisan Iris fixated IOL was designed by Jan Worst in 1979 using the concept that the mid-peripheral iris stroma is largely immobile [6]. Over the following decades the use of this IOL, which was initially only recommended for the correction of aphakia, was extended to include other indications such as phakic IOL correction of myopia, hyperopia and astigmatism. Paradoxically, the phakic IOL was given FDA approval, but the original aphakic IOL for the correction of aphakia did not receive FDA approval. However, several centres in the USA are currently evaluating the use of the Artisan IOL to correct aphakia in children. Outside of the USA, large experience has already been gathered with this lens in the correction of aphakia. It has been used as a primary implant in cases of traumatic lens subluxation, ectopia lentis and also for secondary IOL implantation in cases with insufficient capsular support. This anterior chamber IOL is surgically less challenging than scleral sutured or glued PC IOL's. Table 10.1 compares three types of IOL used for secondary implantation in the absence of capsular support.

Table 10.1 Comparison of three types of secondary IOLs

	Artisan	Angle supported lens	Sclera sutured PC IOL
Safety	Complications limited to technique	Angle related complications	Sutures can erode or brake and unstable refraction
Outcomes	Excellent and predictable	Angle related complications	Lens tilt, hemorrhage and secondary glaucoma
Clinical history	30+ years	Removed from many markets	30+ years
Toric option	Yes	No	No
Suturing IOL required	No	No	Yes
Surgical technique	Easy	Easy	Complicated and extensive
Fixation options	Iris	Angle	Sclera, Sulcus, Iris
Surgical time	10–20 min	10–20 min	Up to 60 + min

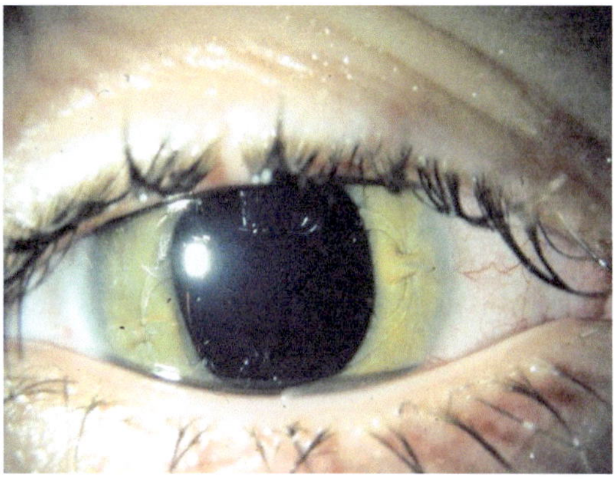

Fig. 10.7 Artisan aphakia IOL 1 day after surgery

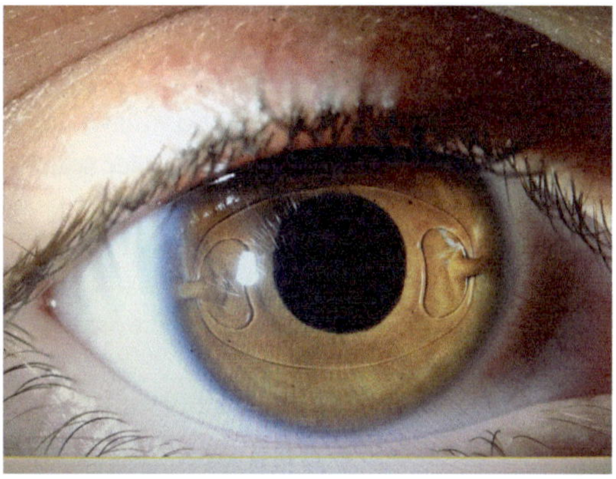

Fig. 10.8 Artisan aphakia IOL 10 years after surgery

The Artisan Aphakia IOL comes in three sizes: the adult lens with an optic size of 5.4 mm and overall diameter of 8.5 mm and two pediatric sizes each with 4.4 mm optic sizes but either a 7.5 or 6.5 mm overall diameter. In the author's experience the pediatric sizes are needed only in cases of microphthalmia. A major advantage of the Artisan IOL over a scleral-sutured PC IOL is that it can be relatively easily removed and exchanged in cases of large myopic shift due to excessive or unanticipated axial elongation (Figs. 10.7 and 10.8).

Before using the Artisan IOL a surgeon needs to become certified by the manufacturer (www.ophtec.com). The technique used for implantation is a delicate bimanual procedure, for which training in a wet lab is required. It is important is to preplan the enclavation sites of the haptics. The IOL is inserted through a corneal incision and

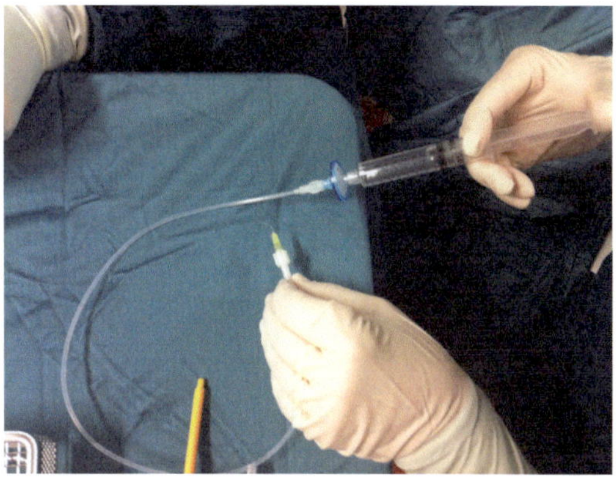

Fig. 10.9 Use of a syringe with extension tube and enclavation needle. Additional suction can facilitate iris enclavation

once it is in the correct position the surgeon holds the IOL for stabilization with forceps while with the other hand uses an enclavation forceps or needle to push midperipheral iris tissue through the slit of the haptics. It is important to ensure that an adequate amount of iris tissue is enclavated. If the iris tissue is stiff, the enclavation needle can be used with additional vacuum from an attached 1 cc or 3 cc syringe with extension tubing. During enclavation an assistant is instructed to withdraw the plunger on the syringe as required, so that the surgeon can simultaneously aspirate a small portion of iris tissue to facilitate enclavation (see Fig. 10.9). Once a small portion of iris tissue is caught between the claws of the haptic, it is easier to enclavate more iris strands as needed. When the enclavation is too large, tissue can be released by pushing on one leg of the claws. My preference is to start with nasal enclavation in non-dyscoric eyes since the pupil is more nasally oriented in most eyes. The nasal enclavation site should be chosen carefully, avoiding larger blood vessels. At the temporal side of the pupil more iris tissue is available to produce a well-centred enclavation. The surgeon should avoid under and over-enclavation of iris tissue. Too little enclavated iris runs the risk of the haptic losing grip and subsequent dislocation of the Artisan IOL, while too much iris enclavation will cause pupil distortion. The second haptic is enclavated 180° across on the other side of the iris. Good centration over the pupil is also crucial. The angulation of the Artisan

Table 10.2 Complications of the Artisan IOL

A. Per-operative:
1. Hyphaema
2. Iris damage
3. Decentration
4. Iris prolapse
B. Postoperative:
1. Uveitis
2. Lens deposits
3. Ocular hypertension/acute glaucoma (particularly if inadequate peripheral iridotomy/iridectomy)
4. Iris depigmentation/atrophy
5. IOL dislocation e.g. traumatic dislocation of haptic(s)
6. Earring phenomenon
7. Corneal endothelial cell loss.
C. Contra indications for Artisan IOL:
Shallow anterior chamber (<2.6 mm)
Endothelium cell count less than 2000 cells/mm^2
Weak iris support
Uveitis
Automutilation
Contact sports
Non certified surgeons

IOL should be checked. When using the Artisan IOL in the anterior chamber, the haptics should have posterior angulation whilst retropupillary use requires anterior angulation (See Table 10.2).

An iridotomy or iridectomy is essential in order to prevent pupillary block glaucoma. This is not required in eyes that have previously undergone a total vitrectomy. Iridotomies can be made with a YAG-laser prior to surgery. The 5 mm corneal wound is sutured either with running or interrupted sutures. In children any induced astigmatism will usually reduce relatively quickly.

I prefer to use the Artisan Aphakia IOL in the anterior chamber, where the whole lens can be observed. If the lens dislocates after blunt trauma, it will remain in the anterior chamber and can thus be retrieved and re-enclavated. Some surgeons advocate retropupillary use of the Artisan Aphakia IOL suggesting that the increased distance of the optic to the corneal endothelium reduces the loss of corneal endothelium cells in the long term. However fixing the Artisan IOL to the posterior surface of the iris makes it difficult to assess the position of the IOL at follow up. This position also leads to chafing of the iris pigment epithelium. In addition, should dislocation occur, the IOL will drop into the vitreous cavity. Retrieval is more complicated warranting the involvement of a vitreo-retinal expert. It could be argued that it is technically easier to perform an endothelial transplant of the cornea for corneal decompensation than to repair a severely damaged retina or macula due to IOL dislocation into the vitreous cavity (Figs. 10.10 and 10.11a–d).

Studies have been published outlining long-term results of Artisan Aphakia IOL implantation in children. However the longest follow up is 10 years. In my own clinics I encounter patients who received Artisan IOL's more than 25 years ago and who still have excellent endothelial cell density (ECD) counts. Some of these patients have Marfan syndrome and request the same procedure for their affected children. Sminia et al. [2] have suggested that a well-placed Artisan IOL in the anterior chamber will have a similar rate of ECD loss as an eye with a PC IOL over a period of 10 years [2].

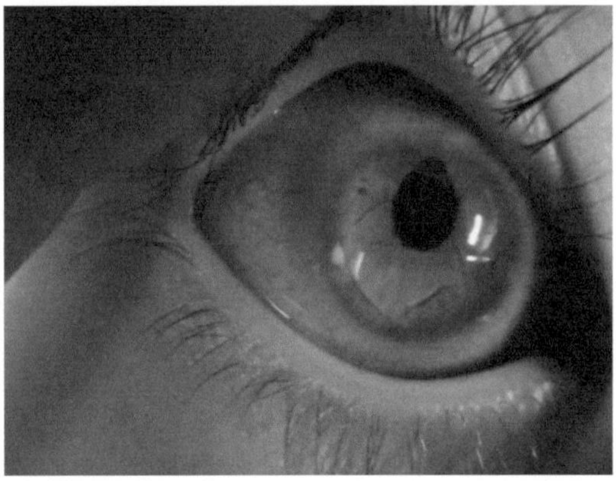

Fig. 10.10 Artisan dislocation after blunt trauma with a loose nasal haptic. Re-enclavation was performed the same day

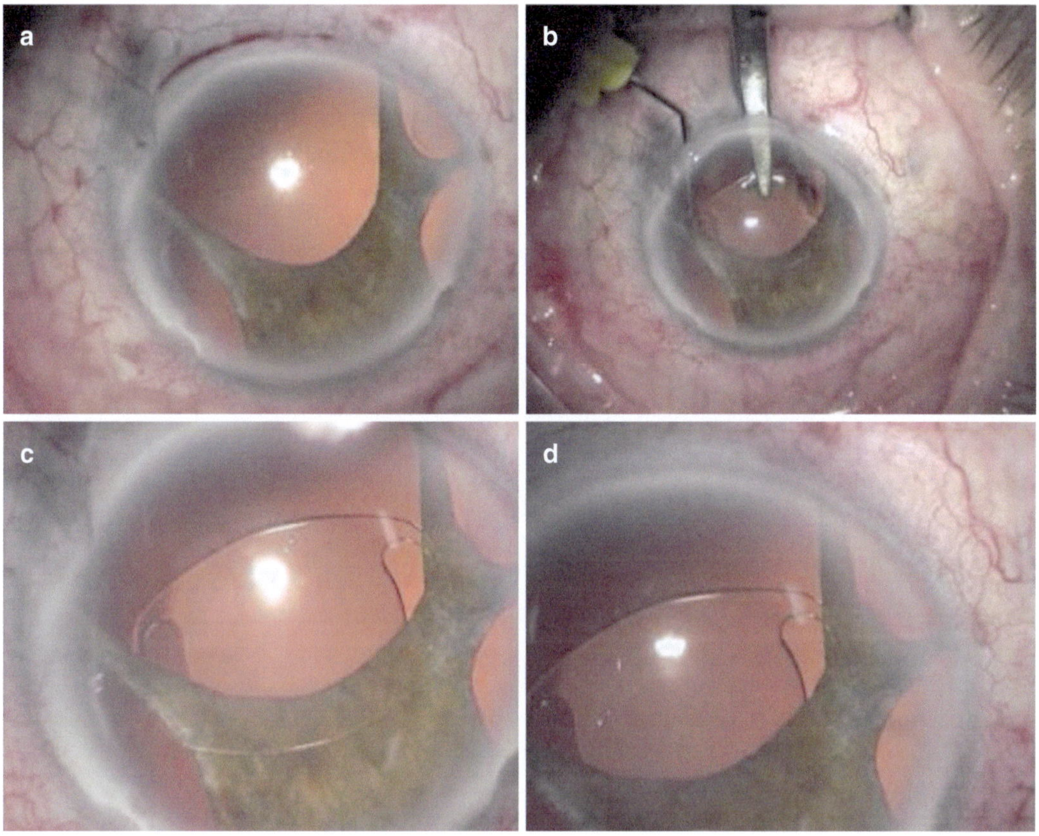

Fig. 10.11 (**a–d**) Artisan IOL in an aphakic eye after traumatic injury. Note how relatively little iris tissue is needed to support this IOL

10.4 Anterior Chamber Angle Supported IOL'S

Although fairly easy to implant in an aphakic eye, AC angle supported IOL's have developed an unfavourable reputation due to the high incidence of complications associated with their use in children. The placement of AC IOL haptics in the anterior chamber angle risks trabecular meshwork damage, angle fibrosis and PAS formation. This in turn can lead to diminished aqueous outflow, elevated IOP and secondary glaucoma. Angle supported anterior chamber lenses are thus not recommended for use as a secondary implant in children [3].

10.5 Posterior Chamber Intraocular Lenses

10.5.1 Iris-Sutured Lenses

Techniques to suture posterior chamber IOLs to the iris have been described by several surgeons [7–9]. Chafing of the iris is a common complication of this technique. Placing sutures within iris tissue to hold an IOL close to its posterior surface could be expected to cause chafing and thus chronic inflammation because of the natural mobility of the iris tissue. Two important factors affecting the likelihood of iris chafe from the sutures are the location of suture placement and the tightness of the sutures. The central iris is most mobile. Central suture placement will not only result in excessive inflammation but will also result in an irregular pupil with peaking at the suture sites. Excessively tight sutures or excessively large bites of iris may also cause peaking of the pupil or bunching of the iris (Table 10.1).

10.5.2 Scleral Sutured Lenses

Scleral sutured PC IOLs have been used for several decades to correct aphakia in cases of lacking sufficient capsular support [4, 10].

Typically the haptics of the PC IOL are sutured to the sclera under partial thickness scleral flaps to prevent suture knot erosion. Erosion of suture knots through the conjunctiva creates a communication between the intra and extra-ocular environments with the subsequent risk of microbial contamination and endophthalmitis. When the technique was first developed IOL fixating sutures were tied under conjunctiva alone. Up to 24 % of cases experienced suture erosion. Even when scleral flaps are used, this problem can occur in around 15 % of cases. This may be an underestimate as longer follow up is likely to reveal that many of the sutures that have eroded through sclera will eventually erode through conjunctiva as well.

Lens stability may become independent of suture integrity if the IOL haptics become encased in fibrous tissue in the ciliary sulcus. However this phenomenon cannot be relied upon (Figs. 10.5 and 10.6).

Partial IOL dislocation into the vitreous as a result of suture loosening/rupture has been reported. IOL dislocation can also occur if there is internal cheese wiring of the suture without disintegration or disruption of the polypropylene knot. Prolene 10.0 sutures tend to break after 5–6 years due to biodegradation and hydrolysis. Even thicker 9.0 Prolene sutures degrade and become brittle in around 10 years. The use of these sutures to fixate an IOL in children will thus theoretically be a "ticking time bomb". An alternative suture to consider is 10.0 Goretex that may be less prone to degradation.

A relatively new alternative is the glued posterior chamber IOL technique. This procedure uses two tunnels through the sclera, under partial thickness scleral flaps. The polypropylene haptics of a 3 piece PC IOL are fed into the sclera tunnels with the lens optic behind the iris. The haptics are then trimmed, glued to the sclera with fibrin glue and covered with a scleral flap. Although promising, this technique does not have long term follow up in children [11, 12].

10.6 Complications of Sutured Posterior Chamber Lenses

10.6.1 Cystoid Macular Edema (CME)

Several factors contribute to the occurrence of CME after scleral fixation of PC IOLs. These cases are invariably associated with vitreous loss, which may have occurred either at the initial event causing aphakia and loss of capsular support, or at the time of scleral fixation (where a careful anterior vitrectomy is required).

Vitreous loss or rupture of the anterior hyaloid has been shown to be associated with vitreomacular traction and CME. This can be prevented, when occurring intraoperatively, by careful anterior vitrectomy. If present postoperatively, Nd:YAG laser vitreolysis of vitreous strands or repeat vitrectomy may be required. OCT monitoring has greatly enhanced the diagnosis and thus treatment of CME although in small children this might not be feasible unless a portable OCT instrument is available.

10.6.2 Endophthalmitis

Endophthalmitis is a serious and dreaded complication, which can occur after any intraocular procedure. Acute cases usually present in the early postoperative period.

Chronic endophthalmitis, caused by organisms of low virulence, may present months to years after the procedure. Although pathogens can be introduced at the time of surgery, they can also gain access to the eye via exposed sutures in cases of suture-fixated PC IOLs. Bacteria probably enter the eye through the suture wick. These cases illustrate the importance of avoiding the creation of exposed suture ends that can gradually erode through partial thickness scleral flaps and the overlying conjunctiva. Methods to prevent this include leaving the suture ends long, rotating knots into the sclera, or tying the knot in the depths of a partial thickness scleral incision.

10.6.3 Hyphaema/Vitreous Hemorrhage

Suturing PC IOLs necessitates a needle passing through vascular uveal tissue with the attendant risk of causing intra-ocular bleeding. Although many cases of intraocular bleeding are believed to be related to direct trauma during needle passes, wicking of extra-ocular blood into the eye may also occur along the suture. Careful attention to haemostasis during the dissection of conjunctiva and Tenon's capsule will help to avoid this complication.

10.6.4 Lens Tilt/Decentration

Without the support of the lens capsule, a PC IOL can potentially tilt around the two points where it is sutured. It can also decentre. Tilt and decentration result in oblique astigmatism and can also cause myopic shift and lateral shift of focus.

10.6.5 Retinal Detachment

Retinal detachment is more common when the anterior hyaloid face has been disturbed (with or without vitreous prolapse) or when there has been trauma to the vitreous base by the needle or lens haptics. Traction may also be exerted on pre-existing vitreo-retinal adhesions during IOL insertion. Damage to the vitreous base may result in giant retinal tears, whilst traction on other adhesions may cause smaller retinal holes or tears.

10.7 Advantages/Disadvantages

AC IOLs are technically easy to insert and involve little intra-ocular manipulation of the eye. They are also generally easier to remove or replace should this become necessary. Early rigid closed-loop angle supported AC IOLs were associated with many problems. These included the uveitis-glaucoma-hyphaema syndrome (UGH) first described by Ellerton [3], increased endothelial cell loss associated with subsequent corneal decompensation, and glaucoma.

Newer AC IOLs have been associated with fewer complications. However, they are still contraindicated in cases of significant loss of iris tissue or in the presence of angle damage. They should be avoided when the anterior chamber is shallow and are not recommended for use in children.

These factors are less applicable to iris-fixated claw lenses. These can in the author's opinion be safely be used in children provided the iris is intact and the AC is deeper than 2.8 mm. Traumatic or accidental dis-enclavation of one or both haptics is a possible risk. Contact sports should thus be avoided by individuals implanted with these lenses and the use of safety glasses is recommended in other sports such as tennis or badminton.

A PC IOL theoretically causes less damage to the cornea, iris and angle structures thereby reducing the chances of corneal decompensation, inflammation, and glaucoma. However, inserting and fixating a PC IOL in the absence of capsular support is technically demanding and can potentially lead to a new spectrum of problems. Suture fixing a PC IOL involves suture passes through uveal tissue, which can cause hyphaema or vitreous hemorrhage. This procedure has also been known to liberate large amounts of uveal pigment intraoperatively.

Suturing a PC IOL directly to the iris produces some of the benefits of posterior chamber fixation and can be less technically demanding than scleral fixation. Importantly it avoids manipulation of posterior uveal tissue. Despite the risk of iris chafing and chronic uveitis, several studies suggest that CME and corneal decompensation are not increased with this fixation method [7, 8]. However there is some restriction of pupillary dilation dependent upon how peripherally the sutures are placed. Scleral sutured lenses carry the risk of knot erosion and exposure. Although atrophy of the overlying scleral flap is relatively common, the sutures do not appear to always erode through the conjunctiva. Patients with sutured PC IOLs certainly require long-term follow-up as prompt recognition and intervention in cases of suture breakage will help to minimize complications associated with subsequent IOL dislocation. Similarly early recognition of suture exposure may prevent the devastating complication of endophthalmitis.

References

1. Por YM, Lavin MJ. Techniques of intraocular Lens suspension in the absence of capsular/zonular support. Surv Ophthalmol. 2005;50:429–62.
2. Sminia ML, et al. Long term follow up of corneal endothelium after aphakic iris fixated IOL implantation for bilateral cataract in children. J Cataract Refract Surg. 2011;37:866–72.
3. Ellerton CR, et al. Secondary implantation of open-loop, flexible anterior chamber intraocular lenses. J Cataract Refract Surg. 1996;22:951–4.
4. Solomon K, et al. Incidence and management of complications of transsclerally sutured posterior chamber lenses. J Cataract Refract Surg. 1993;19:488–93.
5. Wilson ME. In-the-bag secondary intraocular lens implantation in children. J AAPOS. 1997;3:350–5.
6. van der Pol BEA, Worst JGF. Iris-claw intraocular lenses in children. Doc Ophthalmol. 1996;22:29–35.
7. Arkin MS, Steinert RF. Sutured posterior chamber intraocular lenses. Int Ophthalmol Clin. 1994;34:67–85.
8. Hirashima DE, Soriano ES, Meirelles RL, Alberti GN, Nosé W. Outcomes of iris-claw anterior chamber versus iris-fixated foldable intraocular lens in subluxated lens secondary to Marfan syndrome. Ophthalmology. 2010;117:1479–85.
9. Yen KG, Reddy AK, Weikert MP, Song Y, Hamill MB. Iris-fixated posterior chamber intraocular lenses in children. Am J Ophthalmol. 2009;147:121–6.
10. Buckley EG. Scleral fixated (sutured) posterior chamber lens implantation in children. J AAPOS. 1999;3:289–94.
11. Holt G, Young J, Stagg B, Ambati BK. Anterior chamber intraocular lens, sutured posterior chamber intraocular lens, or glued intraocular lens: where do we stand? Curr Opin Ophthalmol. 2012;23:62–7.
12. Kumar DA, Agarwal A. Glued intraocular lens: a major review on surgical technique and results. Curr Opin Ophthalmol. 2013;24:21–9.
13. Kumar M, et al. Scleral-fixated intraocularlens implantation in unilateral aphakic children. Ophthalmology. 1999;106:2184–9.
14. Hannush SB. Sutured posterior chamber intraocular lenses: indications and procedure. Curr Opin Ophthalmol. 2000;11:233–40.

Recommended Books

Budo CJR. The artisan lens. Highlights Ophthalmol Int. 2004;1:20–183.

Wilson ME, Trivedi RH, Pandey SK. Pediatric cataract surgery. Philadelphia: Lippincott Williams and Wilkins; 2005.

11 Management of Congenital Cataract in Sub-Saharan Africa

Richard Bowman and Godfrey Furahini

11.1 Background

Successful control of measles immunization and vitamin A deficiency has seen the prevalence of childhood blindness in Sub Saharan Africa (SSA) fall from 1 in 1000 to between 0.2 and 0.8 per 1000 [1] and has also seen cataract become the leading cause of childhood blindness.

Population based surveys suggest that 15–35 % of childhood blindness is due to congenital or developmental cataract and blind school surveys suggest similar proportions. There may therefore be up to 82,000 children with non-traumatic cataract in Africa, with approximately 19,000 new cases each year [1]. Management of congenital cataracts in SSA remains a challenge and requires a dedicated team effort. Barriers to good outcomes include late presentation and surgery, inadequate training or facilities, and inadequate visual rehabilitation and poor follow-up. Improved early identification and referral of children with congenital cataract by training rural health care workers (who regularly examine children in reproductive and child health clinics as part of successful high coverage vaccination programs) to screen for absence of the eye's red reflex and poor visual functioning in newborn, infants and toddlers is recommended to facilitate timely diagnosis and treatment, but routine screening programs have not been established and experimental projects have met with variable success [2, 3].

11.2 Presentation and Access to Services

In the absence of screening programs, and with long distances to travel to specialist centers, children are likely to present late with leukocoria (Fig. 11.1a), poor vision or nystagmus. In one series of bilateral pediatric cataract from Tanzania, the mean age of surgery was 5 years old and yet a third had nystagmus indicating congenital origin and a huge delay in accessing treatment [4]. Another study from Tanzania showed that lower maternal educational and socio-economic status, longer distance from treating hospital and developmental versus congenital cataract all predicted longer delays [5]. Further qualitative research also implicated gender relations within the family, health beliefs about cataract and trust in health pro-

R. Bowman, MA, MD, FRCOphth
Department of Clinical and Academic Ophthalmology, Great Ormond Street Hospital for Children, London WC1N 3JH, UK
e-mail: richardbowman493@gmail.com

G. Furahini, BSc (ed), MD, MMed, FCOphth.ECSA
Ophthalmologist, Kilimanjaro Christian Medical Centre, Moshi, Kilimanjaro, Tanzania

Department of Ophthalmology, Kilimanjaro Christian Medical University College, Moshi, Kilimanjaro, Tanzania

Department of Clinical Research, Faculty of Infectious and Tropical Diseases, London School of Hygiene and Tropical Medicine, London, UK
e-mail: godfrey_f@hotmail.com

I.C. Lloyd, S.R. Lambert (eds.), *Congenital Cataract*, DOI 10.1007/978-3-319-27848-3_11

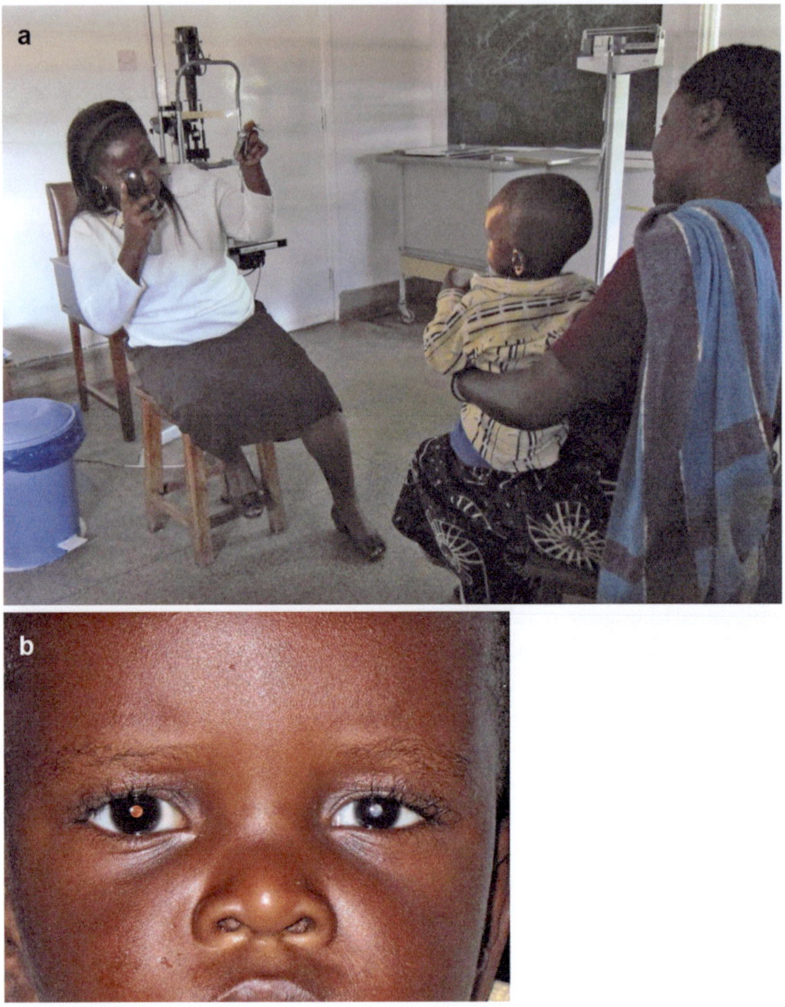

Fig. 11.1 (**a**) Red Reflex examination in a child. (**b**) Child with Cataract in the left eye

fessionals in delayed presentation [6]. Many infants and children do have contact with health workers at different points during infancy and childhood, and this could be utilized given sufficient training and motivation. The 2010 Tanzania Demographic and Health Survey showed that, according to vaccination cards or mother's reports, 75% of children age 12–23 months are fully immunized. With the exception of polio and measles, more than 80% of the reported vaccinations were received by age 12 months, as recommended. Only 3% of children have not received any vaccinations at all [7].

Evidence from Asia has shown that the opportunity is either not taken or when taken the child is not referred for proper surgical management, thus causing long delays before presentation for surgery [8]. Another study from Tanzania indicated quite limited knowledge about childhood blindness among public health workers; only 50% realizing that pediatric cataract needed urgent surgery [9]. Another approach, used very successfully in Bangladesh [10], uses lay people (termed key informants) in the community who volunteer to take responsibility for identifying blind children and receive a short training. This has been replicated in SSA with variable success [2, 11–13]. Screening programs (see Fig. 11.1a) looking for leucocoria (see Fig. 11.1b) may also pick up retinoblastoma and hence save lives

11.3 Etiology

The etiology/causation of most congenital cataract seen in SSA is unclear/idiopathic. One series suggested a family history in about 20% similar

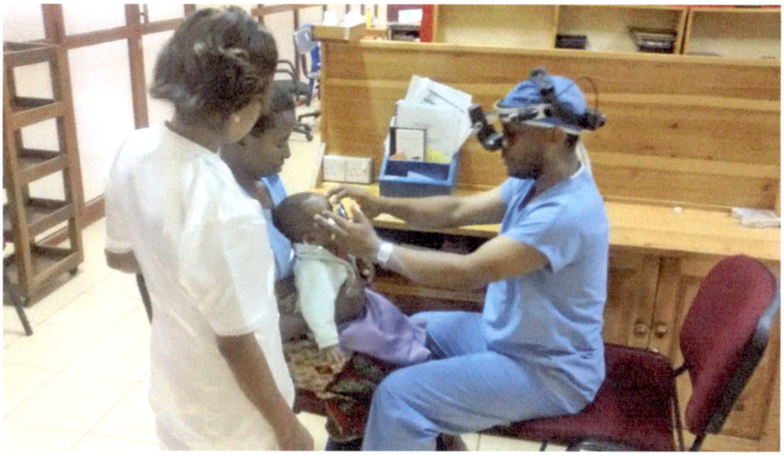

Fig. 11.2 Dr. Furahini Godfrey Mndeme examining 1 year old with bilateral cataract

to western populations [14]. There is also some clinical evidence for the importance of congenital rubella [15–17]. There are no rubella vaccination programs in SSA or any facilities for serological testing for evidence of congenital rubella. Rubella has also been reported as a common cause (15–20 %) in other developing countries [18].

Congenital cataracts that occur in both eyes are associated with a systemic disease approximately 5–10 % of the time [19]. For bilateral cataracts, it is important to determine if there is a systemic association that may need to be treated and that may increase anesthetic risk.

11.4 Clinical Assessment

History and examination are performed as anywhere in the world and include questions about family history, age of onset, any infections during pregnancy and questions about general health and development.

11.4.1 Examining the Eye

Although B-scan ultrasonography is increasing available, if there is dense leukocoria with calcific anterior capsule changes plus or minus partial resorption of the lens, a differential diagnosis of retinoblastoma may need to be considered. Evidence of traction on the ciliary processes, present in persistent fetal vasculature associated with cataract, and not seen in retinoblastoma can be helpful here. If portable slit lamps are not available an indirect ophthalmoscope (see Fig. 11.2) can be used with the condensing lens head close to the eye for a reasonably good anterior segment examination

11.4.2 Visual Assessment

Visual assessment in milder cataracts is essential in determining whether surgery is needed and doctors and other health professionals need to be trained in the basics of visual acuity assessment in preverbal children such as preferential looking. For older children, logMAR, Snellen, Allen, Lea, HOTV, numbers, tumbling E have all been used. Kay's pictures are acuity tests that depend on the child recognition and naming, which may depend on previous cultural and educational exposure. Pictures tests such as LEA symbols, have been found to be culturally relevant to most cultures and can be used for older illiterate children. Smartphone apps to test visual acuity have been utilised successfully in adults and children (both recognition and detection acuity tests) in rural African settings also aiding data collection and geographic monitoring of patient location using linked GPS facilities [20]

11.4.3 Examining the Child

General examination should include assessment of hydration status, nutritional status, posture and gait, color of mucous membranes, lymph node assessment, pattern of breathing, temperature, presence of finger clubbing and any other obvious clinical abnormality. Children suspected of an underlying systemic disorder should be assessed by a pediatrician. All children must be assessed by an anesthetist. Most generally healthy children require only a full blood count (to look for malaria related anemia). Otherwise only clinically indicated investigations are needed with appropriate treatment provided where necessary. Specific investigations for suspected systemic diseases should be taken by the pediatrician/anesthetist carrying out this assessment.

11.5 Surgical Treatment

The same principles of management apply as elsewhere: early surgery, early optical rehabilitation, and maintenance of a clear visual axis. However these can be more difficult to achieve in SSA. Problems caused by late presentation have already been discussed. In addition contact lenses are not a feasible option for optical rehabilitation leaving a choice of intraocular lenses or glasses. Sometimes, because of geographic remoteness, surgery is carried out by adult cataract surgeons who do not have access to foldable lenses, vitrectomy machines or children's glasses, making early optical rehabilitation and maintenance of a clear visual axis (for which primary posterior capsulotomy and anterior vitrectomy is essential) impossible. The World Health Organization has encouraged referral of children with cataract to specialist centers which they term Childhood Eye Health Tertiary Facilities (CEHTFs) [21] but the scarcity of these centers throughout the continent means that this is not often possible.

The following are technique modifications that the authors have found helpful in a setting of restricted financial resources and limited follow up.

Wound Construction and Closure Use a scleral tunnel instead of a clear corneal incision. This enables the use of non-absorbable sutures, which are cheaper and more widely available. These can then be covered by the conjunctiva to avoid exposure. Corneal paracenteses can be sealed with hydro-inflation. In this way repeated anaesthetic exposure to remove exposed corneal sutures or the alternative risk of infectious keratitis and endophthalmitis from suture abscesses is reduced. The scleral tunnel and pars plana/plicata incision for anterior vitrectomy (if this approach is used) can be closed with a single cross suture.

Capsulorhexis Creation of a continuous curvilinear capsulorhexis (CCC) is ideal but can be difficult in the absence of high quality viscoelastics, capsule dyes and squeeze handle rhexis forceps. If these are not available and CCC proves challenging, vitrectorhexis is a useful alternative. The quality/consistency of the anterior capsule in late presenting mature pediatric cataracts can also be an obstacle to CCC and again vitrectorhexis can be helpful.

The anterior capsule is breached with an MVR blade and then the vitrector is used at low cut rate and aspiration rate, either from above the capsule (with the port downwards) or from below the anterior capsule (with the port upwards) and a near circular capsulotomy is slowly nibbled outwards. Sometimes with mature cataracts this technique is not possible because the anterior capsule which can be under some tension splits out peripherally in a linear fashion as soon as it is punctured with an MVR blade. However this split usually provides an adequate capsulotomy itself – when the IOL is inserted the leaves of the anterior capsule retract backwards leaving an adequate gap. This can then be enlarged with the vitrector if necessary.

Use an IOL Wherever Possible Long term use of contact lenses is not feasible and glasses quickly lost or broken, therefore IOLs represent the best chance of optical rehabilitation in this setting. A study in Tanzania showed that the use of foldable lenses was associated with less postoperative astigmatism [4].

Primary Posterior Capsulotomy and Anterior Vitrectomy Because return for followup is usually uncertain, we are more aggressive and perform this on all children under age 10 years (unless they live locally, are likely to attend for follow-up and would be compliant with a table mounted YAG capsulotomy). Surgical capsulotomy and anterior vitrectomy can be performed, as anywhere else, before or after IOL implantation and via an anterior or posterior approach. Vitrectomy machines are not as readily available or as well maintained as in more developed settings, but this situation is improving. Pediatric cataract surgery should not be performed without a functioning vitrector. The authors have successfully used a budget vitrector made by Geuder (Vitron 2020), which has a manual syringe driven suction mechanism when conducting pediatric cataract surgery in an outreach setting.

The placement of the sclerotomy site for pars plana posterior capsulotomies is shown here.

Sclerotomy sites for par plana vitrectomy port (measured in mm from the limbus) [22].

Table 11.1

Less than 6 months	1.5
6–12 months	2
1–2 years	2.5
2–6 years	3
>6 years	3.5

11.6 Biometry

Several options can be used to calculate the dioptric strength of the intraocular implant required. The most accurate involves keratometry and A-scan ultrasound. If keratometry is not available, the Ks can be estimated using either the axial length measurements or the child's age. Alternatively an average K can be used (see Tables). It is possible to use the axial length measurements alone and if all else fails the age of the child, but this should only be as a last resort. It is important to under-correct the child to allow for growth of the eye. The following are taken from the paediatric ophthalmology fellowship handbook [22] at CCBRT.

Intraocular lens calculation by age alone (least favoured method)

Table 11.2

Age	Power
3 months	27
6 months	26
1 year	24
2 year	22
3 year	22
4 year	22
5 year	21

Intraocular lens calculation using axial length

Table 11.3

AL	IOL power
17	+28
18	+27
19	+26
20	+24
21	+22

Intraocular lens power calculation using biometry and SRK formula

Table 11.4

Age	Desired outcome (dioptres)
<10 weeks	+8.0
1 year	+4.0
2 years	+2.0
3 years	+1.0

Secondary IOL calculation

Aphakic retinoscopy divided by 0.67 (this usually results in under correction, so add 1 to 2D)

Average K readings (in dioptres)
Estimated Ks to be used for biometry calculation if a keratometer is unavailable

Table 11.5

Less than 6 months	47.5 D
12–18 months	45.5 D
5 years	42.5 D
Average K for child with cataract	45.0 D

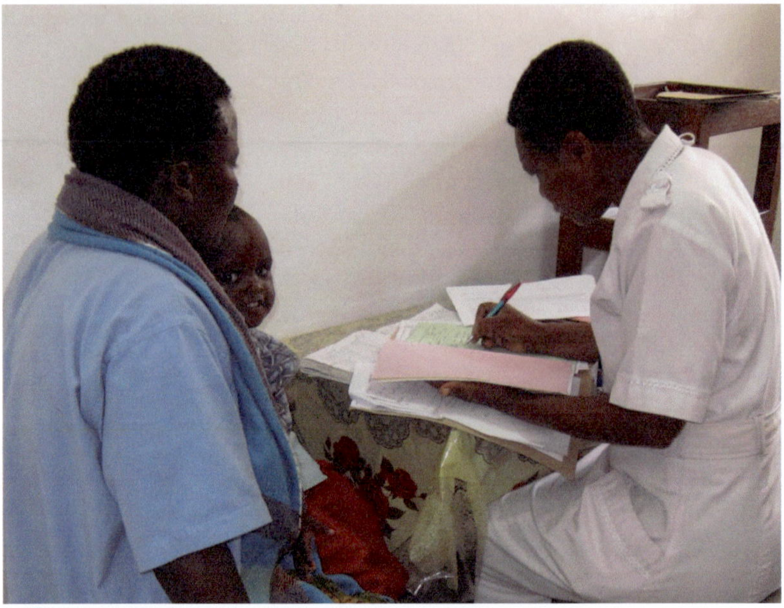

Fig. 11.3 Counselling after cataract surgery in a child

K calculation formula:

Table 11.6

Predicted K using age	=46.27 – (0.02 × age in months)
Predicted K using axial length	=57.98 – (0.61 × AL)

11.7 Post-operative Follow-Up

Encouraging families to bring their children back for follow-up has always been a problem in SSA because of long distances involved and the costs of travel. In Kenya 23 % [14], in Senegal 30 % [23], and in Nigeria 73 % [24] of patients failed to return for follow-up at 3 months. In Madagascar 72 (83.7 %) were lost to follow-up 5 weeks after surgery; although 64 (74.4 %) of children underwent refraction during their encounters with the eye care facility, only 3 (3.5 %) were actually provided with glasses [25]. In a prospective study of 154 children with cataract (a mixture of congenital, developmental and traumatic) from Tanzania, 57 % were lost to follow-up 10 weeks after surgery. Multivariate analysis revealed that male gender, close proximity to a hospital, and minimal delay in presentation for surgery all independently predicted good follow-up at 2 weeks. Closer distance to a hospital and better preoperative vision (not blind in operated eye) predicted good 10 week follow-up [26]. Recruiting a dedicated childhood blindness coordinator (see Fig. 11.3) to provide special counselling and to track families and use mobile phone reminders has been shown to improve follow up rates [27]. Mobile phones are now commonly used to transfer money in SSA and this method can be utilized to pay for transport and to provide incentive for follow up.

11.8 Visual Results and Complications

Reports from SSA are characterized by late presentation, poor follow up and difficulty in knowing the exact time of onset of the cataract (e.g. whether they are congenital or developmental). All of these factors influence visual results and complications and hence the interpretation of published series. In our experience glaucoma is relatively uncommon – this is likely to be due to the older age at surgery but may also have an additional genetic basis.

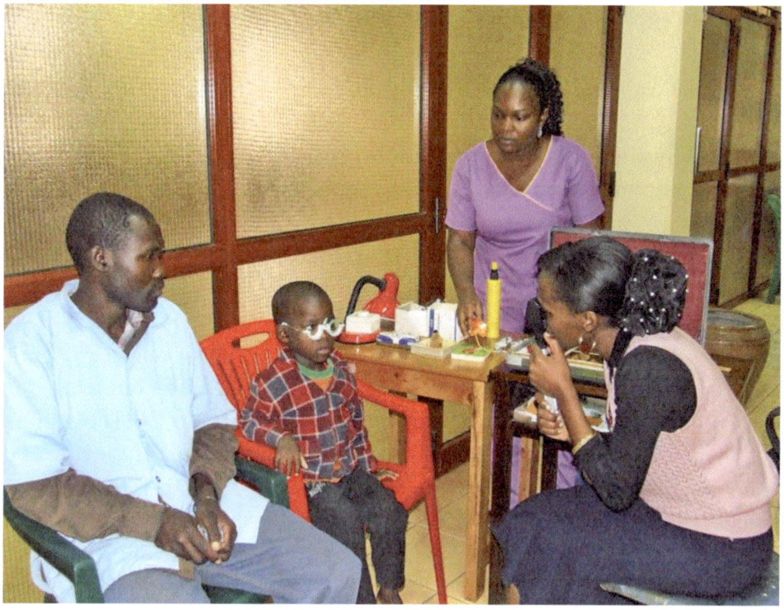

Fig. 11.4 Refraction after cataract surgery in a child

In a follow-up study that included developmental and congenital cataract from Tanzania cumulative incidence of glaucoma at 3 years was 6.5 % (95 % CI, 2.5–16.0), and the annual incidence rate was 2.0 cases per 100 operated eyes. Total time of follow-up and absence of primary intraocular lens implantation correlated with risk for postoperative glaucoma, but multivariate analysis could not confirm independent associations [28]. In another series of 232 children with bilateral cataract from Tanzania (a mixture of congenital and developmental with 25 nystagmus prevalence at presentation [4]), 62 % of a subset of children with follow-up quantitative visual acuities recorded in the notes had an acuity of at least 20/60 in the better eye, allowing a chance of mainstream education. In this series acute fibrinous uveitis occurred in 30 cases (12 %), transient corneal haze occurred in 20 cases (8 %), 27 (11 %) had chronic complications, 69 (28 %) underwent a further general anaesthetic procedure, and 9 (4 %) underwent YAG capsulotomy. Most of the second GA procedures were suture removal procedures since 10-0 vicryl was unavailable. We later changed our practice to hydroinflate paracenteses preventing the later development of exposed corneal sutures and thus reducing the need for repeated GA procedures. Thirteen of 131 children (10 %) with more than 3 months follow-up required a secondary posterior capsulotomy even though six of them had undergone primary posterior capsulotomy and anterior vitrectomy.

In a retrospective review of 181 eyes of 102 patients with congenital or developmental cataract from Nigeria, 71.2 % of the eyes had moderate vision (between <20/60 and 20/200) 12 weeks postoperatively. The most common complication was posterior capsular opacification which occurred in 65 eyes of 43 children [24]. Another retrospective survey of 118 eyes in 71 children with bilateral cataract from Kenya reported 44 % of the eyes had a latest corrected visual acuity of 6/18 (20/60) or better (42 % of these had nystagmus at presentation). In those patients followed up for a minimum of 6 months, 10 % still exhibited nystagmus. Severe fibrinous uveitis occurred in 36 (30.5 %) eyes. 35.7 % of a subset of eyes, which did not undergo intraoperative capsulotomy, developed significant posterior capsular opacification within 2 years postoperatively [14]. In a retrospective case series of 86 children (114 eyes) with cataract from Madagascar (a mixture of congenital, developmental and traumatic) only 2.7 % of the children had 20/60 vision or better at last documented follow-up [25].

11.9 Cost Effectiveness

One study estimated the costs of pediatric cataract surgery in Zambia (US$277) and Malawi (US$202) using labor cost allocations proportional to employee time allocated to treatment of pediatric cataract. One-time costs of equipment were US$179,832 for Zambia and US$178,121 for Malawi [29]. A survey of Child Eye Health Tertiary Facilities (CEHTFs) across SSA showed a mean charge to patients of US$117 per eye. This may be a considerable financial barrier even though it does not cover the real cost [30]. It is recommended that CEHTFs be attached to high volume adult cataract centers where there is a greater chance of cost recovery. There are considerable health economic benefits from operating on children with cataract. When Vision 2020 was originally launched the five priority conditions were cataract, childhood blindness, trachoma, onchocerciasis, refractive error and low vision. Of these, childhood blindness came second only to adult cataract in terms of the burden of blind person years.

A recent long term follow-up study of children operated with cataract in Bangladesh (similar to SSA in terms of economic development and late presentation) showed that better visual outcomes predicted school attendance showing the potential for this intervention to promote the Millennium Development Goals [31].

11.10 Distribution and Productivity of Child Eye Health Tertiary Facilities (CEHTFs)

The Vision 2020 campaign targets included a CEHTF for every 10 million of the population in SSA by the year 2020. In 2010 we published a survey of questionnaires sent out to the 27 CEHTFs in SSA known to the authors (this will since have significantly increased) [30]. The mean catchment area of the 21 who replied was 9.4 million, thus complying with the Vision 2020 target. The mean number of cataract surgeries performed per year was 72, compared to 37 squint surgeries. A more detailed study of different regions across Tanzania developed the concept of the childhood cataract surgical rate (CCSR) [32]. Cataract surgical rate (CSR) has long been used as a marker of medical eye care activity in a population (number of adult cataract operations performed per million population per year) but this was adapted to create the CCSR – number of children receiving cataract surgery per million population per year. Overall, the CCSR (2006) in Tanzania was 9.9 per million populations, ranging from 32.3 for regions where CEHTFs are located to 5.4 for regions not adjacent to CEHTF regions. There were, on average, 148 boys for every 100 girls receiving surgery.

Higher productivity of CEHTFs in terms of numbers of pediatric cataract surgeries was associated with the presence of a dedicated anesthetist, optometrist and childhood blindness co-ordinator [30].

11.11 Training

The above survey indicated that there were 20 countries in SSA with a population of at least 10 million, which lacked a CEHTF, indicating the need for training. At the time of the survey there were two pediatric ophthalmology fellowship programs in SSA one providing high volume pediatric cataract exposure and one with more emphasis on strabismus. A team of professionals is required to manage this condition in addition to the pediatric ophthalmologist. Thus team training has been advocated when establishing a new service for a population. This team should include pediatric anesthesia, orthoptics and visual assessment, pediatric optometry, low vision optometry, theatre nursing and a coordinator or program manager role.

There are alternatives to undergoing fellowship or team training programs within the continent. ‘Sandwich’ training has been used effectively where experienced expatriate pediatric ophthalmologists plus their team come into a unit in SSA for short intense periods of training. During these visits, the local team manages and operates on children who have been pre-identified for surgery and treatment while the trainers provide demonstrations, supervision and advice.. Between visits ongoing support can subsequently be provided through telemedicine and email. Reverse visits where the local surgeon and team visit the trainers' home institution can also be helpful.

India has for some years offered some high volume pediatric ophthalmology fellowship programs which African ophthalmologists have benefited from. The UK based Vision 2020 Links program (*iceh.lshtm.ac.uk/vision-2020-links-programme*) has successfully paired up training units in the UK with service providers in SSA and some of these links have focused on pediatric eye care and cataract in particular.

Conclusions

In a recent multicounty blind school survey from east and southern Africa of over 1000 children, cataract was found to be the main cause of visual impairment in about 18 % [33]. Only 16 % of children with cataract had not undergone surgery, a great improvement on previous surveys. It was shown that the quality of surgery had also improved with only 10 % of children having visual loss due to surgical complications. The majority had undergone IOL insertion which was associated with better visual outcomes.

This along with some of the other data presented in this chapter shows that the situation has improved in SSA over the last 20 years or so. However huge challenges remain including the development of programs to promote early detection and treatment of cataract and to train and equip the teams of professionals needed to provide successful treatment and a chance of sighted education for affected children.

References

1. Courtright P. Childhood cataract in sub-Saharan Africa. Saudi J Ophthalmol. 2012;26(1):3–6.
2. Shija F, Shirima S, Lewallen S, Courtright P. Comparing key informants to health workers in identifying children in need of surgical eye care services. Int Health. 2012;4(1):1–3. doi:10.1016/j.inhe.2011.09.003.
3. Mwakalimba F. Understanding and reducing the barriers to presentation of pediatric cataract in Tanzania. Dissertation, Kilimanjaro Christian Medical University College/Tumaini University; 2012.
4. Bowman RJ, Kabiru J, Negretti G, Wood ML. Outcomes of bilateral cataract surgery in Tanzanian children. Ophthalmology. 2007;114(12):2287–92.
5. Mwende J, Bronsard A, Mosha M, Bowman R, Geneau R, Courtright P. Delay in presentation to hospital for surgery for congenital and developmental cataract in Tanzania. Br J Ophthalmol. 2005;89:1478–82.
6. Bronsard A, Shirima S. Cataract surgery: ensuring equal access for boys and girls. Community Eye Health. 2009;22(70):28–9.
7. National Bureau of Statistics (NBS) [Tanzania] and ICF Macro. Tanzania demographic and health survey 2010. Tanzania: Dar es Salaam; 2011.
8. Muhit MA. Childhood cataract: home to hospital. Community Eye Health. 2004;17(50):19–22.
9. Kishiki E, Hogeweg M, Dieleman M, Lewallen S, Courtright P. Is the existing knowledge and skills of health workers regarding eye care in children sufficient to meet needs? Int Health. 2012;4(4):303–6.
10. Murthy G, Mactaggart I, Mohammad M, et al. Assessing the prevalence of sensory and motor impairments in childhood in Bangladesh using key informants. Arch Dis Child. 2014;99(12):1103–8.
11. Kalua K, Tionenji Ng'ongola R, Frank Mbewe F, Gilbert C. Using primary health care (PHC) workers and key informants for community based detection of blindness in children in Southern Malawi. Hum Resour Health. 2012;10:37.
12. Demissie BS, Solomon AW. Magnitude and causes of childhood blindness and severe visual impairment in Sekoru District, Southwest Ethiopia: a survey using the key informant method. Trans R Soc Trop Med Hyg. 2011;105(9):507–11.
13. Muhammad N, Maishanu NM, Jabo AM, Rabiu MM. Tracing children with blindness and visual impairment using the key informant survey in a district of North-Western Nigeria. Middle East Afr J Ophthalmol. 2010;17(4):330–4.
14. Yorston D, Wood M, Foster A. Results of cataract surgery in young children in east Africa. Br J Ophthalmol. 2001;85:267–71.
15. Maselle SY, Haukenes G, Rutahindurwa A. Preliminary observations on rubella infection in Tanzania and the challenge for its control. East Afr Med J. 1988;65(5):319–24.
16. Bloom S, Rguig A, Berraho A, Zniber L, Bouazzaoui N, Zaghloul Z, Reef S, Zidouh A, Papania M, Seward J. Congenital rubella syndrome burden in Morocco: a rapid retrospective assessment. Lancet. 2005;365(9454):135–41.
17. Ge XL, Zhang Y, Wu Y, Lv J, Zhang W, Jin ZB, Qu J, Gu F. Identification of a novel GJA8 (Cx50) point mutation causes human dominant congenital cataracts. Sci Rep. 2014;4:4121. doi:10.1038/srep04121.
18. WHO. Rubella vaccines: WHO position paper. Wkly Epidermiol Rec. 2000;75:161–9.

19. Junk AK, Morris DA. Cataracts and systemic disease. In: Tasman W, Jaeger EA, editors. Duane's ophthalmology. 15th ed. Philadelphia: Lippincott Williams & Wilkins; 2009.
20. Bastawrous A, Rono HK, Livingstone IA, Weiss HA, Jordan S, Kuper H, Burton MJ. Development and validation of a smartphone-based visual acuity test (peek acuity) for clinical practice and community-based fieldwork. JAMA Ophthalmol. 2015;133(8):930–7.
21. World Health Organization. Preventing blindness in children: report of a WHO/IAPB Scientific Meeting. WHO/PBL/00.77; 2000.
22. Hughes F. http://www.cybersight.org/data/1/rec_docs/2208_Fellowship_Handbook.pdf.
23. Lam A, Seck CM, Gueye NN, Faye M, Pintart D. Cataract surgery with posterior chamber lens implantation in Senegalese children less than 15 year-old. J Fr Ophtalmol. 2001;24(6):590–5.
24. Umar MM, Abubakar A, Achi I, Alhassan MB, Hassan A. Pediatric cataract surgery in National Eye Centre Kaduna, Nigeria: outcome and challenges. Middle East Afr J Ophthalmol. 2015;22(1):92–6.
25. Randrianotahina HC, Nkumbe HE. Pediatric cataract surgery in Madagascar. Niger J Clin Pract. 2014;17(1):14–7.
26. Eriksen JR, Bronsard A, Mosha M, Carmichael D, Hall A, Courtright P. Predictors of poor follow-up in children that had cataract surgery. Ophthalmic Epidemiol. 2006;13(4):237–43.
27. Kishiki E, Shirima S, Lewallen S, Courtright P. Improving postoperative follow-up of children receiving surgery for congenital or developmental cataracts in Africa. J AAPOS. 2009;13(3):280–2.
28. Baden C, Shija F, Lewallen S, Courtright P, Hall A. Glaucoma after pediatric cataract surgery in a population with limited access to care. J AAPOS. 2013;17(2):158–62.
29. Evans CT, Lenhart PD, Lin D, et al. Cost analysis of pediatric cataract surgery at two child eye health tertiary facilities in Africa. J AAPOS. 2014;18(6):559–62.
30. Agarwal PK, Bowman R, Courtright P. Child eye health tertiary facilities in Africa. J AAPOS. 2010;14(3):263–6.
31. Negretti GS, Ayoub T, Ahmed S, et al. Cataract surgery outcomes in Bangladeshi children. Ophthalmology. 2015;122(5):882–7.
32. Courtright P, Williams T, Gilbert C, et al. Measuring cataract surgical services in children: an example from Tanzania. Br J Ophthalmol. 2008;92(8):1031–4.
33. Msukwa G, Njuguna M, Tumwesigye C, Shilio B, Courtright P, Lewallen S. Cataract in children attending schools for the blind and resource centers in eastern Africa. Ophthalmology. 2009;116(5):1009–12.

12 Surgical Management of Pediatric Cataract in India

Virender Sachdeva and Ramesh Kekunnaya

12.1 Magnitude of the Problem in India

Childhood blindness due to pediatric cataract is one of the major causes of avoidable blindness in children in developing countries (including India) [1]. It has been estimated that out of 1.4 million blind children globally, 190,000 (14 %) are due to lens-related conditions [2, 3]. India may have the largest burden of avoidable childhood blindness in the world, most of which is due to congenital and developmental cataracts [4–6]. The high incidence of pediatric cataracts in India has been attributed to maternal infections, especially rubella, malnutrition and consanguinity. Within India, the magnitude of the problem is believed to be greater in south India due to a high prevalance of consanguineous marriages. Hence, pediatric cataract management is one of the highest priority issues of government authorities and non-governmental organisations (NGOs) focused on ophthalmological conditions.

Electronic supplementary material The online version of this chapter (doi:10.1007/978-3-319-27848-3_12) contains supplementary material, which is available to authorized users.

V. Sachdeva, MS • R. Kekunnaya, FRCS (Ophthal) (✉)
Paediatric Ophthalmology and Strabismus Services, Child Sight Institute, Jasti V Ramanamma Children's Eye Care Center, Hyderabad, India
e-mail: rameshak@lvpei.org; drrk123@gmail.com

12.2 Other Co-existing Challenges

The availability of facilities, infrastructure and trained human resources remains uneven in India. According to a survey by Murthy and coworkers [7] of 1204 institutions providing ophthalmic care in India, only 192 (28.7 %) provided pediatric eye care services. In addition, they reported that tertiary eye care hospitals and NGOs were more likely to have separate pediatric ophthalmology units compared to primary and secondary level hospitals. Similarly, there are few institutions that provide pediatric eye care and training in pediatric ophthalmology. Thus, in India, it is not uncommon that pediatric cataract surgery is performed by both trained pediatric ophthalmologists and anterior segment surgeons.

Indian pediatric ophthalmologists face the challenge of managing children with pediatric cataracts with delayed presentation and co-existing strabismus and amblyopia. Another challenge is that there is often a poor follow-up rate postoperatively. Gogate et al. [8] reported that only about 20 % of children who underwent cataract surgery in Maharashtra came for regular follow-up examinations postoperatively, which likely contributed to their poor visual outcomes.

I.C. Lloyd, S.R. Lambert (eds.), *Congenital Cataract*, DOI 10.1007/978-3-319-27848-3_12

12.3 Aetiology of Pediatric Cataracts in India

Infantile cataracts may be caused by intrauterine infections, genetic and metabolic disorders, trauma and prematurity [9, 10]. However, the aetiology is labelled idiopathic in a large percentage of patients [10, 11].

Traumatic cataracts account for a minority of pediatric cataracts in India (12–30 %), tend to occur in children greater than 6 years of age and are usually unilateral. Penetrating and open globe injuries (bow and arrow, stick, and fire-cracker injuries) are the most frequent cause of traumatic cataracts in children [10–12].

Among children with non-traumatic cataracts, Eckstein et al. reported that 25 % were hereditary and 15 % secondary to congenital rubella syndrome (CRS) [10]. Lenhart et al. [13], reported that rubella vaccination rate remains inadequate in India (only 50–60 %) despite recent efforts to increase vaccination rates. There are some reports that suggest there might be an increase in the rubella seropositivity in the mothers of children with non-traumatic pediatric cataracts [14]. Hence, it is believed familial (Fig. 12.1a) and CRS (Fig. 12.1b) still continue to be the most common etiologies of non-traumatic pediatric cataracts.

12.4 Clinical Features and Associations Noted in Pediatric Cataracts in India

Nuclear, zonular, membranous and total cataracts are the most commonly observed morphologies. In a study from Nepal, Adhikari and coworkers [15] the reported mean age at presentation was 5.63 ± 3.59 years for non-traumatic cataracts and 7.39 ± 3.94 years for traumatic cataracts. Only about 10 % of patients with non-traumatic cataract were brought for consultation below the age of 1 year. The situation is very similar on the Indian subcontinent. A child's cataract may be noticed by parents, community health care workers, friends, or other family members early in life, but more often than not parents wait until their child is older before seeking treatment. As a result, many children with infantile cataracts have strabismus and nystagmus when they finally seek medical attention.

12.5 Laboratory Test Findings in Children with Pediatric Cataracts in India

Little is known regarding the laboratory findings in these children for two reasons: firstly, pediatric cataract care is often provided by anterior segment surgeons who do not perform extensive laboratory studies; and secondly, many patients cannot afford laboratory investigations. Hence,

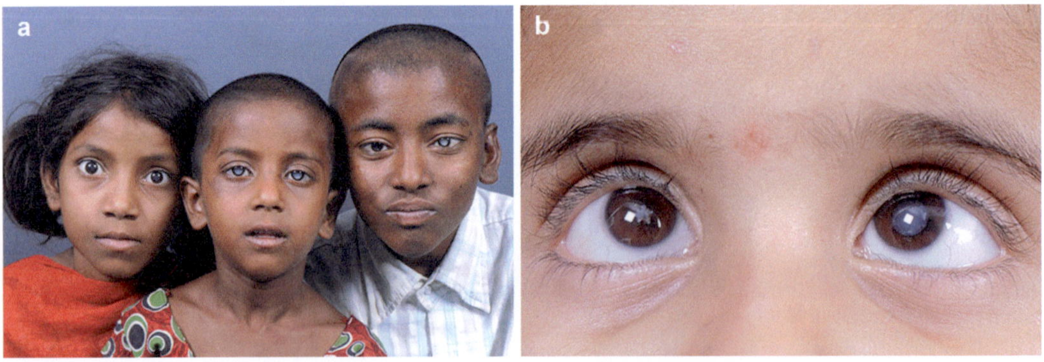

Fig. 12.1 (**a**) Clinical photograph of three siblings anterior with bilateral familial cataract. (**b**) Clinical picture of a child with bilateral rubella cataracts (note presence of dirty looking capsule with multiple posterior synechiae)

patients are usually classified simply as having familial or non-familial cataracts. In familial cases, further investigations are rarely performed. For non-familial cataracts, TORCH titers, serum calcium, and urine for reducing sugars may be performed. In patients with delayed development, failure-to-thrive, and seizures, further systemic work-up is recommended to rule out underlying metabolic conditions.

12.6 IOL Power Calculation

Axial lengths are usually measured in older and cooperative children using partial coherence interferometry because of its greater repeatability and reliability [16, 17]. However, in younger or uncooperative children, contact or immersion A scan biometry is preferred. Ben Zion et al. [18], reported that biometry done using immersion A scan has better test-retest reliability than applanation biometry. However, the difference between the two techniques is clinically and statistically significant only in children less than 2 years of age. In India most pediatric ophthalmologists' tend to use contact A scan biometry in younger or uncooperative patients due to its ease of use and availability. We recommend the following when performing biometry and keratometry for IOL calculations:

- Keratometry mires should be round, circular, complete and centered over the cornea,
- When performing applanation biometry, careful attention should be paid to the retinal, scleral and choroidal echoes. They should have a gain of over 90 % without notches.
- Multiple readings should be taken and the standard deviation for measurements should be <0.10 mm.

12.7 IOL Implantation

12.7.1 Decision to Implant or Not to Implant

Most pediatric ophthalmologists in India prefer primary intraocular lens (IOL) implantation in children 12–18 months of age. For children <1 year, most pediatric ophthalmologists prefer primary IOL implantation only if there are no contraindications, such as axial length <17.0 mm, horizontal corneal diameter <10.0 mm, or co-existing glaucoma or anterior segment dysgenesis.

IOL Types

Most pediatric ophthalmologists in India prefer a hydrophobic acrylic IOL rather than a PMMA IOL because they are associated with a reduced incidence and density of visual axis opacification (VAO, Fig. 12.2a, b), postoperative inflammation, and glaucoma. Aasuri and colleagues reported that, the incidence of clinically significant VAO was only 12 % after hydrophobic acrylic IOL implantation in children vs. 75 % after PMMA implantation with a median onset at 2.9 ± 0.7 months [19].

In addition, both the incidence of postoperative inflammation (26 %) and presumed non-infectious postoperative endophthalmitis (8 %) were increased in children after PMMA IOL implantation. Pehere et al. [20] reported an increased incidence of calcium and phosphate deposits on *hydrophilic* single piece IOLs (Fig. 12.3). Hence, we recommend the use of hydrophobic acrylic lenses wherever possible; however, if the parents cannot afford them, PMMA IOLs may be used in children older than 1 year. In infancy, we recommend a hydrophobic acrylic IOL or leaving the child aphakic.

IOL Power Undercorrection

Most pediatric ophthalmologists in India target an undercorrection in children when an IOL is implanted in anticipation of a later myopic shift. The undercorrection is calculated using either Dahan's formula [21] or Enyedi's rule of seven. We have found Enyedi's rule of seven to be a simple way of calculating the desired undercorrection.

Amount of Undercorrection = 7   age in years.

Thus, if a child is 3 years old and an IOL power of + 30 D is calculated for emmetropia,

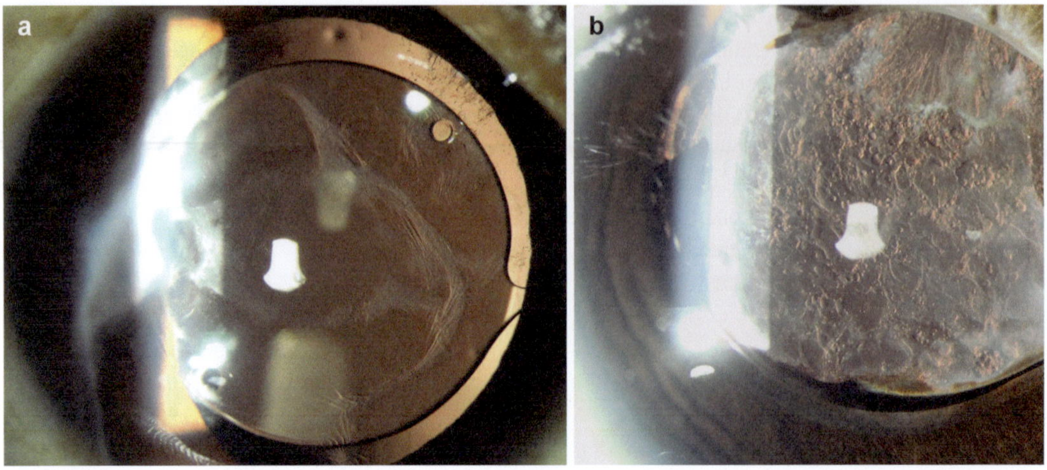

Fig. 12.2 Slit lamp photograph of children showing the pattern of the visual axis opacification after polymethylmethacrylate (PMMA) IOL implantation: (**a**) Dense fibrotic plaques; (**b**) Elschnig's pearls. Children with PMMA IOLs tend to have denser and thicker PCO

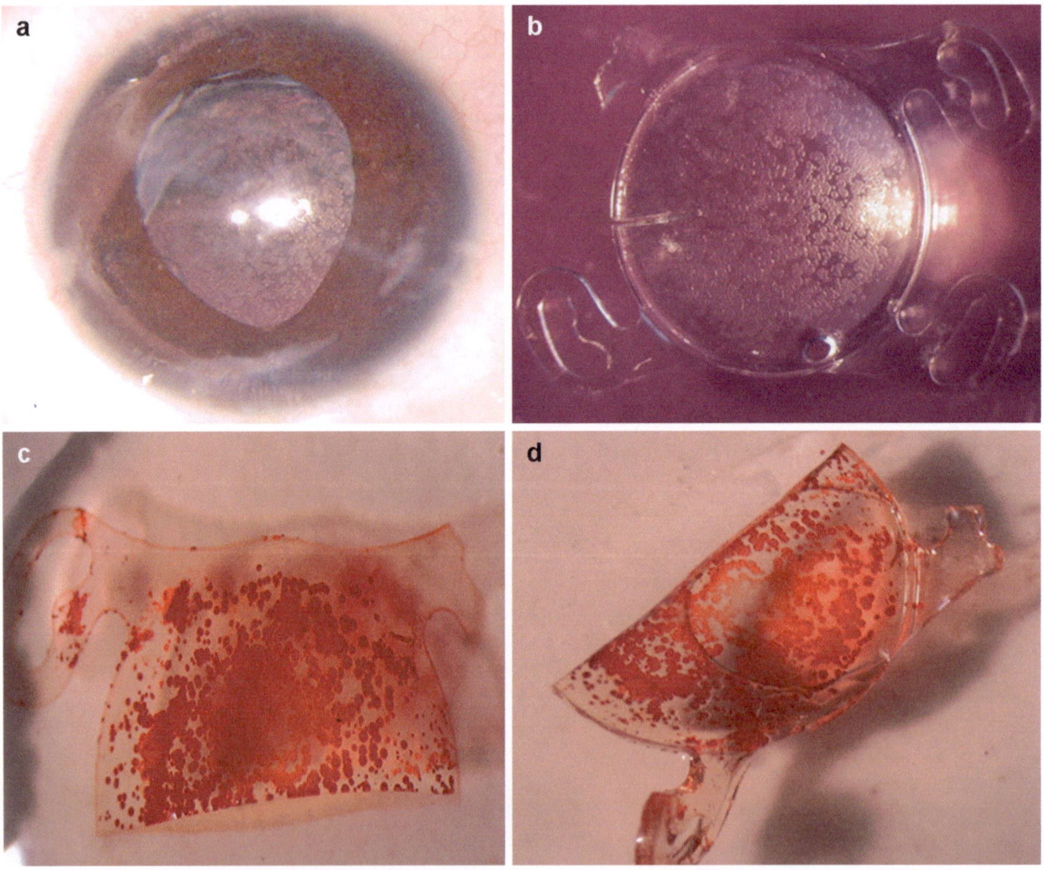

Fig. 12.3 Clinical photograph of a child with multiple pigmentary deposits on a hydrophilic acrylic IOLs in situ (**a**) and an explanted IOL (**b**). (**c**, **d**) Show the typical appearance of these deposits after staining with alizarin (Courtesy: Dr. Niranjan Pehere, Consultant, David Brown Children's Eye Care Centre, LV Prasad Eye Institute, Vijayawada)

we would reduce the IOL power by 4 D to +26 D. Although there is no published data reporting long-term outcomes with this technique, in unpublished data from our institute, we have noted a mean refractive error ranging from −1.38 to +1.4 D when these patients are 7 years of age. We have also noted that the results are more unpredictable in children younger than 2 years of age.

Although most surgeons' target an undercorrection, some believe a large undercorrection may itself be amblyogenic and therefore prefer to target a smaller undercorrection.

We take into account the likelihood of a patient returning for follow-up and wearing contact lenses when choosing the magnitude of the undercorrection. If we deem it unlikely that parents will bring their child back for follow-up and if it is not likely that they can afford contact lenses, we target emmetropia or a small undercorrection.

12.8 Surgical Technique

12.8.1 Lens Aspiration + Primary Posterior Capsulotomy + Anterior Vitrectomy + PCIOL Implantation (LA + PPC + AV + PCIOL)

We perform cataract surgery as soon as a child is healthy enough to undergo general anesthesia. We wait 1 week before performing surgery on the second eye for children with bilateral cataracts. Cataract surgery is performed using either a scleral or clear corneal incision. A scleral tunnel incision with two side port incisions is preferred while implanting a PMMA IOL. Since, many children in India have total or membranous cataract; most pediatric ophthalmologists stain the anterior capsule with 0.5 % trypan blue. Many surgeons use a high molecular weight viscoelastic agent such as hyaluronic acid (Healon or Healon GV, Pharmacia). However, 2 % Methylcellulose is used for patients who cannot afford Healon or Healon GV. Muralidhar et al. [22] reported an anterior and posterior capsulorrhexis completion rate of 81.8 % and 90.9 % respectively in children <6 years undergoing pediatric cataract surgery using 2 % methylcellulose.

After injecting a viscoelastic into the anterior chamber, a continuous curvilinear capsulorhexis is initiated with a cystitome and completed with pediatric capsulorrhexis forceps (23 G, Model no. IG- 3984, Pediatric Capsulorhexis forceps; Indo-German, Mumbai, India) (Video 12.1). Lens aspiration is performed through two corneal incisions using an automated bimanual irrigation and aspiration cannula or an anterior chamber maintainer and an aspiration cannula. The targeted size of the anterior capsulorhexis is 5.0–5.5 mm and 4.0–4.5 mm for the posterior capsulotomy (Fig. 12.4).

Another commonly used surgical technique is using a vitrector to perform the anterior capsulorhexis, lens aspiration, and primary posterior capsulotomy prior to lens implantation (Video 12.2). This approach is particularly useful in children less than 1 year of age, in whom it can be difficult to control a manual capsulorhexis, as well as in older children with thick fibrosed anterior capsules.

As mentioned previously, our preferred implants are hydrophobic acrylic IOLs (Acrysof SA60 AT, MA60AC, or SN60WF; Alcon Laboratories) with an optic diameter of 6 mm and overall diameter of 13 mm or a rigid PMMA IOL (Ocular Vision SF 102; Eye Care, Vadodara, India) with an optic diameter of 5.5 mm and overall diameter of 12 mm.

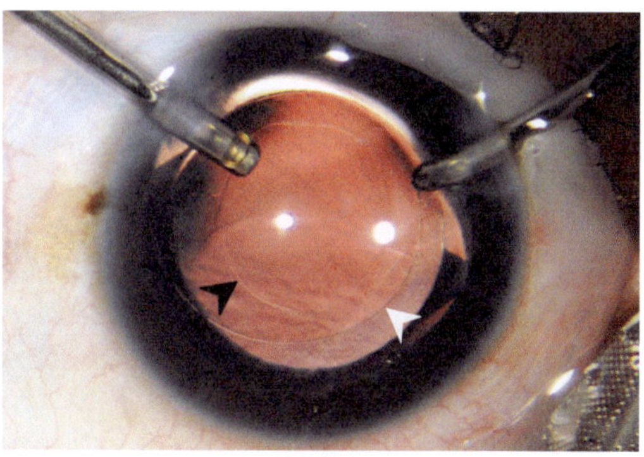

Fig. 12.4 Intra-operative photograph of an adequate sized anterior capsulorhexis (*white arrowhead*) and posterior capsulorhexis (*black arrowhead*)

Primary Posterior Capsulotomy (PPC) In accordance with the surgeon's preference, primary posterior capsulotomy (PPC) is performed before or after IOL implantation. In cases, where the primary capsulotomy is performed after IOL implantation, a vitrector is passed under the edge of the IOL edge to create a PPC. Some surgeons prefer to nick the posterior capsule using a 26G cystitome or a MVR knife, and then enlarge the posterior capsular opening using a vitrector with a cut rate of 150 cuts per minute and vacuum of 80–100 mmHg. This is typically followed by an anterior vitrectomy. Although most pediatric ophthalmologists perform a manual posterior capsulorhexis using microrhexis or utrata forceps, less experienced surgeons often prefer a posterior vitrectorhexis. In a study of 50 eyes, Kochgaway et al. [23] reported that a posterior vitrectorhexis is easier, has a shorter learning curve, and is more associated with in-the-bag IOL implantation compared to manual capsulorhexis.

Anterior Vitrectomy An anterior vitrectomy is performed in all pediatric cases. After completing the PPC, an anterior vitrectomy is performed with settings of 800 cuts per minute and aspiration of 80–100 mmHg. The end point of the vitrectomy is when the remnants of the posterior capsule fall backwards with a smooth margin. Some pediatric ophthalmologists use adjuncts such as intravitreal triamicinolone acteonide [24, 25] or an external endoilluminator [26] to visualise remnants of the vitreous.

Wound Closure Most pediatric ophthalmologists suture all wounds closed in children <7 years of age. For children >7 years, surgeons typically assess the integrity of the wound/scleral tunnel and then decide whether sutures are needed. Non-absorbable 10-0 nylon sutures are most commonly used. These are removed 7–10 days postoperatively either in the office or during an examination-under-anesthesia in young children.

12.8.2 Standard Surgical Technique of Lens Aspiration + Primary Posterior Capsulotomy + Anterior Vitrectomy (LA+ PPC + AV) in Infants

When primary IOL implantation is not indicated, lens aspiration is coupled with a primary posterior capsulotomy and anterior vitrectomy. The technique is similar to that described previously, except an IOL is not implanted. Usually the surgeon operates from two side-port incisions. The anterior capsule is stained using trypan blue, an anterior capsulorrhexis is made, and lens cortex is aspirated. A primary posterior capsulotomy is performed either using forceps or a vitrector as described above. Importantly, the anterior and posterior capsulotomies are made equal sizes so that in-the-bag secondary IOL implantation may be attempted at a later age by re-opening the capsular bag and aspirating the Sommerring's ring. The side port wounds are then closed with 10-0 nylon sutures.

12.9 Intra-operative Challenges and Management

Although surgical management is standardized in children with nuclear and zonular cataracts, thick anterior capsules, membranous cataracts, posterior lenticonus, and persistent fetal vasculature (PFV) may require different techniques. Listed below are ways that we address some of these intraoperative challenges:

(a) Dense anterior capsular plaques:

An attempt may be made to peel off these plaques using pediatric rhexis forceps. However, when this is unsuccessful, they can be managed using a vitrector (Video 12.3).

(b) Partially absorbed cataracts:

An attempt may be made using pediatric capsulorhexis forceps to create an anterior capsulorrhexis in order to aspirate the lens matter. However, if this is unsuccessful, a vitrector can be used to perform these steps (Video 12.4).

(c) Posterior lenticonus

Care should be taken to make a small ACC and to aspirate the nuclear matter first if it is suspected that there is a pre-existing rent in the posterior capsule. If a pre-existing posterior capsular rent is encountered, an IOL can still be implanted into the capsular bag or sulcus after performing an anterior vitrectomy (Video 12.5).

(d) Persistent Fetal vasculature (PFV) cataracts:

PFV is usually unilateral and is frequently associated with microphthalmos. Posterior capsular plaques can usually be excised with a vitrector at a cut-rate of 300–400 cuts per minute and vacuum of 150–200 mmHg. Patent anterior hyaloid blood vessels should be cauterized with endo-diathermy (Video 12.6a, b).

12.10 Postoperative Management and Follow-Up

We examine all children on the first postoperative day, at which time we prescribe topical tobramycin 0.3 % four times a day for a week, atropine sulfate 1 % eye ointment twice a day (for children less than 1 year of age), or homatropine bromide 2 % eye drops two times a day (for children >1 year of age) and prednisolone acetate 1 % eight to ten times a day. Tobramycin is continued for 2 weeks and prednisolone acetate for 6 weeks at a tapering dose.

Sutures are removed 1–2 weeks after cataract surgery either in the office or during an examination-under-anesthesia in young children. After the sutures are removed, retinoscopy is performed and glasses (Fig. 12.5a) or contact lenses are prescribed (Fig. 12.5b). Parents are encouraged to perform visual stimulation exercises to stimulate visual development.

Follow-up examinations are performed at 3 month intervals during the first postoperative year. Visual acuity, clarity of the visual axis, cycloplegic refractive error, tonometry, and ocular motility are assessed during these examinations. Amblyopia is managed by prescribing the appropriate glasses or contact lenses and patching or penalization therapy. Most children are followed by pediatric ophthalmologists for their long-term care.

12.11 Reported Visual Outcomes from India

Visual outcomes following pediatric cataract surgery have been reported from South, entral and Western India. Khanna et al. [2], reported that 269 out of 430 eyes (62.6 %) had successful IOL implantation, and more importantly, that at a mean follow-up of 13.1 months, 40 % had visual acuity >6/18. Gogate et al. [27] described visual outcomes in 258 eyes of 129 children aged 7 weeks to 15 years from western India. They reported 109 (42.2 %) eyes had best corrected visual acuity (BCVA) >6/18 and 157 (60.9 %) had BCVA >6/60 3–8 years after surgery. In both these studies, factors associated with worse outcomes were congenital onset total cataract type of cataract, type of cataract surgery, type of IOL, age at surgery, absence of postoperative uveitis and pre-operative vision.

Sukhija et al. [28] reported long-term visual outcomes (mean follow-up, 102 months) in 26 eyes of 13 children operated at age <2 years. They noted that 92 % achieved a final visual acuity (VA) ≥6/18 at last follow-up with 19/26 (73 %) having acuity of ≥6/12. They found elevated intraocular pressure in one eye only. We have studied 174 eyes of 104 children who underwent secondary IOL implantation. Best corrected visual acuity improved from 1.08 ± 0.65 LogMAR (20/200, 6/60) pre-operatively to 0.55 ± 0.51 LogMAR (20/70, 6/48) at last post-operative follow-up. 51 eyes (35 %) had a BCVA of 20/40 or better at the final follow-up visit. The most significant postoperative complications observed were secondary membranes (17 eyes, 9.77 %), optic capture (15 eyes, 8.6 %), IOL de-centration (9 eyes, 5.17 %) and secondary glaucoma (11 eyes, 5 %).

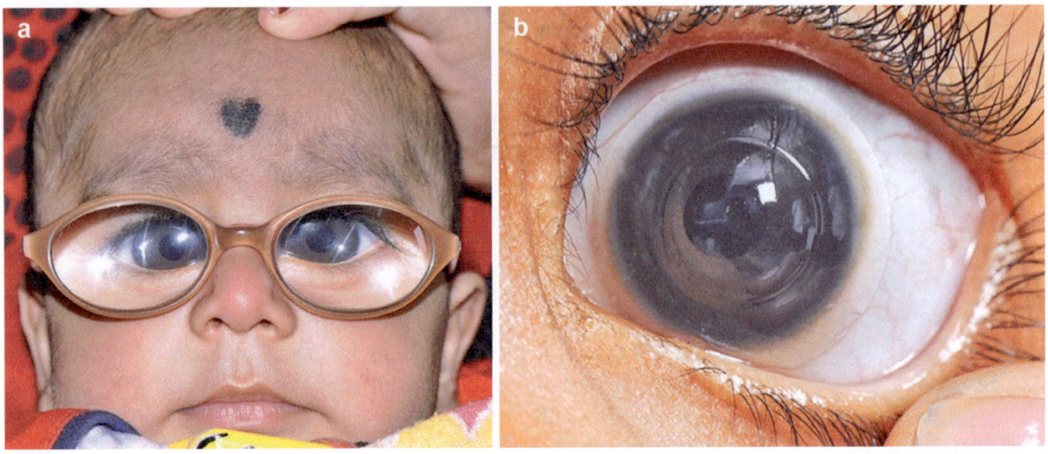

Fig. 12.5 Aphakic child wearing glasses (**a**) or contact lenses (**b**)

12.12 Current Challenges to Pediatric Cataract Management in India

The major challenges limiting good outcomes for the Indian population of children with pediatric cataracts are inadequate availability of services, especially in rural areas, delay in seeking medical care, the poor socioeconomic status of many of the patients, irregular follow-up examinations, and poor compliance with glasses and contact lenses.

It is not unusual that the first ophthalmology consultation for these children occurs when they are 5 years of age or older. Often the child is taken to an adult ophthalmologist, and cataract surgery is performed without IOL implantation. Aphakic glasses are prescribed postoperatively, but most families cannot afford them and they are thus not worn on a consistent basis.

The financial means of the parents often influences the surgical technique, materials and type of IOL implanted. While some parents may be able to afford high quality treatment, these may not be available at the eye hospital where their child is treated. Moreover, many Indian hospitals do not have access to the supplies required for high quality pediatric cataract surgery, such as acrylic IOLs, cohesive viscoelastic materials, and contact lenses.

In most reported studies from India, follow-up rates are poor. Gogate et al. [8] noted that only 53 (20.6 %) of 262 children who underwent cataract surgery between 2004 and 2008, had regular postoperative follow–up. Poor follow-up was directly associated with older age ($P<0.001$), decreased maternal education ($P=0.012$), father's occupation ($P=0.031$), increased cost of travel ($P=0.033$) and whether the surgery was free ($P=0.001$). The cost and distance of travel were major barriers to adequate follow-up, as was inability of the eye care centre to communicate the importance of follow up. Gogate et al. [27] reported a cohort of Indian children examined prospectively after bilateral cataract surgery and noted that 93 needed Nd YAG LASER capsulotomy, 5 needed low vision aids, 4 contact lenses, and 162 a change of spectacles. They also reported a mean improvement in BCVA by 1 line in these children after these treatments.

Lastly, it is not uncommon that spectacles are either not worn, or not replaced when they are lost or broken. In unpublished data from our institute, we noted that glasses were changed 1.8 times (range 1–5) over a 3 year period [29]. In addition, aphakic patients had their glasses changed more often than pseudophakic patients (mean: aphakic, 2.05 times; pseudophakic, 1.54 times). Poor compliance with wearing aphakic glasses may result in dense amblyopia in these children.

Although contact lenses are preferred in the western world for the optical correction of aphakic children, parents in India cannot usually afford them.

12.13 Pediatric Ophthalmologists Training

In the last decade there has been a significant increase in the number of fellowship trained pediatric ophthalmologists in India [7]. Most large teaching institutions now have a structured training program, and there are currently over 200 trained pediatric ophthalmologists in India. However, they are distributed unevenly across the county, with the majority based in urban areas.

Conclusion

In conclusion, most pediatric ophthalmologists in India manage cataracts in children using techniques similar to those used in other parts of the world. However pediatric cataract surgery is performed by both pediatric ophthalmologists and adult anterior segment surgeons. Improved peri- and post-operative care is needed from paediatricians, rehabilitation teams, and community eye care workers.

Currently pediatric cataract surgery is in a period of transition in India. There is great need for earlier identification of patients and funds to cover the costs of surgical consumables, IOLs, travel expenses, and medications for economically underprivileged children. Improvements in healthcare provision to aid early diagnosis and better transportation to urban eye centres, together with the training of more ophthalmologists to work in rural areas, will help improve visual outcomes in these children.

References

1. WHO. Preventing blindness in children: report of WHO/IAPB scientific meeting. Programme for prevention of blindness and deafness and International Agency for prevention of blindness. Geneva: WHO; 2000.
2. Khanna RC, Foster A, Krishnaiah S, et al. Outcome of bilateral congenital and developmental cataract in young children in south India and causes of poor outcome. Indian J Ophthalmol. 2013;61(2):65–70.
3. Rogers NK, Gilbert CE, Foster A, Zakhidov BO, McCollum CJ. Childhood blindness in Uzbekistan. Eye (Lond). 1999;13:65–70.
4. Gogate P, Deshpande M, Sudrik S, Taras S, Kishore H, Gilbert C. Changing pattern of childhood blindness in Maharashtra, India. Br J Ophthalmol. 2007;91:8–12.
5. Gilbert CE, Rahi JS, Quinn GE. Visual impairment and blindness in children. In: Johnson GJ, Weale R, Minassian DC, West SK, editors. The epidemiology of eye disease. 2nd ed. London: Arnold; 2003.
6. Neena J, Rachel J, Praveen V, Murthy GV, Rapid Assessment of Avoidable Blindness India Study Group. Rapid assessment of avoidable blindness in India. PLoS One. 2008;3:e2867.
7. Murthy GVS, John N, Gupta SK, Vashist P, Rao GV. Status of pediatric eye care in India. Indian J Ophthalmol. 2008;56(6):481–8.
8. Gogate P, Patil S, Kulkarni A, Mahadik A, Tamboli R, Mane R, et al. Barriers to follow-up for pediatric cataract surgery in Maharashtra, India: how regular follow-up is important for good outcome. The Mirahj Pediatric Cataract Study II. Indian J Ophthalmol. 2014;62:327–32.
9. Lambert SR, Drack AV. Infantile cataracts. Surv Ophthalmol. 1996;40:427–58.
10. Eckstein M, Vijayalakshmi P, Killedar M, Gilbert C, Foster A. Aetiology of childhood cataract in south India. Br J Ophthalmol. 1996;80:628–32.
11. Kaid Johar SR, Savalia NK, Vasavada AR, Gupta PD. Epidemiology based etiological study of pediatric cataracts in Western India. Indian J Med Sci. 2004;58:115–21.
12. Khokhar S, Gupta S, Yogi R, Gogia V, Agarwal T. Epidemiology and intermediate-term outcomes of open- and closed-globe injuries in traumatic childhood cataract. Eur J Ophthalmol. 2014;24(1):124–30.
13. Lenhart PD, Courtright P, Wilson ME, Lewallen S, Taylor DS, et al. Global challenges in the management of congenital cataract: proceedings of the 4th International Congenital Cataract Symposium held on March 7, 2014, New York, New York. J AAPOS. 2015;19(2):e1–8.
14. Chandy S, Abraham AM, Jana AK, Agarwal I, Kekre A, et al. Congenital rubella syndrome and rubella in Vellore, South India. Epidemiol Infect. 2011;139(6):962–6.
15. Adhikari S, Badu BP, Bhatta NK, Jha CB, Baral N, Kumari N. Etiology and clinical profile of pediatric cataract in a tertiary care centre of Eastern Nepal. JNMA J Nepal Med Assoc. 2007;46(167):94–8.
16. Connors III R, Boseman III P, Olson RJ. Accuracy and reproducibility of biometry using partial coherence interferometry. J Cataract Refract Surg. 2002;28:235–8.

17. Hussin HM, Spry PGD, Majid MA, et al. Reliability and validity of the partial coherenceinterferometry for measurement of ocular axial length in children. Eye (Lond). 2006;20:1021–4.
18. Ben-Zion I, Neely DE, Plager DA, Ofner S, Sprunger DT, Roberts GJ. Accuracy of IOL calculations in children: a comparison of immersion versus contact A-scan biometry. J AAPOS. 2008;12(5):440–4.
19. Aasuri MK, Fernandes M, Pathan PP. Comparison of acrylic and polymethyl methacrylate lenses in a pediatric population. Indian J Ophthalmol. 2006;54(2):105–9.
20. Pehere NK, Bojja S, Vemuganti GK, et al. Opacification of intraocular lenses implanted during infancy: a clinicopathologic study of 4 explanted intraocular lenses. Ophthalmology. 2011;118(11):2128–2132.e1.
21. Dahan E. Pediatric cataract surgery. In: Yanoff M, Ducker JS, editors. Ophthalmology. St Louis: Mosby-Yearbook; 1998. p. 30.1–6.
22. Muralidhar R, Siddalinga Swamy GS, Vijayalakshmi P. Completion rates of anterior and posterior continuous curvilinear capsulorhexis in pediatric cataract surgery for surgery performed by trainee surgeons with the use of a low-cost viscoelastic. Indian J Ophthalmol. 2012;60(2):144–6.
23. Kochgaway L, Biswas P, Paul A, Sinha S, Biswas R, Maity P, Banerjee S. Vitrectorhexis versus forceps posterior capsulorhexis in pediatric cataract surgery. Indian J Ophthalmol. 2013;61(7):361–4.
24. Shah SK, Vasavada V, Praveen MR, Vasavada AR, Trivedi RH, Dixit NV. Triamcinolone-assisted vitrectomy in pediatric cataract surgery. J Cataract Refract Surg. 2009;35:230–2. 15.
25. Praveen MR, Shah SK, Vasavada VA, Dixit NV, Vasavada AR, Garg VS, et al. Triamcinolone-assisted vitrectomy in pediatric cataract surgery: intraoperative effectiveness and postoperative outcome. J AAPOS. 2010;14:340–4.
26. Matalia J, Anaspure H, Shetty BK, Matalia H. Intraoperative usefulness and postoperative results of the endoilluminator for performing primary posterior capsulectomy and anterior vitrectomy during pediatric cataract surgery. Eye (Lond). 2014;28:1008–13.
27. Gogate PM, Sahasrabudhe M, Shah M, Patil S, Kulkarni AN, Trivedi R, et al. Long term outcomes of bilateral congenital and developmental cataracts operated in Maharashtra, India. Miraj pediatric cataract study III. Indian J Ophthalmol. 2014;62(2):186–95.
28. Sukhija J, Ram J, Gupta N, Sawhney A, Kaur S. Long-term results after primary intraocular lens implantation in children operated less than 2 years of age for congenital cataract. Indian J Ophthalmol. 2014;62:1132–5.
29. Adio A, Sachdeva V, Kekunnaya R. The aphakia versus pseudophakia dilemma in pediatric cataracts: a developing world perspective. J AAPOS. 2014;18(4):e25.

Part IV

Perioperative Care

13 Perioperative Care of the Child with Congenital Cataract-Intraoperative and Post-operative Medication

Jane Ashworth and Susmito Biswas

Complications such as severe postoperative inflammation or infection may limit the visual outcome following surgery for congenital cataract, and on rare occasion may have devastating consequences. Postoperative inflammation and related complications such as pupillary membranes, posterior synechiae, intraocular lens (IOL) deposits or decentration are more common following surgery in infants and young children than adults (Chap. 16). It is imperative to take measures therefore to limit the postoperative inflammatory response and to minimise the risk of endophthalmitis. Intra- and postoperative medication may in addition aid pain relief following cataract surgery in children. The regime for peri- and postoperative medication must be tailored with regard to the pre-existing ocular and systemic status of the child, the surgical technique and complications, and surgeon preference. This chapter discusses the available options for the use of intra- and post-operative medication in order to reduce postoperative inflammation, reduce risk of infection and help alleviate postoperative pain.

J. Ashworth, PhD, FRCOphth (✉)
S. Biswas, FRCOphth
Department of Paediatric Ophthalmology, Manchester Royal Eye Hospital, University of Manchester, Manchester, UK
e-mail: Jane.Ashworth@cmft.nhs.uk; Susmito.Biswas@cmft.nhs.uk

13.1 Reduction of Postoperative Inflammation

Severe postoperative inflammation is recognised as a significant potential complication following cataract surgery in children and especially in infants; see Chap. 16. Occurrence of inflammation can be reduced by careful surgical technique and minimising tissue manipulation (particularly of the iris). The use of peri-operative intracameral heparin, steroids (intracameral, intravitreal, subconjunctival, orbital floor) and postoperative corticosteroids (intravenous, oral or topical) can also minimise inflammation; the risks and benefits of each needs to be considered in order to optimise the management plan for a child undergoing congenital cataract surgery.

13.1.1 Intracameral Heparin

Intracameral heparin reduces the rate of postoperative inflammation when used in the irrigation solution during surgery or when flushed into the anterior chamber at the end of the procedure. Infusion of heparin into the anterior chamber during paediatric cataract surgery has been shown to reduce the incidence of complications such as anterior chamber inflammation, fibrin formation, lens precipitates, synechiae, membrane formation, and IOL decentration [1–3]. In a prospective, randomised controlled trial of congenital cataract surgery in 80 eyes using balanced salt solution (BSS)

I.C. Lloyd, S.R. Lambert (eds.), *Congenital Cataract*, DOI 10.1007/978-3-319-27848-3_13

Table 13.1 Suggested per and post-operative medications for a child undergoing routine congenital cataract surgery

Intraoperative medication	Intracameral heparin
	Intracameral antibiotic
	Subconjunctival corticosteroid (Orbital floor corticosteroid)
	Topical anaesthetic
Postoperative medication	Topical antibiotic for 2 weeks
	Topical corticosteroid, tapered over 4–6 weeks
	Topical cycloplegics

alone as an irrigating solution, or with 40 mg, 20 mg or 10 mg enoxaparin (a low molecular weight heparin) added to 500 ml BSS, the mean number of inflammatory cells and IOL precipitates were significantly higher in the BSS alone group at a mean follow-up period of up to 19.20 months, and the anti-inflammatory effect was dose-dependent [4]. There was also less fibrin and synechiae formation in the heparin groups. However, another study of 40 eyes randomised into having irrigating solution with and without heparin did not show any difference in early postoperative inflammation 3 months following surgery [5].

In our experience, a reduction in postoperative inflammation in congenital cataract surgery can be achieved with the addition of heparin to the irrigating solution (1:1000 is sufficient) and/or washout of the anterior chamber at the end of the procedure with the BSS/heparin solution (Table 13.1).

13.1.2 Intracameral Tissue Plasminogen Activator

A prospective, double-masked, randomised trial in 26 patients (34 eyes) having cataract surgery at age 3–14 years compared the outcomes of 20 ug of intracameral recombinant tissue plasminogen activator (r-TPA) injected intracamerally at the end of surgery with eyes having BSS alone; the r-TPA group showed significantly less intraocular fibrin formation up to days 14 but no difference at day 30 and 90. The incidence of pigmented IOL deposits was significantly lower in the r-TPA group [6].

Intracameral r-TPA can also be used postoperatively to treat severe fibrinous membranes following paediatric cataract surgery [7].

13.1.3 Peroperative Corticosteroids

There are many potential methods of administration of corticosteroids at the time of surgery, in order to reduce inflammation and postoperative complications. The methods selected depend on surgeon preference and experience, pre-existing systemic and ocular conditions of the patient, and surgical technique and complications.

13.1.3.1 Intracameral Corticosteroids

Some surgeons advocate the use of preservative-free intracameral corticosteroids in congenital cataract surgery in order to reduce the risk of postoperative anterior membranes. Several studies have shown that intracameral triamcinolone used at the time of childhood cataract surgery reduces the incidence of anterior chamber inflammation, posterior synaechae, deposits on the IOL and visual axis re-opacification [8,9]. A prospective randomised study of children having cataract surgery at age less than 2 years compared an intracameral injection of 1.2 mg/0.03 ml of triamcinolone acetonide (31 eyes) or 1 mg/kg per day of oral prednisolone for 15 days postoperatively (29 eyes) and found no difference in the incidence of cell deposits and posterior synaechae [10], suggesting that intracameral corticosteroids are as effective as oral in controlling post-operative inflammation.

Intracameral triamcinolone may also be used to allow visualisation of the anterior vitreous, to ensure adequate vitreous removal from the anterior chamber [11].

Children are at significant risk of ocular hypertension and glaucoma related to corticosteroid use. However, in a case series of 24 eyes in which intracameral dexamethasone was used at the time of infantile cataract surgery, no cases of glaucoma were reported at follow-up ranging from 20 to 48 months [12].

13.1.3.2 Intravitreal Corticosteroids

Intraoperative intravitreal steroids may be used in paediatric cataract surgery in selected cases (for example children with uveitis and refractory macular oedema). However caution needs to be made with regard to the risk of postoperative ocular hypertension and secondary glaucoma.

13.1.3.3 Subconjunctival Corticosteroids

Sub-conjunctival corticosteroids may reduce postoperative inflammation. A half dose of subconjunctival short-acting dexamethasone may be used in infants, increased to full adult dose in older children. Subconjunctival use of long acting corticosteroids such as triamcinolone and depomedrone may precipitate a corticosteroid-related IOP rise, which occasionally necessitates removal of the corticosteroid deposit. Conjunctival necrosis has also been reported following subconjunctival corticosteroid injection in a child [13].

13.1.3.4 Orbital Floor Corticosteroids

Long acting corticosteroids (triamcinolone or depomedrone) can be given as an orbital floor injection at the end of surgery [14]. This is particularly helpful when there is a high risk of severe post-operative inflammation such as in infantile cataract surgery requiring iris hooks or in eyes with uveitis, or in situations when instillation of post-operative drops may be difficult (due to cooperation of the child, or parental compliance issues). There is a risk however of post-operative IOP rise.

13.1.4 Postoperative Corticosteroids

13.1.4.1 Topical Corticosteroids

Topical corticosteroids are routinely used following childhood and adult cataract surgery to reduce postoperative inflammation. There is evidence however that systemic absorption of topical corticosteroids may cause growth suppression [15] and suppression of endogenous adrenal function [16]. Synacthen testing of 26 children who had cataract surgery at less than 5 years of age followed by topical dexamethasone treatment found that seven children (27 %) had adrenal insufficiency, which was severe in five children [17]. Cushing syndrome may be manifest as facial fullness, growth suppression, thin skin with bruising, and striae. Adrenal insufficiency reduces the physiological response to fever, infection, trauma and general anaesthesia; although the effects are reversible, hydrocortisone supplementation may be necessary during intercurrent infection or during further anaesthesia.

A significant number of children using topical corticosteroids have an ocular hypertensive response, and secondary glaucoma due to topical corticosteroids may occur even in infancy after a short course of topical corticosteroids [18].

High strength hourly topical corticosteroids can be used when the risk of severe inflammation is high (such as infantile cataract surgery with iris hooks, in cases with pre-operative uveitis) but risks systemic side effects in an infant. Topical corticosteroids are frequently used in a combined drop with antibiotics; six times a day maxitrol (dexamethasone, neomycin sulphate and polymixin B; Alcon UK) is usually sufficient following routine surgery, tapered over a 4–6 week period (combined with maxitrol ointment at night for the first few weeks) [19].

13.1.4.2 Systemic Corticosteroids

Oral corticosteroids have been advocated by some surgeons [10] in the postoperative period. Intracameral triamcinolone has been shown to be as effective as oral corticosteroids in children having cataract surgery at less than 2 years of age in prevention of IOL deposits and posterior synechiae [10]. However, the use of careful operative technique, periocular corticosteroid and postoperative corticosteroid drops has meant that oral corticosteroids and their associated side effects can be avoided in most cases. Intravenous corticosteroids are reserved for children with active uveitis prior to the cataract surgery.

13.1.4.3 Topical Cycloplegics

Topical cycloplegics are usually given for 2 weeks following uncomplicated paediatric cataract surgery (for example cyclopentolate 0.5 or

1 % three times a day, topical phenylephrine 2.5 % two times a day).

13.2 Reduction of Risk of Infection

Endophthalmitis, although rare, has potentially devastating consequences following childhood cataract surgery, as in adults. The risk of endophthalmitis in paediatric cataract surgery is similar to that in adults; approximately 7 per 10,000 cases for paediatric anterior segment surgery [20]. Options for reducing the risk of endophthalmitis include use of pre-operative skin preparation, subconjunctival or intracameral peri-operative antibiotics, and topical post-operative antibiotics (as a sole drop or as a combination with a steroid). Systemic antibiotics are not usually necessary.

13.2.1 Pre-operative Skin and Conjunctival Disinfection

Pre-operative periocular skin disinfection (with 10 % povidone-iodine or polyvinyl alcohol-iodine) or conjunctival disinfection (with 5 % PI) significantly reduces the risk of endophthalmitis [21].

13.2.2 Peri-operative Antibiotics

13.2.2.1 Subconjunctival Antibiotics

Half adult dose of subconjunctival antibiotics can be used at the end of the surgery (cefuroxime, vancomycin).

13.2.2.2 Intracameral Antibiotics

The use of intracameral antibiotics at the end of the surgery has significantly reduced the incidence of endophthalmitis in adult cataract surgery [22–25] and so has been widely adopted in paediatric cataract surgery also. The relative risk of endophthalmitis is 0.12 when intracameral antibiotics are used [25]. The standard adult dose of antibiotic (1 mg cefuroxime, cefazolin, moxifloxacin) can be instilled into the anterior chamber following placement and tying of the sutures. Any excess in the syringe can be washed onto the surface of the eye. Intracameral cefuroxime is safe to use in the presence of non-severe (non-IgE mediated anaphylaxis) penicillin allergy. Caution would be advised in cases of IgE mediated anaphylaxis to penicillin and an alternative agent such as intracameral vancomycin may be substituted.

13.2.3 Post-operative Antibiotics

13.2.3.1 Topical Antibiotics

It is standard practice to use topical antibiotics following cataract surgery in adults and children, usually in a combination drop with a steroid (dexamethasone, neomycin sulphate and polymixin B; prednisolone and gentamicin; prednisolone and sulfacetamide or tobramycin). These are usually used four times daily for 2 weeks postoperatively, although there is no evidence that post-operative antibiotics alone are effective in reduction of endophthalmitis [25].

13.3 Reduction in Post-operative Pain

Topical anaesthetics are commonly given at the end of the cataract procedure in infants and children. Administration of a subtenon's block following induction of anaesthesia has been shown to improve postoperative analgesia compared to intravenous fentanyl during cataract surgery in infants [26]. Postoperative analgesia can be given as necessary; paracetamol or non-steroidal anti-inflammatory medications are usually sufficient.

13.4 Miscellaneous Adjuncts to Cataract Surgery

13.4.1 Intra-cameral Mydriatics

Cataract surgery is facilitated by optimal pupillary dilation. Pre-operative preparation of the patient involves the use of topical mydriatics, but some infants and children may be sub-optimally dilated, or whilst undertaking surgery, the pupil may become constricted, making surgery more hazardous. The use of intracameral mydriatics (phenylephrine 0.5 %, epinephrinc 0.5 cc/500 cc BSS, has been adopted for adult cataract surgery, particularly in the context of intra-operative floppy iris syndrome (IFIS). Concerns regarding the safety of intracameral phenylephrine in adult cataract surgery, particularly to the corneal endothelium, toxic anterior segment syndrome, and endophthalmitis, have been allayed by 6 year follow up demonstrating no significant difference in endothelial cell loss, IOP control, and PCO rates compared with controls only receiving topical mydriatics [27]. Systemic adverse effects are rare, although a small rise in mean arterial pressure has been described in adults [28]. A combination of intracameral phenylephrine and ketorolac (Omeros) has been shown to maintain mydriasis and reduce post-operative pain in adult cataract surgery [29]; a randomised controlled trial is underway to study its use in paediatric cataract surgery. Until data is available on the safety and efficacy of intracameral mydriatics in the paediatric population, they should be used with caution.

13.4.2 Subconjunctival Mydriatics (Mydricaine)

There are two formulations of Mydricaine prepared by Moorfields Pharmaceuticals. Mydricaine No. 1 contains 0.5 mg atropine, 0.06 mg of adrenaline and 3 mg procaine, whilst Mydricaine No. 2 contains twice the amount in the same volume. Sub-conjunctival injections of mydricaine in the perilimbal area per-operatively can achieve rapid dilation of the pupil. However, both formulations of mydricaine are associated with systemic adverse effects including elevated heart rate [30,31], cardiac arrhythmias, and myocardial ischaemia [32,33], necessitating caution with its use and close consultation with the anaesthetist/anesthesiologist.

13.4.3 Intracameral Acetylcholine (Miochol-E®)

This is used for intra-operative pupillary constriction. This may be useful during paediatric cataract surgery for ensuring complete removal of vitreous in the anterior chamber, preventing lens optic capture by the iris, and potentially lowering the IOP in the immediate post-operative period. In addition, it aids performing an intra-operative peripheral iridotomy by allowing rapid pupil constriction, even after using intracameral phenylephrine. In adult cataract surgery, however, use of Miochol-E® has been associated with bradycardia, bronchospasm and hypotension, so its use in paediatric cataract surgery requires caution.

Conclusions

There are a multitude of methods to reduce post-operative inflammation, infection risk and post-operative pain and the surgeon must chose the optimal per- and postoperative regime based on experience, individual patient factors and risk/benefit of each method. Table 13.1 is a standard suggested per and postoperative medication protocol for routine congenital cataract surgery. The surgeon must adjust the methods however based on each individual case; the pre-operative risk factors, the surgical technique and any perioperative complications, and the general health of the child.

References

1. Ozkurt YB, Taşkiran A, Erdogan N, Kandemir B, Doğan OK. Effect of heparin in the intraocular irrigating solution on postoperative inflammation in the pediatric cataract surgery. Clin Ophthalmol. 2009;3:363–5.
2. Rumelt S, Stolovich C, Segal ZI, Rehany U. Intraoperative enoxaparin minimizes inflammatory reaction after pediatric cataract surgery. Am J Ophthalmol. 2006;141(3):433–7.
3. Bayramlar H, Totan Y, Borazan M. Heparin in the intraocular irrigating solution in pediatric cataract surgery. J Cataract Refract Surg. 2004;30(10):2163–9.
4. Çaça I, Şahin A, Cingü AK, Ari S, Alakuş F, Çinar Y. Effect of low molecular weight heparin (enoxaparin) on congenital cataract surgery. Int J Ophthalmol. 2012;5(5):596–9.
5. Vasavada VA, Praveen MR, Shah SK, Trivedi RH, Vasavada AR. Anti-inflammatory effect of low-

molecular-weight heparin in pediatric cataract surgery: a randomized clinical trial. Am J Ophthalmol. 2012;154(2):252–8.
6. Siatiri H, Beheshtnezhad AH, Asghari H, Siatirit N, Moghimi S, Piri N. Intracameral tissue plasminogen activator to prevent severe fibrinous effusion after congenital cataract surgery. Br J Ophthalmol. 2005; 89(11):1458–61.
7. Mehta JS, Adams GG. Recombinant tissue plasminogen activator following paediatric cataract surgery. Br J Ophthalmol. 2000;84(9):983–6.
8. Dixit NV, Shah SK, Vasavada V, Vasavada VA, Praveen MR, Vasavada AR, Trivedi RH. Outcomes of cataract surgery and intraocular lens implantation with and without intracameral triamcinolone in pediatric eyes. J Cataract Refract Surg. 2010;36(9): 1494–8.
9. Gupta R, Ram J, Sukhija J, Singh R. Outcome of paediatric cataract surgery with primary posterior capsulotomy and anterior vitrectomy using intra-operative preservative-free triamcinolone acetonide. Acta Ophthalmol. 2014;92(5):e358–61.
10. Ventura MC, Ventura BV, Ventura CV, Ventura LO, Arantes TE, Nosé W. Outcomes of congenital cataract surgery: intraoperative intracameral triamcinolone injection versus postoperative oral prednisolone. J Cataract Refract Surg. 2014;40(4):601–8.
11. Praveen MR, Shah SK, Vasavada VA, Dixit NV, Vasavada AR, Garg VS, Trivedi RH. Triamcinolone-assisted vitrectomy in pediatric cataract surgery: intraoperative effectiveness and postoperative outcome. J AAPOS. 2010;14(4):340–4.
12. Mataftsi A, Dabbagh A, Moore W, Nischal KK. Evaluation of whether intracameral dexamethasone predisposes to glaucoma after pediatric cataract surgery. J Cataract Refract Surg. 2012;38(10):1719–23.
13. Ying-Jiun C, Chee-Kuen W, Shatriah I. Conjunctival necrosis following a subconjunctival injection of triamcinolone acetonide in a child. Middle East Afr J Ophthalmol. 2015;22(1):125–8.
14. Taravati P, Lam DL, Leveque T, Van Gelder RN. Postcataract surgical inflammation. Curr Opin Ophthalmol. 2012;23(1):12–8.
15. Wolthers OD. Growth suppression caused by corticosteroid eye drops. J Pediatr Endocrinol Metab. 2011;24(5-6):393–4.
16. Krupin T, Mandell AI, Podos SM, Becker B. Topical corticosteroid therapy and pituitary-adrenal function. Arch Ophthalmol. 1976;94(6):919–20.
17. Haargaard B, Bangsgaard R, Main K, Boberg-Ans G, Meldgaard Lund A, la Cour M. Adrenal gland functionin children below 5 years of age after treatment with Dexamethasone eye drops after congenital cataract surgery. BIPOSA Annual Meeting abstract Barcelona. 2014.
18. Hutcheson KA. Steroid-induced glaucoma in an infant. J AAPOS. 2007;11(5):522–3.
19. Lambert SR, Plager DA, Buckley EG, Wilson ME, DuBois L, Drews-Botsch CD, Hartmann EE, Lynn MJ. The Infant Aphakia Treatment Study: Was the high rate of intraoperative and postoperative adverse events in the intraocular lens group preventable? J AAPOS. 2015;19:101–3.
20. Wheeler DT, Stager DR, Weakley Jr DR. Endophthalmitis following pediatric intraocular surgery for congenital cataracts and congenital glaucoma. J Pediatr Ophthalmol Strabismus. 1992;29(3): 139–41.
21. Wu PC, Li M, Chang SJ, Teng MC, Yow SG, Shin SJ, Kuo HK. Risk of endophthalmitis after cataract surgery using different protocols for povidone- iodine preoperative disinfection. J Ocul Pharmacol Ther. 2006;22(1):54–61.
22. Gower EW, Lindsley K, Nanji AA, Leyngold I, McDonnell PJ. Perioperative antibiotics for prevention of acute endophthalmitis after cataract surgery. Cochrane Database Syst Rev. 2014;7:CD006364. Author manuscript; available in PMC 2014 December 10.
23. Braga-Mele R, Chang DF, Henderson BA, Mamalis N, Talley-Rostov A, Vasavada A; ASCRS Clinical Cataract Committee. Intracameral antibiotics: safety, efficacy, and preparation. Cataract Refract Surg. 2014;40(12):2134–42.
24. Wejde G, Samolov B, Seregard S, Koranyi G, Montan PG. Risk factors for endophthalmitis following cataract surgery: a retrospective case-control study. J Hosp Infect. 2005;61(3):251–6.
25. Kessel L, Flesner P, Andresen J, Erngaard D, Tendal B, Hjortdal J. Antibiotic prevention of postcataract endophthalmitis: a systematic review and meta-analysis. Acta Ophthalmol. 2015;93(4):303–17.
26. Sethi S, Ghai B, Sen I, Ram J, Wig J. Efficacy of subtenon block in infants – a comparison with intravenous fentanyl for perioperative analgesia in infantile cataract surgery. Paediatr Anaesth. 2013;23(11):1015–20.
27. Lundberg B, Behndig A. Intracameral mydriatics in phaco-emulsification cataract surgery – a 6 year follow up. Acta Ophthalmol. 2013;91:243–6.
28. Bekir OA, Toufeeq S, Woods E, Jabir M. Effect of intracameral phenylephrine on systemic blood pressure. Eye (Lond). 2014;28:1267–8.
29. Lindstrom RL, Loden JC, Walters TR, Dunn SH, Whitaker JS, Kim T, Demopulos GA, Tjia K. Intracameral phenylephrine and ketorolac injection (OMS302) for maintenance of intraoperative pupil diameter and reduction of postoperative pain in intraocular lens replacement with phacoemulsification. Clin Ophthalmol. 2014;8:1735–44.
30. Steel DH, Thorn J. The incidence of systemic side effects following subconjunctival Mydricaine No 1 Injection. Eye (Lond). 1999;13:720–2.
31. Jayamanne DGR, Ray-Chaudhuri N, Wariyar R, Cottrell DG. Haemodynamic responses to subconjunctival mydriatic agents (Mydricaine) used for maintenance of perioperative mydriasis in patients undergoing vitreoretinal surgery. Eye (Lond). 1998;12:792–4.
32. Keembiyage RD, Raymond GL, Newland HS. Atrial fibrillation following subconjunctival injection of mydricaine number 02. Clin Experiment Ophthalmol. 2006;34:806–8.

33. Keembiyage RD, Newland HS, Lai C. Tachycardia and myocardial ischaemia following subconjunctival injection of mydricaine (number 02) for vitrectomy procedure. Clin Experiment Ophthalmol. 2005;33:105–6.
34. Sukhija J, Kaur S, Ram J. Minimizing inflammation after congenital cataract surgery. J Cataract Refract Surg. 2014;40(6):1056–7.
35. Hertle RW, Wilson MC. Adjunctive use of alpha-chymotrypsin during infantile lensectomy and vitrectomy. J Pediatr Ophthalmol Strabismus. 2001;38(2):109–11.
36. Sukhija J, Ram J. Anti-inflammatory effect of low-molecular-weight heparin in pediatric cataract surgery. Am J Ophthalmol. 2012;154(6):1003–4; author reply 1004-5.
37. Wilson Jr ME, Trivedi RH. Low molecular-weight heparin in the intraocular irrigating solution in pediatric cataract and intraocular lens surgery. Am J Ophthalmol. 2006;141(3):537–8.
38. Dada T. Intracameral heparin in pediatric cataract surgery. J Cataract Refract Surg. 2003;29(6):1056.
39. Dada T, Dada VK, Sharma N, Vajpayee RB. Primary posterior capsulorhexis with optic capture and intracameral heparin in paediatric cataract surgery. Clin Experiment Ophthalmol. 2000;28(5):361–3.

14 Amblyopia Therapy and Occlusion Regimens

Carey Drews-Botsch

14.1 Introduction

Children born with visually significant unilateral congenital cataracts often have poor visual outcomes. Previous reports have suggested that achieving a good visual outcome requires early surgical removal of the cataract, consistent optical correction of the aphakia or residual refractive errors, and good adherence to a regimen of occlusion of the fellow eye [1–5].

Chak and colleagues found that poor adherence to occlusion was the factor most strongly associated with poor acuity in children following treatment for unilateral cataract [6]. However, others have noted that good visual acuity can be achieved among infants with good adherence to patching in the first year of life, but lower levels of adherence thereafter [7, 8].

However, occlusion therapy is often difficult for caregivers [9–11]. For example, Allen et al reported that occlusion therapy was abandoned prior to 4 years of age in nearly one-third of children treated for unilateral cataract [11]. Earlier studies reported that language barriers, parental education and socioeconomic status [12–16] were related to adherence to occlusion therapy in children with amblyopia. However, it is unclear the extent to which this information is applicable to adherence to patching in infants as most of the children in these studies were older and because the amount of patching achieved is affected by the developmental level of the child and the child's visual acuity [7]. Further, it is difficult to disentangle the impact of these three factors on patching in children with long-standing amblyopia and the developmental capacity to resist patching. In contract, adherence to patching in early infancy relies primarily on the caregiver since infants are less able to resist occlusion or to remove the patch themselves, and since these children likely start with similar visual abilities.

It is likely that achieving good visual acuity in an eye treated for unilateral congenital cataract depends on adherence to occlusion therapy, but that adherence also depends on visual acuity because patching becomes more difficult in children with poorer visual acuity [9]. The impact of good adherence to occlusion therapy on visual outcome is, therefore, likely to be somewhat difficult to disentangle from the impact of visual acuity on adherence to occlusion. Data from the Infant Aphakia Treatment Study (IATS) can be used to shed light on some of these questions. Specifically, we use data from IATS to understand factors that predict early adherence to patching in infants treated for unilateral congenital cataracts, to describe the amount of patching to which these children are exposed, and to assess

C. Drews-Botsch, PhD, MPH
Department of Epidemiology, Rollins School of Public Health, Emory University, Atlanta, GA, USA
e-mail: cdrews@emory.edu

I.C. Lloyd, S.R. Lambert (eds.), *Congenital Cataract*, DOI 10.1007/978-3-319-27848-3_14

the relationship between patching and visual acuity in these children. We also describe the methods used in IATS to assess adherence to patching.

14.2 Infant Aphakia Treatment Study

IATS is a multi-center, randomized, controlled clinical trial of treatment for unilateral congenital cataract in infants between 1 and 7 months of age sponsored by the National Eye Institute. The objective of the study is to compare the visual outcome in children with a unilateral congenital cataract if an IOL is implanted at the time of cataract extraction with the visual outcome in children left aphakic [17]. Earlier reports from the Infant Aphakia Treatment Study suggest there is wide variation in the visual outcome of children treated for unilateral congenital cataract, but that the treatment choice is not significantly associated with visual acuity at either 12 months of age or at 4½ years of age [18, 19].

In IATS, patching was prescribed for all patients throughout the first five years of life. Starting the second week after cataract surgery, caregivers were instructed to have the child wear an adhesive occlusive patch over the fellow eye 1 h/day/month of age until the child was 8 months old. Thereafter, patching was prescribed for half of waking hours either by patching full time every other day or by daily patching one-half of the time that the child was awake.

14.3 Methods of Assessing Occlusion Among Infants and Young Children Treated for Unilateral Congenital Cataract

It is difficult to accurately assess adherence to patching. Patching adherence has been assessed using parental diaries, recall interviews and Occlusion Dose Monitors (ODM). Fielder has reported significant discrepancies between reported adherence and the objective assessment of adherence using ODMs. He reported that parents reported patching children for 50 % more time than is objectively shown on ODM [20]. However, while ODMs are likely the most accurate way to assess patching adherence, they are only currently available on an investigational basis. Additionally, as currently configured, ODM's have difficulty assessing adherence to patching at certain ambient temperatures and have limitations related to battery life [21, 22]. Therefore, many studies using ODM's also employ diaries. In IATS, adherence to prescribed refractive correction and patching were reported by caregivers to staff from the IATS Data Coordinating Center (DCC) using two different methodologies: a retrospective telephone interview every 3 months and an annual prospective diary. The telephone interview and 7-day patching diary collected similar information. In the diary parents reported sleep patterns, patch use, contact lens wear and spectacle wear over a 7 day prospective period (see Fig. 14.1). Diaries were completed 2 months after surgery and at 14, 26, 38, and 50 months of age. The diary was mailed to the caregiver, who mailed the diary back following completion. The telephone interviews were completed quarterly, starting 3 months after surgery, until the child was 5 years of age, and used a semi-structured interview to elicit information for the previous 48-h similar to that reported in the diary. The timing of the interview was determined using an algorithm that distributed the preferred day of the call evenly throughout the week since patching has been reported to differ on weekdays and weekend days [23]. Caregivers were not informed in advance about the specific day or times of the interview. The interviews were conducted by one of three trained interviewers (one English-speaking, one Spanish-speaking, and one Portuguese-speaking) in the caregiver's primary language so that the caregiver was interviewed by the same person on each occasion. The vast majority of interviews (>95 %) were performed by the English-speaking interviewer.

Measures of adherence were derived from caregivers' reports of sleep/wake times, as well as the times that the caregiver reported that the

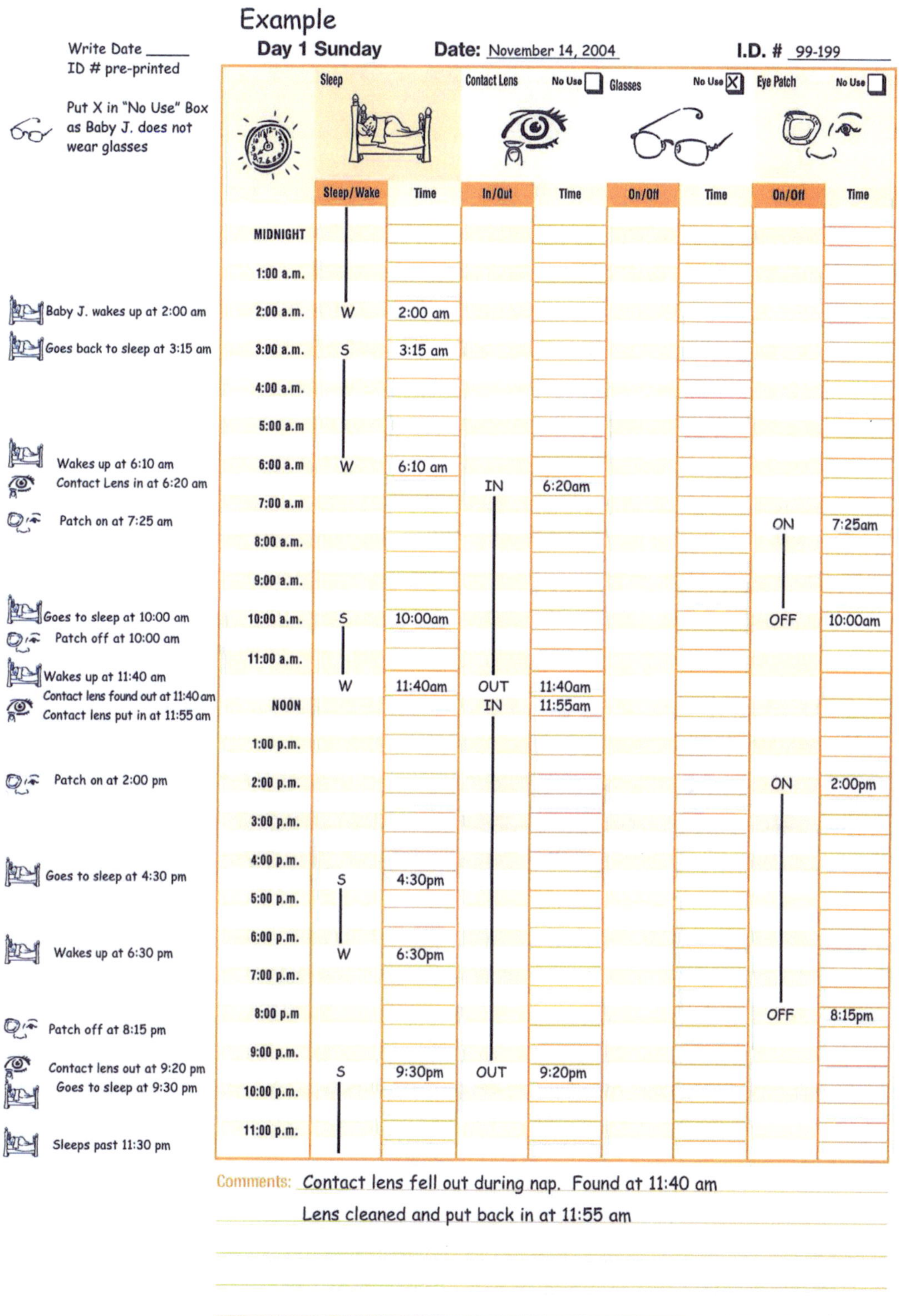

Example

Day 1 Sunday Date: November 14, 2004 I.D. # 99-199

Write Date _____
ID # pre-printed

Put X in "No Use" Box as Baby J. does not wear glasses

Sleep | Contact Lens No Use ☐ | Glasses No Use ☒ | Eye Patch No Use ☐

	Sleep/Wake	Time	In/Out	Time	On/Off	Time	On/Off	Time
MIDNIGHT								
1:00 a.m.								
2:00 a.m.	W	2:00 am						
3:00 a.m.	S	3:15 am						
4:00 a.m.								
5:00 a.m								
6:00 a.m	W	6:10 am	IN	6:20am				
7:00 a.m							ON	7:25am
8:00 a.m.								
9:00 a.m.								
10:00 a.m.	S	10:00am					OFF	10:00am
11:00 a.m.	W	11:40am	OUT	11:40am				
NOON			IN	11:55am				
1:00 p.m.								
2:00 p.m.							ON	2:00pm
3:00 p.m.								
4:00 p.m.	S	4:30pm						
5:00 p.m.								
6:00 p.m.	W	6:30pm						
7:00 p.m.								
8:00 p.m							OFF	8:15pm
9:00 p.m.	S	9:30pm	OUT	9:20pm				
10:00 p.m.								
11:00 p.m.								

Baby J. wakes up at 2:00 am
Goes back to sleep at 3:15 am
Wakes up at 6:10 am
Contact Lens in at 6:20 am
Patch on at 7:25 am
Goes to sleep at 10:00 am
Patch off at 10:00 am
Wakes up at 11:40 am
Contact lens found out at 11:40 am
Contact lens put in at 11:55 am
Patch on at 2:00 pm
Goes to sleep at 4:30 pm
Wakes up at 6:30 pm
Patch off at 8:15 pm
Contact lens out at 9:20 pm
Goes to sleep at 9:30 pm
Sleeps past 11:30 pm

Comments: Contact lens fell out during nap. Found at 11:40 am
Lens cleaned and put back in at 11:55 am

Fig. 14.1 Data collection instrument used to collect adherence data child wore a patch, contact lenses and spectacles. We used this information to calculate the number of hours per day that the caregiver reported that the patch was worn, the percentage of waking hours that the child was wearing refractive correction and the number of hours that the child slept each day. Thus, these measures of adherence were derived using an approach designed to provide a *quantitative* estimate of the average number of hours that caregivers report patching every day, rather than a *qualitative* assessment of adherence. Further, the caregivers were aware that these data were collected independently of the clinical staff monitoring their children's visual acuity and ocular health data. Central data collection helped to assuage concerns about social desirability bias relative to data obtained in other contexts. Further, these data are unlikely to be comparable to qualitative data assessed by clinicians in an office context where both social desirability and the results of visual acuity assessments might impact the assessment.

14.4 Quality of Data on Adherence to Patching

On average, completion rates were higher for the 48-h recall interviews than for the prospective diaries. For example, 87 % of caregivers completed the first diary 2 months after surgery; while a month later the completion rate for the 48-h interview was 10 % higher (97 %). The completion rates of both interviews and diaries declined over time (see Table 14.1). Even so, nearly 5 years after surgery, telephone interviews were completed by almost three-quarters of caregivers. Half of the caregivers returned the diary when the children were 4 years of age. Forty-three (38 %) of the caregivers completed all five diaries and an additional 24 (21 %) completed four of the five diaries. Eight (7.0 %) caregivers did not complete any of the diaries. All of the caregivers completed at least four of the 48-h recall interviews and nearly two-thirds (n=71, 62.2 %) completed 17 or more interviews. All participants had adherence data available for the first year following surgery with three-quarters (n=89, 78.1 %) completing all five possible assessments in this first year. Although there was some tendency for caregivers who did not provide adherence data at subsequent time points to report less adherence with occlusion than parents who did provide data, these differences were neither consistent nor did they approach statistical significance (data not shown).

Table 14.1 also documents the effort required to collect these data. Half of all interviews were completed within two phone calls, regardless of the time since surgery. However, numerous attempts were required to successfully collect data on some participants. For example, at nearly all time points, more than ten contact attempts were required in order to collect data on one or more participants.

Overall, caregivers report patching consistently. For example, the number of hours of patching reported in one interview was strongly correlated with patching reported 3 months later. Further, reports of adherence to patching show excellent reliability, particularly after the first year (see Table 14.2). Further, although caregivers reported slightly more patching on the prospective diaries than on telephone interviews, the amount of patching reported on the diaries correlates well with the amount of patching reported in interviews (see Table 14.3).

A number of investigators have reported that adherence to patching is more accurately estimated using Occlusion Dose Monitors (ODM) than using parental report [24] although others have found good correspondence between adherence reported on diaries and ODM's [21]. They further suggest that parental reports overestimate adherence to occlusion, are not free from bias and require observation of entire treatment period [20]. However, IATS data suggest that caregivers can report adherence to prescribed occlusion. Further, our methods can be used in situations in which ODMs might not be appropriate or acceptable. In IATS, for example, ODMs were not deemed acceptable for use with infants and other young children because of parental and IRB concerns about risks associated with the devices. Additionally, we monitored adherence over a nearly 5 year period. It may be difficult to use ODMs over this extended time. Finally, using

Table 14.1 Completion of reports of adherence to patching and visual correction in the Infant Aphakia treatment study by method of collection and time

Assessment time point	Method of collection	Completion rate[a] (n=114)	Number of contacts[b]
3 months after surgery	48-h interview	97.4% (111)	2 (1–10)
6 months after surgery	48-h interview	97.4% (111)	2 (1–14)
9 months after surgery	48-h interview	93.0% (106)	2 (1–14)
12 months after surgery	48-h interview	93.0% (106)	2 (1–15)
15 months after surgery	48-h interview	86.8% (99)	2 (1–21)
18 months after surgery	48-h interview	92.1% (105)	2 (1–12)
21 months after surgery	48-h interview	91.2% (104)	2 (1–16)
24 months after surgery	48-h interview	86.9% (99)	2 (1–11)
27 months after surgery	48-h interview	84.2% (96)	2 (1–9)
30 months after surgery	48-h interview	85.1% (97)	2 (1–14)
33 months after surgery	48-h interview	83.3% (95)	2 (1–10)
36 months after surgery	48-h interview	83.3% (95)	2 (1–10)
39 months after surgery	48-h interview	86.9% (99)	2 (1–16)
42 months after surgery	48-h interview	82.4% (94)	2 (1–16)
45 months after surgery	48-h interview	77.2% (88)	2 (1–10)
48 months after surgery	48-h interview	79.8% (91)	3 (1–9)
51 months after surgery	48-h interview	80.7% (92)	2 (1–11)
54 months after surgery	48-h interview	79.8% (91)	2 (1–9)
57 months[c] after surgery	48-h interview	73.2% (82)	2 (1–6)
2 months after surgery	Diary	87.7% (100)	N/A
13 months of age	Diary	72.8% (83)	N/A
25 months of age	Diary	66.7% (76)	N/A
37 months of age	Diary	56.1% (64)	N/A
49 months of age	Diary	54.4% (62)	N/A

[a]Number of completed adherence assessment/number of participants
[b]Median (Range)
[c]112 Expected because the other two participants reached their fifth birthday less than 57 months after surgery

parental reports, we were able to successfully monitor adherence on both occlusion and use of contact lenses and spectacles. Although methods to separately monitor adherence to spectacle use and occlusion are under development [25], as currently configured, ODMs are only able to monitor adherence to the use of eye patches for occlusion.

In summary, we believe that our findings show that adherence to patching and visual occlusion can be successfully reported by caregivers of infants and young children over an extended period of time. We further conclude that, although either prospective diaries or retrospective telephone interviews may be used to gather data on adherence to patching, obtaining data via quarterly telephone interview may be preferred given the higher completion rates obtained. Additionally, the frequent telephone contact may have an added benefit of enhancing retention in clinical research.

14.5 Amount of Patching That Caregivers Report

There was substantial inter- and intra-subject variation in the amount of patching reported. For example, in the first twelve months after surgery, caregivers reported patching their children from 0.37 to 7.63 h/day with an interquartile range from 2.7 to 4.7 h/day. Half of all caregivers reported patching their children less than 3.7 h/day in the first year of life (see Fig. 14.2). Between 12 and 48 months of life, caregivers

Table 14.2 Consistency of reporting hours waking hours patched and hours sleep per day by method of data collection

	N	Waking hours patched per day	
		Median (IQR)	Cronbach's alpha (95% CI)
Interviews conducted in 1st year post surgery	96	4.07 (2.69,5.37)	0.69 (0.58,0.80)
Interviews conducted in 2nd year post surgery	87	3.32 (1.37,4.95)	0.85 (0.79,0.90)
Interviews conducted in 3rd year post surgery	72	3.50 (1.91,5.34)	0.88 (0.83,0.90)
Interviews conducted in 4th year post surgery	63	3.41 (1.73,5.52)	0.87 (0.80,0.91)
All diaries	43	3.78 (2.92,5.00)	0.86 (0.78,0.92)

[a]Interviews conducted 3, 6, 9 and 12 months after surgery
[b]Interviews conducted 15, 18, 21 and 21 months after surgery
[c]Interviews conducted 24, 27, 30, and 33 months after surgery
[d]Interviews 36, 39, 42 and 45 months after surgery
[e]Diaries 2 months after surgery and at 14, 26, 38 and 50 months of age

Table 14.3 Comparison[a] between adherence reported on the 7-day prospective diary and adherence reported on the 48-h telephone recall interview closest in time to the diary

	N	Days between diary and interview[b] Mean ± SD (range)	Correlation between interview and diary data	Reported hours of patching per day		Difference in reported hours of patching per day mean (95 % CI)
				Interview	Diary	
2 months after surgery	98	−19.07 ± 13.03 (−64, 33)	0.384*	4.27 ± 2.03	3.91 ± 1.65	0.36 (−0.05, 0.77)
14 months of age	84	−1.00 ± 30.41 (−50, 54)	0.765*	3.68 ± 2.36	4.22 ± 1.87	−0.54 (−0.88, −0.21)
26 months of age	73	−8.30 ± 22.42 (−57, 46)	0.752*	3.64 ± 2.66	4.15 ± 2.32	−0.59 (−0.93, −0.09)
38 months of age	56	−1.84 ± 25.34 (−45, 53)	0.848*	4.10 ± 2.98	3.89 ± 2.35	0.21 (−0.22, 0.63)
50 months of age	55	−3.96 ± 27.30 (−57, 58)	0.647*	3.22 ± 2.79	3.51 ± 2.49	−0.29 (−0.91, 0.32)

[a]With the exception of sleep hours reported at 50 months of age, all correlations were statistically significant, p <0.001
[b]Diary – interview, *p < 0.05

reported patching their children an average of 3.39 h/day, with 75 % of caregivers reporting patching their children 1.86–4.91 h/day (see Fig. 14.3).

These data demonstrate that caregivers can continue to successfully patch their young children throughout the preschool years. However, our data also suggest that the amount of patching parents report varies over time. For example, in Fig. 14.4, we show the amount of patching reported on each interview by the five children whose caregiver reported patching 3.8–4.2 h/day averaged over the entire 5 year study period. This figure shows that patterns of patching vary over time for different individuals. Additionally a number of these caregivers reported very little patching at some points, but reported being able to successfully occlude their child on subsequent assessments. This is an important message for caregivers, particularly during the second and third years of life when young children may express more resistance to patching [11, 26].

14.6 Predictors of Adherence to Patching

IATS provided the opportunity to identify factors that affect patching shortly after cataract surgery, early in the first year of life when caregiver char-

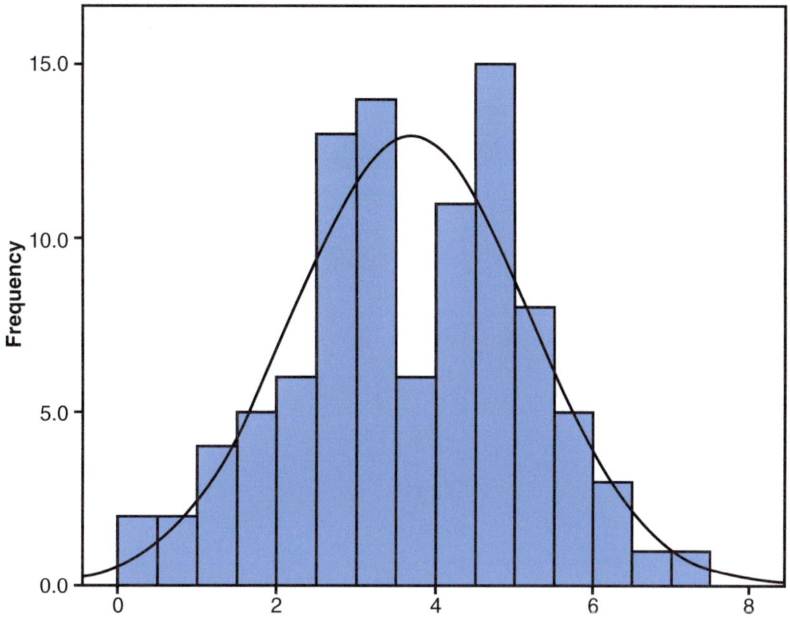

Fig. 14.2 Average hours of patching reported per day before 12 months of age

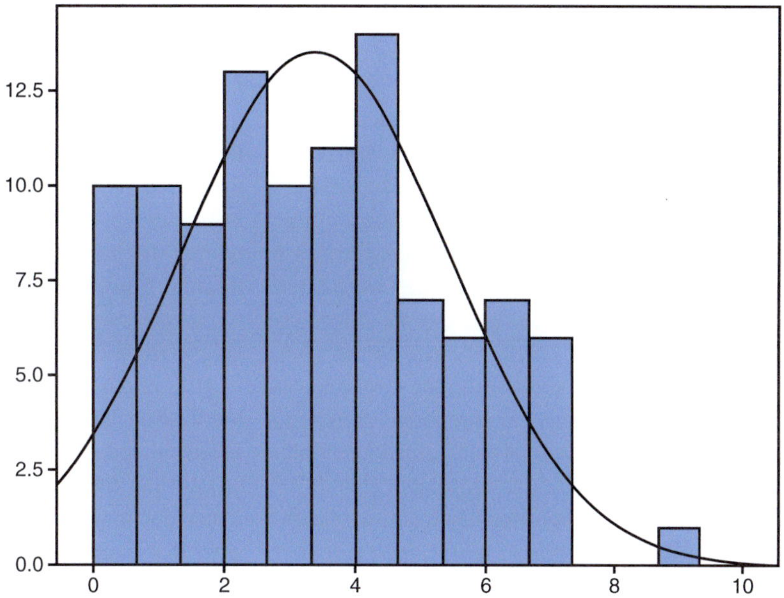

Fig. 14.3 Average hours of patching reported per day between 12 and 48 months of age

acteristics are most likely to influence adherence and when child behavior and differences in vision are less likely to play a substantial role.

For these analyses we assessed the percentage of prescribed patching that caregivers reported being able to achieve 3 months after surgery. Adherence was defined in this way, rather than hours of patching per day, because patching was prescribed for 1 h/day for each month of life. Thus, in young children, the amount of patching prescribed depended on the child's age. More than 40 % (n = 48) of the children were under 5 months of age at the time the information on adherence was obtained 3 months after surgery; two-thirds (65.4 %) were under 6 months of age. The oldest child was 10 months

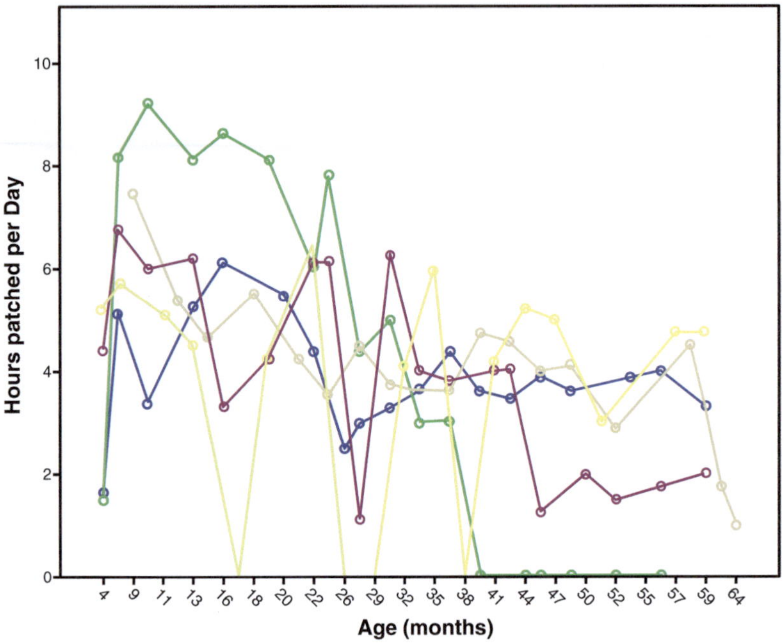

Fig. 14.4 Average reported hours of patching per day by assessment for the five IATS participants with reported average patching between 3.8 and 4.2 h/day over the 5 year study period

of age. Thus, most of the children were neither walking nor talking.

Adherence to patching 3 months after surgery was similar in children who were randomized to receive an IOL and those randomized to remain aphakic. Caregivers with higher socioeconomic status, measured as higher maternal education and availability of private insurance, were more likely to adhere to patching 3 months after surgery than were other caregivers (see Tables 14.4, 14.5, and 14.6). Those reporting the lowest levels of total parenting stress also reported achieving the highest percentage of prescribed patching. Total parenting stress was correlated ($r=-0.22$, $p=0.03$) with the proportion of prescribed patching that caregivers reported achieving, but neither life stress ($r=-0.11$, $p=0.26$) nor age at surgery (measured in days) ($r=-0.07$, $p=0.48$) were. Although the mean adherence to patching did not differ by age at surgery, children who were older at the time of surgery were less likely to be patched at least 90 % of the prescribed time than were those who were younger when the cataract was removed.

These results suggest that most caregivers are able to adhere to prescribed patching shortly after extraction of a unilateral congenital cataract. The type of correction (IOL versus contact lens) does not seem to significantly influence the amount of patching achieved, but the age at cataract extraction may. Additionally, socioeconomic status, measured as the availability of private health insurance, and parenting stress appear to be related to adherence to occlusion therapy in infancy. Thus, clinicians should be alert to levels of caregiver stress and the support systems available to them.

It should be noted that the directionality of the association between adherence and parenting stress is unclear because stress was reported around the time of the 3 month 48-h telephone interview to assess patching adherence. It is possible that parenting stress influenced the amount of patching achieved by caregivers, but it is also possible that caregivers who found it difficult to patch had increased levels of stress as a result of this difficulty. The observed association may also result from a combination of these two effects. One earlier study found that patching did not produce psychological distress among caregivers [27], but other studies have found measures of caregiver stress to be associated with patching in children with amblyopia [28, 29]. Our study is unique in that we used a well-validated measure

Table 14.4 Relationship between treatment, demographic characteristics and stress levels and adherence to patching 3 months after cataract extraction in IATS patients

Variable		N	% of prescribed patching	
			Mean ± SD	P[a]
Overall		104	82.5 ± 42.9	
Treatment	IOL	51	81.0 ± 47.9	0.73
	CL	53	84.0 ± 37.9	
Age at surgery	28–48 days	46	91.0 ± 47.9	0.18
	49 days to 3.0 months	30	78.4 ± 36.6	
	3.1 to <7 months	28	73.1 ± 38.9	
Gender	Male	50	76.9 ± 48.0	0.20
	Female	54	87.8 ± 37.2	
Race	White	89	80.55 ± 41.8	0.25
	Other	16	93.74 ± 46.8	
Hispanic	Yes	15	85.6 ± 59.6	0.77
	No	89	82.0 ± 39.8	
Insurance	Private	64	**90.6 ± 39.4**	**0.01**
	Other	40	**69.6 ± 45.5**	
Maternal education	<High school	10	60.1 ± 41.2	0.07
	High school grad	23	79.7 ± 48.1	
	Some college	41	78.7 ± 41.1	
	College grad	29	98.0 ± 38.3	
Parenting stress	Lowest third	37	**97.1 ± 43.4**	**0.03**
	Middle third	33	**75.9 ± 38.4**	
	Highest third	34	**73.1 ± 43.4**	
Life stress	Lowest third	39	91.2 ± 40.47	0.06
	Middle third	33	68.2 ± 36.9	
	Highest third	32	86.7 ± 48.4	

[a]T-test or ANOVA

Table 14.5 Spearman's correlation coefficient (and 95 % confidence intervals) between reported adherence to prescribed occlusion therapy 2, 3 and 6 months after surgery and grating acuity at 12 months of age

	N	$R_{spearman}$ (95 % CI)
Overall	108	−0.26 (−0.43, −0.08)
By treatment		
IOL	55	−0.41 (−0.61, −0.16)
CL	53	−0.03 (−0.30, 0.24)

of stress associated with the parenting role that was not specific to stress related to patching.

14.7 The Association Between Patching and Visual Acuity

Previous reports have suggested that achieving a good visual outcome requires early surgical removal of the cataract, consistent optical correction of the aphakia or residual refractive errors, and good adherence to a regimen of occlusion of the fellow eye [1–5]. Chak and colleagues found that poor adherence to occlusion was the factor most strongly associated with poor acuity in children following treatment for unilateral cataract [6]. However, others have noted that good visual acuity can be achieved among infants with good adherence to patching in the first year of life, but lower levels of adherence thereafter [7, 8]. It is likely that good visual acuity depends on adherence to occlusion therapy, but that adherence also depends on visual acuity because patching becomes more difficult in children with poorer visual acuity [9]. The impact of good adherence to occlusion therapy on visual outcome is, therefore, likely to be somewhat difficult to disentangle from the impact of visual acuity on adherence to occlusion.

14.7.1 Association Between Adherence and Grating Visual Acuity Measured at Twelve Months of Age

Infants whose caregivers reported better adherence to patching within the first year of life tend to have better logMAR grating visual acuity than children whose parents reported less patching in the first six months after surgery. However, the association appeared to be somewhat stronger among those treated with an IOL than among infants who were left aphakic. The association was also stronger, and statistically significant among children with an adverse event ($r_{Spearman} = -0.35$), than among children who did not experience an adverse event ($r_{Spearman} = -0.10$).

Table 14.6 Odds of achieving graing visual acuity within normal limits at 12 months of age by the proportion of adherence reports of patching at least 75 % of prescribed time

	Vision WNL	Poor vision	Crude OR		Adjusted OR[a]	
Never report ≥75 % adherence	8	13	0.36	(0.12, 1.05)	0.45	(0.15, 1.38)
Sometimes report ≥75 % adherence	25	21	0.69	(0.29, 1.62)	0.83	(0.33, 2.06)
Always report ≥75 % adherence	26	15	1.0	Ref	1.0	Ref

[a]Adjusted for age at surgery, IOL implantation, and having either an additional surgery or an adverse event in first year

The odds of achieving visual acuity within normal limits at 12 months of age depended on the amount of time that caregivers reported patching their child 2, 3 and 6 months after surgery. For example, after adjusting for whether or not an IOL was implanted, the age at surgery, experiencing an adverse event in the first year, infants whose caregiver never reported patching 75 % of the prescribed time were less than half as likely to achieve vision within normal limits as infants whose caregivers always reported patching at least 75 % of the prescribed time.

14.7.2 Association Between Adherence and Optotype Visual Acuity Measured at Fifty Four Months of Age

Although it is important to know the association between patching and visual acuity assessed at 12 months of age, the utility of this information is limited by the fact that grating acuity is generally not believed to be strongly predictive of visual acuity later in life [30–32]. On the other hand, optotype acuity at 4½ years of age is likely predictive of later visual acuity. We assessed the relationship between visual acuity and average hours of patching during two time intervals: (1) throughout the first year of life and (2) between the child's first and fourth birthdays because visual acuity assessment at 12 months of age may have affected subsequent patching and because it has previously been observed that patching is higher in the first year of life than thereafter [16].

Reported patching behaviors did, in fact, differ for children with measured visual acuity at 12 months of age that was within normal limits and those with poorer visual acuity. As shown in Fig. 14.5, approximately half of children with grating acuity estimated to be better than 20/200 at 12 months of age were patched a similar amount before and after 12 months of age. Twenty percent patched at least 1 h more per day after 12 months of age, with thirty percent reporting patching an average of at least 1 h less per day than they had in the first year of life. In contrast, among those with poorer visual acuity measured at 12 months of age, relatively few continued the same level of patching and approximately half patched at least 1 h/day less after 12 months of age than before. This suggests that caregivers give up on patching because they believe that patching is not benefitting their child and/or because children with poor vision become more difficult to patch.

Patching during both the first and subsequent years of life was associated with visual acuity. For example, children who were patched at least 4 h/day throughout the first four years of life had the best visual acuities and those patched fewer than 1 h/day throughout this period had, on average, the worst vision (Fig. 14.6) [33]. Further, among the children who were patched relatively few hours per day during the first year of life, patching more than 4 h/day during the later period was associated with better vision. Similarly, among those children patched at least 4 h/day in the first year of life, those who continued to be patched at least this amount per day ended up with better vision, on average, than those who received less patching in the subsequent 3 years. However, a fixed amount of reported patching was associated with a wide

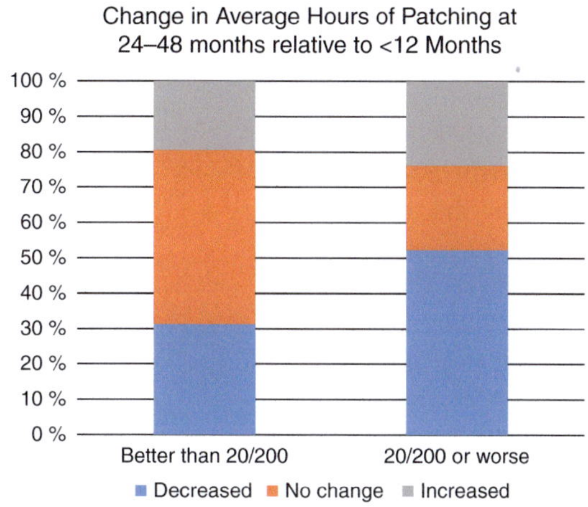

Fig. 14.5 Change in reported hours of patching per day before and after 12 months of age by grating visual acuity measured at 12 months of age

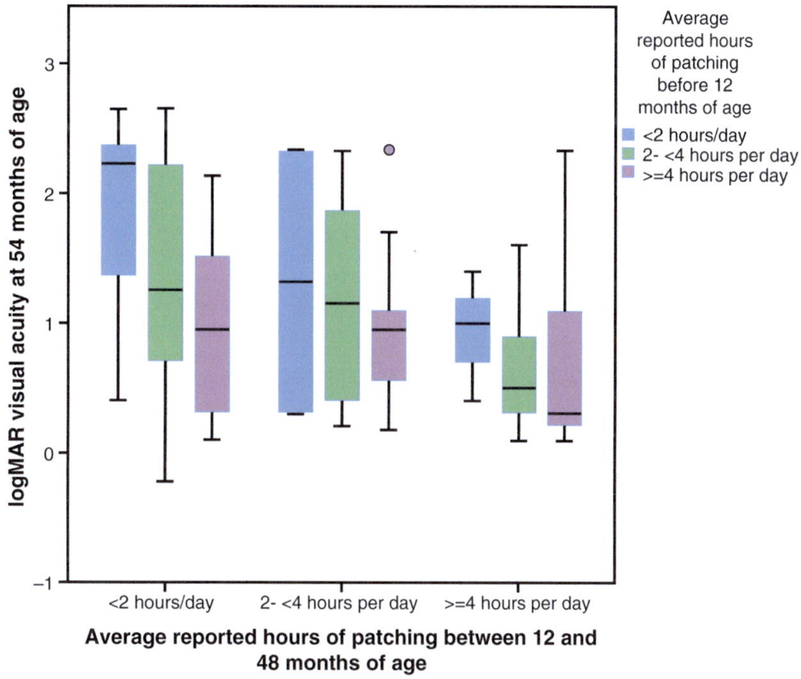

Fig. 14.6 Optotype visual acuity measured at 4½ years of age by average hours of patching reported in the 1st year of life and in the 2nd, 3rd and 4th years of life

range of visual acuity outcomes suggesting that factors other than patching influence visual outcomes in these children [33].

Regression analyses provide evidence of a similar association between visual acuity and patching. The average number of hours of patching that caregivers reported both in the first year of life and in the second, third and fourth years of life combined was significantly associated with optotype visual acuity at 4.5 years of age ($r_{pearson} = -0.324$ and −0.359, respectively). The association between visual acuity and patching was similar for children left aphakic ($r_{pearson} = -0.368$ for adherence in the first year of life and −0.295 for patching between 12 and 48 months of age) and for those receiving an IOL ($r_{pearson} = -0.275$ for adherence in the first year of life and -0.413 for patching between 12 and 48 months of age) [33]. However, average hours of patching predicted only about 10% of the observed variance in optotype visual acuity at age 4½ years of age.

14.8 Summary

In summary, the Infant Aphakia Treatment Study has demonstrated that adherence to patching predicts visual acuity, particularly at 4½ years of age. This finding supports the hypothesized association and that observed among children with other types of amblyopia. However, our findings also confirm that the relationships between patching and visual acuity are complicated. Specifically, our findings suggest that early adherence to patching predicts visual acuity which, in turn, predicts caregivers' later ability and/or willingness to patch. Thus, patching in the first year after cataract extraction may be particularly important as it may set the stage for the ability to patch later, when children may be more able to participate in patching, or resist efforts to patch. Further, our data suggest that parents who are stressed and those with lower socioeconomic status may have the most difficulty in adhering to prescribed patching, and therefore may benefit from support for these efforts. Finally, we found that, although information regarding adherence to patching can be reliably reported by parents, the amount of occlusion achieved by many families can be quite variable over time. Thus, parents should be reassured in their efforts to provide occlusion therapy that they can continue to achieve adequate amounts of patching even if there are periods in which they can achieve only minimal levels of adherence to patching.

References

1. Beller R, Hoyt CS, Marg E, Odom JV. Good visual function after neonatal surgery for congenital monocular cataracts. Am J Ophthalmol. 1981;91(5):559–65.
2. Birch EE, Stager DR. Prevalence of good visual acuity following surgery for congenital unilateral cataract. Arch Ophthalmol. 1988;106(1):40–3.
3. Birch EE, Stager DR, Wright WW. Grating acuity development after early surgery for congenital unilateral cataract. Arch Ophthalmol. 1986;104(12):1783–7.
4. Pratt-Johnson J, Tillson G. Visual results after removal of congenital cataracts before the age of 1 year. Can J Ophthalmol. 1981;16(1):19–21.
5. Lewis TL, Maurer D, Brent HP. Effects on perceptual development of visual deprivation during infancy. Br J Ophthalmol. 1986;70(3):214–20.
6. Chak M, Rahi JS. The health-related quality of life of children with congenital cataract: findings of the British Congenital Cataract Study. Br J Ophthalmol. 2007;91(7):922–6.
7. Lloyd IC, Dowler J, Kriss A, Speedwell L, Thompson D, Russell-Eggitt I, Taylor D. Modulation of amblyopia therapy following early surgery for unilateral congenital cataracts. Br J Ophthalmol. 1995;79(9):802–6.
8. Lambert SR, Plager DA, Lynn MJ, Wilson ME. Visual outcome following the reduction or cessation of patching therapy after early unilateral cataract surgery. Arch Ophthalmol. 2008;126(8):1071–4.
9. Dixon-Woods M, Awan M, Gottlob I. Why is compliance with occlusion therapy for amblyopia so hard? A qualitative study. Arch Dis Child. 2006;91(6):491–4.
10. Webber AL, Wood JM, Gole GA, Brown B. Effect of amblyopia on self-esteem in children. Optom Vis Sci Off Pub Am Acad Optometry. 2008;85(11):1074–81. doi:10.1097/OPX.0b013e31818b9911.
11. Allen R, Speedwell L, Russell-Eggitt I. Long-term visual outcome after extraction of unilateral congenital cataracts. Eye. 2010;24(7):1263–7.
12. Loudon SE, Passchier J, Chaker L, de Vos S, Fronius M, Harrad RA, Looman CW, Simonsz B, Simonsz HJ. Psychological causes of non-compliance with electronically monitored occlusion therapy for amblyopia. Br J Ophthalmol. 2009;93(11):1499–503. doi:10.1136/bjo.2008.149815.
13. Newsham D. Parental non-concordance with occlusion therapy. Br J Ophthalmol. 2000;84(9):957–62.
14. Searle A, Norman P, Harrad R, Vedhara K. Psychosocial and clinical determinants of compliance with occlusion therapy for amblyopic children. Eye. 2002;16(2):150–5.
15. Smith L, Thompson J, Woodruff G, Hiscox F. Factors affecting treatment compliance in amblyopia. J Pediatr Ophthalmol Strabismus. 1994;32(2):98–101.
16. Nucci P, Alfarano R, Piantanida A, Brancato R. Compliance in antiamblyopia occlusion therapy. Acta Ophthalmol. 1992;70(1):128–31.
17. Group IATS. The infant aphakia treatment study: design and clinical measures at enrollment. Arch Ophthalmol. 2010;128(1):21.
18. Group IATS. A randomized clinical trial comparing contact lens to intraocular lens correction of monocular aphakia during infancy: HOTV optotype acuity at age 4.5 years and clinical findings at age 5 years. JAMA Ophthalmol. 2014;132(6):676.
19. Group IATS. A randomized clinical trial comparing contact lens to intraocular lens correction of monocular aphakia during infancy: grating acuity and adverse events at age 1 year. Arch Ophthalmol. 2010;128(7):810.
20. Fielder A, Irwin M, Auld R, Cocker K, Jones H, Moseley M. Compliance in amblyopia therapy: objective monitoring of occlusion. Br J Ophthalmol. 1995;79:585–9.
21. Chopovska Y, Loudon S, Cirina L, Zubcov A, Simonsz H, Lüchtenberg M, Fronius M. Electronic recording of occlusion treatment for amblyopia: potential of the new technology. Graefes Arch Clin

Exp Ophthalmol. 2005;243(6):539–44. doi:10.1007/s00417-004-1067-8.
22. Fronius M, Chopovska Y, Nolden J, Loudon S, Lüchtenberg M, Zubcov A, Pepler L. Occlusion treatment for amblyopia: assessing the performance of the electronic occlusion dose monitor. Strabismus. 2006;14(2):65. doi:10.1080/09273970600700962.
23. Wallace M, Stewart C, Moseley M, Stephens D, Fielder A. Compliance with occlusion therapy for childhood amblyopia. Invest Ophthalmol Vis Sci. 2013;54:6158–66.
24. Simonsz H, Polling J, Voorn R, Van Leeuwen J, Meester H, Romijn C, Dijkstra B. Electronic monitoring of treatment compliance in patching for amblyopia. Strabismus. 1999;7(2):113–23.
25. Januschowski K, Bechtold TE, Schott TC, Huelber-Januschowski MS, Blumenstock G, Bartz-Schmidt KU, Besch D, Schramm C. Measuring wearing times of glasses and ocular patches using a thermosensor device from orthodontics. Acta Ophthalmol. 2013;91(8):e635–40.
26. Chua BEG, Johnson K. A retrospective review of the associations between amblyopia type, patient age, treatment compliance and referral patterns. Clin Experiment Ophthalmol. 2004;32(2):175–9.
27. Choong Y, Lukman H, Martin S, Laws D. Childhood amblyopia treatment: psychosocial implications for patients and primary carers. Eye. 2004;18(4):369–75.
28. Carlton J, Kaltenthaler E. Amblyopia and quality of life: a systematic review. Eye. 2011;25(4):403–13.
29. Hrisos S, Clarke M, Wright C. The emotional impact of amblyopia treatment in preschool children: randomized controlled trial. Ophthalmology. 2004;111(8):1550–6.
30. Dobson V, Quinn G, Siatkowski R, Baker J, Hardy R, Reynolds J, Trese M, Tung B. Agreement between grating acuity at age 1 year and Snellen acuity at age 5.5 years in the preterm child. Cryotherapy for Retinopathy of Prematurity Cooperative Group. Invest Ophthalmol Vis Sci. 1999;40(2):496–503.
31. Hall HL, Courage ML, Adams RJ. The predictive utility of the Teller acuity cards for assessing visual outcome in children with preterm birth and associated perinatal risks. Vision Res. 2000;40(15):2067–76.
32. Prager TC, Zou YL, Jensen CL, Fraley JK, Anderson RE, Heird WC. Evaluation of methods for assessing visual function of infants. J Am Asso Pedi Ophthalmol Strab. 1999;3(5):275–82.
33. Drews-Botsch C, Celano M, Cotsonis G, Hartmann EE, Lambert SR. The relationship between occlusion therapy and optotype visual acuity at 4 1/2 years using data from a randomized clinical trial, the Infant Aphakia Treatment Study. In press, JAMA Ophthalmology.

15 The Refractive Management of Infantile Aphakia and Pseudophakia

Cindy Tromans and Helen Wilson

15.1 Introduction

Successful management of children following congenital and infantile cataract surgery involves early surgical intervention together with accurate and intensive optical rehabilitation with spectacles or contact lenses in conjunction with occlusion therapy.

The use of intraocular lenses (IOLs) in the management of these patients has now become accepted by paediatric ophthalmologists as microsurgical techniques and IOL technology has improved, together with an increased knowledge and understanding of the refractive rate of growth of the human eye. To obtain a satisfactory long-term refractive result allowances must be made for growth of the eye, so pseudophakic eyes are left hypermetropic to allow for the axial elongation with corresponding myopic shift [14].

This chapter will look at the optical rehabilitation options available in the care of both aphakic and pseudophakic patients.

C. Tromans, PhD, MCOptom, DipTp(IP) (✉)
H. Wilson, BSc(Hons), MCOptom, Dip Tp(IP)
Manchester Royal Eye Hospital,
Oxford Road, Manchester M13 9WL, UK
e-mail: Cindy.Tromans@cmft.nhs.uk; Helen.Wilson@cmft.nhs.uk

15.2 Aphakia

Surgery for congenital and infantile cataract is usually within the first six weeks of life, to minimize deprivation amblyopia and to give the eye the optimum chance of visual development [3]. When optically managing the resultant aphakia following surgery, it is vital to be aware of rapid changes in the ocular dimensions that occur within the first few months of life. The average radius of curvature of the cornea in a newborn is around 6.90 mm [8] to 7.18 mm [19] and this will flatten rapidly in the first 6 months of life. Corneal diameter is approximately 10 mm at birth [19]. Axial length will also increase rapidly from around 17.00 mm in neonates to 21.00 mm within the first 6 months of life and then more slowly during infancy and childhood [13]. The Infant Aphakia Treatment Study (IATS) group found that eyes with unilateral cataract were shorter than the fellow eye and that the rate of axial elongation was less in eyes that were corrected using a contact lens for aphakia compared to those eyes corrected with an IOL [11]. These changes to axial length cause a 'myopic shift', with the average aphakic optical correction decreasing from approximately +35.00 to +20.00 D in the first few years of life. However, eyes with congenital cataract can also have associated disorders such as persistent fetal vasculature and microphthalmos, which can result in an optical correction with powers in excess of +50.00 D.

I.C. Lloyd, S.R. Lambert (eds.), *Congenital Cataract*, DOI 10.1007/978-3-319-27848-3_15

The refractive management of bilateral aphakia can be successfully achieved with spectacles (Fig. 15.1). Spectacles are easily worn and are non-invasive. They also provide the infant with additional magnification thereby helping to improve visual acuity. However, due to the high plus prescription required, the lenses are often heavy and bulky and even in lenticulated form are only available up to around +26.00D [20]. It is often difficult to achieve a good spectacle frame fit in babies and young infants, even with specially designed plastic frames. The spectacles can look cosmetically poor and slip down the nose if not fitted correctly. High plus lenticulated lenses also cause a restricted field of view, a ring scotoma and peripheral distortion. The lenses need to be fitted as close to the eye as possible, taking care to adjust the strength to take in to consideration the back vertex distance which is critical when dispensing such high prescriptions.

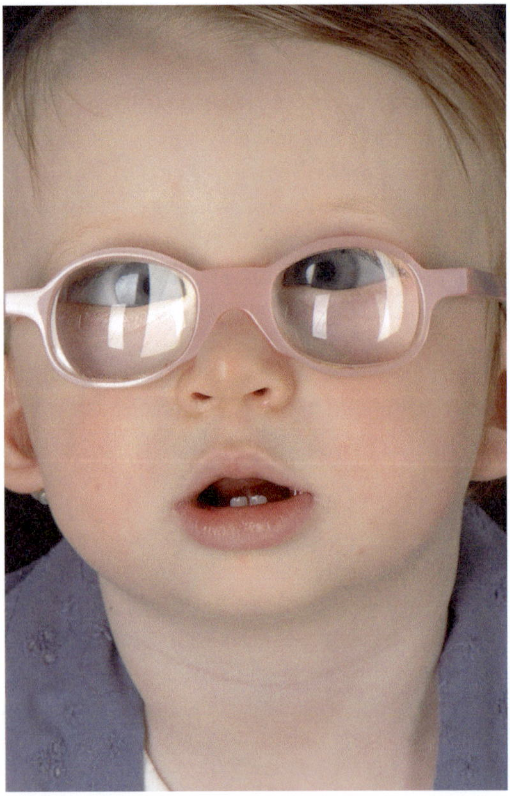

Fig. 15.1 An infant wearing aphakic spectacles

In cases of unilateral aphakia, spectacles are not an option due to aniseikonia and prismatic imbalance between the eyes [17]. In these cases correction with a contact lens provides optimal management of the anisometropia. In certain circumstances, however, spectacles can be prescribed if the parents are struggling with contact lens handling, with the spectacles only to be worn whilst undergoing occlusion therapy.

15.3 Pseudophakia

As previously described the use of IOLs in the management of congenital cataract has now become more common. Pseudophakic eyes are deliberately left hypermetropic to allow for axial elongation with the corresponding myopic shift. The desired refractive result for infants undergoing surgery under the age of 10 weeks should be 8–9 dioptres of hypermetropia, reducing to 4 dioptres at 12 months of age and 2 dioptres by 24 months. The final refractive status, following cessation of axial elongation, is aimed at emmetropia or low myopia [14]. The recent IATS group under corrected the IOL power by 8 dioptres for those infants operated between 4 and 6 weeks, and by 6 dioptres for infants aged 7 weeks but less than 7 months [10]. The residual refractive error can then be corrected with either spectacles, or in cases of unilateral pseudophakia, a contact lens in the early months, gradually reducing the lens power until the eye reaches an emmetropic state and refractive correction is no longer required or spectacles can be prescribed.

A retrospective case review was carried out at Manchester Royal Eye Hospital [22] of infants 6 months and younger fitted with contact lenses following IOL implantation in 23 eyes of 17 infants, with six infants having bilateral IOLs. About one-half of eyes operated on achieved a best sphere residual refraction of +8.00 to +9.00 dioptres, 35 % had a best sphere of +7.00 dioptres and the remainder had a best sphere greater than +9.00DS but not exceeding +11.50DS. The median refractive error was +9.00DS. At age 1 year the median refractive error was +3.00DS with a range of plano to +8.00DS, resulting in a myopic shift of the median refractive error of −6.00D.

By 2 years of age, 25 % of eyes had a best sphere refractive error of plano to −3.00DS, 45 % of eyes had a refractive error of +0.25DS to +3.00DS, and 20 % of eyes were +3.25DS to +4.50DS. The remaining two eyes had no recorded refractive error, however these eyes also demonstrated 'no interest' when assessing visual acuity with one of these eyes diagnosed with anterior segment dysgenesis and the other with persistent fetal vasculature. Both cases had multiple systemic health issues. All the infants were fitted with contact lenses to correct the residual refractive error, by 1 year of age 48 % of eyes were still corrected with a contact lens with the other 52 % discontinuing lens wear as the refractive error had reduced to a level that did not require correction (plano to −2.00DS) or could be corrected with spectacles (plano to +5.00DS). There were no infants still wearing a contact lens by the age of two.

15.4 Examination Techniques and Contact Lens Fitting

15.4.1 Case History

A detailed history is very important in the fitting of contact lenses to these patients. If the baby was born prematurely then they will most likely have steeper corneal curvatures [8] and smaller overall corneal diameters [16]. Many of these infants often have systemic co-morbidity with the parents having to deal with multiple hospital appointments, and making contact lens wear less successful. It is also very important to know whether or not the parents have had experience with handling and maintaining contact lenses for themselves, and whether or not they themselves have any visual impairment making contact lens handling more difficult. The IATS examined the impact of parental stress associated with caring for an infant who had undergone IOL treatment compared to contact lens correction for unilateral aphakia. They expected the main issues to be associated with lens insertion and removal, however found that there was no statistical difference to stress levels between the two treatment groups [5].

15.4.2 Anterior-Segment Examination

As with the adult patient, examination of the anterior segment is an important aspect of contact lens fitting and aftercare. A very simple method to determine the presence of corneal staining or ulceration is to use an ultraviolet lamp with fluorescein to determine the location and extent of the lesion. In babies, a major slit lamp can be used with the 'flying baby' technique and in infants and young children a hand-held slit lamp can be used to examine the anterior segment in more detail. Older children, from 3 or 4 years of age, can usually sit at a slit lamp, kneeling on a chair and grasping the headrest support bars.

15.4.3 Keratometry

A hand-held automated keratometer can be used to determine the corneal radius of curvature in young infants and children too young to sit at a conventional keratometer (Fig. 15.2).

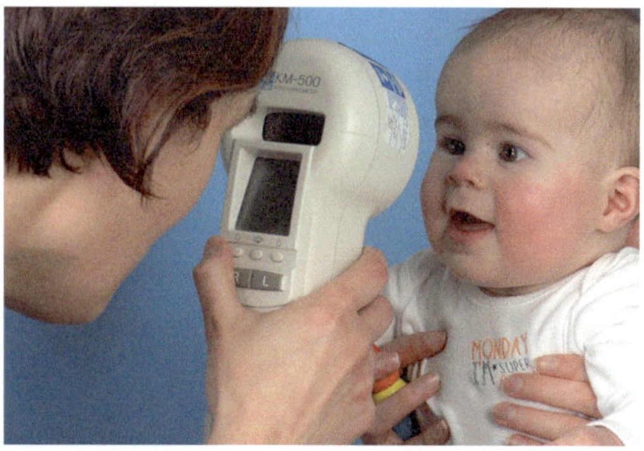

Fig. 15.2 Hand held keratometry

15.4.4 Refraction

Determination of the refractive error or a contact lens over-refraction is performed with retinoscopy using hand-held lenses or a paediatric trial frame in an older child. The use of a cycloplegic drug is recommended in those children with normal accommodative function in the fellow eye. It is also useful to dilate the pupil in aphakes and pseudophakes where there is a small or displaced pupil or where significant media opacity is apparent, e.g., posterior capsular thickening.

Since infants in the early stages of visual development require a focal length of around 30–50 cm to see a face, the power of the selected contact lens is usually 2–3 D greater than the ocular refraction. This over-correction should be reduced at 18 months to 2 years when the toddler becomes more mobile and aware of distant objects. A reading correction or bifocals can be prescribed from around 3–4 years of age when the child starts preschool education.

15.4.5 Biometry

Prior to cataract surgery, the axial length of the eye can be measured with ultrasound and the corneal radius of curvature by keratometry. These measurements can be used to determine the power of the contact lens required post-operatively by using an IOL calculation formula, e.g., Holladay, which can determine the ocular power at the corneal plane postoperatively. This is particularly useful as it allows more or less correct specifications to be ordered, which alleviates the need for many lenses to be used at the initial fitting and allows for fewer lenses to be kept in stock.

15.4.6 Measurement of Corneal Diameter

This is usually done at the time of surgery whilst the infant is under general anaesthesia so that an accurate measurement can be taken. This measurement aids the optometrist in selecting the appropriate contact lens total diameter.

15.5 Contact Lens Selection

Contact lens technology and lens availability has changed dramatically over the past 10–15 years, providing many more choices in terms of lens selection in the care of aphakic and pseudophakic infants. Contact lens types include soft lenses, both hydrogel and silicone hydrogel lenses, rigid lenses and silicone elastomer lenses.

15.5.1 Hydrogel Soft Lenses

High water content hydrogel lenses were traditionally the most frequently used lens types in paediatric contact lens fitting as they are easy to fit, comfortable to wear, can be manufactured in a wide range of parameters to fit any size and shape of eye and are readily available. Parents tend to be less apprehensive about inserting and removing a hydrogel lens and daily wear should always be actively encouraged to reduce the risk of infection as oxygen transmission is reduced through high-powered lenses used to correct aphakia [1]. However, as babies and young children sleep during the daytime, the lenses can remain in the eye during these periods.

Soft hydrogel lenses do, however have some disadvantages including dehydration caused by dry eyes due to the relatively low blink rate of infants. They do not correct any corneal astigmatism. Insertion may be difficult particularly in infants where there is excessive lid squeezing or a small palpebral aperture causing frequent lens loss and damage. There may be a degree of corneal hypoxia due to the combination of the low oxygen permeability of the lens material and the increased central thickness. Long term corneal hypoxia can lead to corneal vascularization, stromal oedema and chronic endothelial dysfunction [4].

Lenses are usually fitted according to age or based on keratometry readings and corneal diameter. Table 15.1 shows appropriate contact lens parameter selection for each age.

15.5.2 Silicone Hydrogel Lenses

Silicone hydrogel lenses are now readily available and can be custom made in the range of base curves, diameters and powers that are required for fitting aphakic and pseudophakic eyes. These lenses are now often the lens of first choice (Fig. 15.3).

Silicone hydrogel lenses have many advantages including an increased modulus, or stiffness, making handling and lens insertion much easier with reduced risk of loss or damage to the lens. They also tend to stabilize and centre much better than hydrogel lenses but do have to be fitted more precisely as they do not drape over the cornea like a hydrogel lens [9]. There is also the added advantage of reduced risk of corneal hypoxia due to the increased oxygen permeability of these materials [6]. They are, however still prone to dehydration and also increased lipid deposition [7].

15.5.3 Silicone Elastomer Lenses

Silicone elastomer lenses are often used in the correction of refractive errors in babies and young children, and are particularly useful where there is frequent lens loss or a dry ocular surface. The lens fit can be checked using fluorescein and ultraviolet light. A period of settling, for example 30 min, is required [21]. In the IATS 70% of eyes corrected with a contact lens were fitted with silicone

Table 15.1 Hydrogel lens specifications based on age for an aphakic eye of normal size

Age (months)	BOZR (mm)	TD (mm)	Power (D)
1	7.00	12.00	+35.00
2	7.20	12.50	+32.00
3	7.50	13.00	+30.00
6	7.80	13.50	+25.00
12	8.10	13.50	+20.00

BOZR back zone optic radius, *TD* total diameter

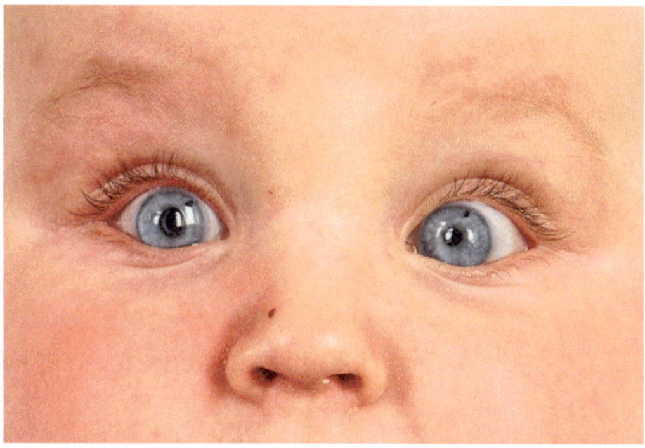

Fig. 15.3 An infant wearing +32.00DS silicone hydrogel contact lenses

elastomer lenses due to its ease of fitting and increased oxygen permeability [18].

The main advantages of silicone elastomer lenses are the very high oxygen permeability and less susceptibility to dehydration. They are less easily rubbed out and therefore less prone to loss and damage [20].

The range of parameters and availability of silicone elastomer lenses is however limited. They are only available up to +32.00DS and limited to three dioptre steps in power. Only three base curves are available over +20.00DS with the steepest base curve being 7.5 mm, which is considerably flatter than most infantile cataract corneal curvatures [15]. They need to be precisely fitted and take longer to fit due to the settling periods required. Negative pressure effects can cause adhesion to the cornea if the lens is too tight [20]. Lenses have a relatively short life span due to surface coating degeneration so need to be replaced more frequently. They are also more expensive than hydrogel and rigid lenses.

These lenses are becoming increasing difficult to obtain as silicone hydrogel materials have developed and become more readily available in the parameters required.

15.5.4 Rigid Lenses

The development of automated hand-held keratometry and rigid lens design has led to the increased use of rigid lenses for paediatric use. They have been successfully used for the management of aphakia in infants and can be fitted without the need for general anaesthesia [2]. Rigid lenses were also used in the IATS as an alternative to silicone elastomer lenses.

Rigid lenses are available in a large range of parameters and very high oxygen permeability materials reducing corneal hypoxia. They correct any corneal astigmatism and the fitting can be easily assessed with the use of fluorescein. The rigidity makes them durable and easier to insert and remove however there is an increased risk of corneal abrasion if insertion is difficult. Older children may find adapting to rigid lenses more difficult due to the initial discomfort.

15.6 Handling of Lenses

Daily insertion and removal of contact lenses is the preferred option for the management of these patients to minimize the risk of complications associated with extended wear including microbial keratitis, corneal hypoxia and neovascularisation.

A modified technique for insertion and removal is required in the young eye (Fig. 15.4).

Parents are counselled on the importance of lens cleaning and disinfection which is to be carried out daily usually with a daily cleaning solution, sterile saline and a hydrogen peroxide system.

Any topical medication used following surgery should be changed to preservative-free varieties so can still be used with the contact lenses in situ.

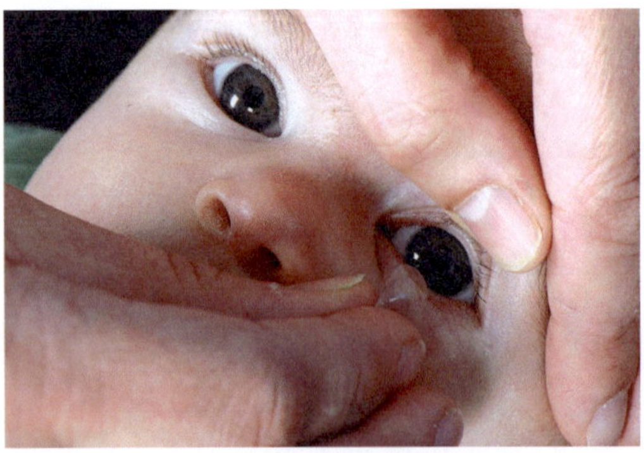

Fig. 15.4 A hydrogel soft lens being inserted into an infant's eye

Some points to consider when handling contact lenses in babies and young children are as follows:

- Lenses are easier to insert and remove with the child lying down on a firm, flat surface, e.g., examination couch, so that the lens can be slid under the upper eyelid using the forefinger whilst the lens is kept in alignment with the corneal surface.
- Babies can be swaddled in a blanket to make handling easier and prevent the interference of the infants' arms and hands.
- It is far easier to learn how to handle lenses on a young infant than on a more active baby or toddler. It is therefore important to encourage parents and carers to undertake lens handling from the outset of lens fitting.
- Parents/carers should be advised to keep to regular times for handling, so that it becomes accepted as part of daily routine. Twelve hours per day is usually acceptable e.g., 7 am–7 pm.
- If handling is difficult in young infants, lenses can always be inserted or removed during sleep, just before the infant wakes or about an hour after they fall asleep.
- Infants should be discouraged from eye rubbing from the outset to minimize lens breakage and loss.
- To aid lens removal a drop of sterile saline can be inserted in to the eye.
- Soft lenses are easiest to remove by manipulating the lids similar to rigid lens removal in adults.
- Handling often becomes more difficult from 18 months onward. Bilateral aphakes can start to use spectacles at this point and anisometropes can use a spectacle correction when occluded.
- Co-operation may be extremely limited in children aged between 2 and 5 years when fitting lenses for the first time. Spectacles may have to suffice in this age if the benefits of contact lenses are outweighed by the distress caused to the child by handling.

15.7 Aftercare

Frequent contact lens aftercare of these patients is essential. The following elements should always be assessed at the aftercare visits:

15.7.1 History

Questions to ask the parents or carers should include the wearing schedule: what time are the lenses inserted and removed? Have there been any episodes of redness or discharge? Has the infant been rubbing the lenses out? Have the lenses remained central over the pupil? Has there been any difficulty with inserting or removing the lenses?

The parents or carers should be asked to demonstrate their cleaning regime to ensure compliance and understanding.

15.7.2 Assessment of the Contact Lens Fitting

The centration and movement of the lens should be assessed either by direct observation in very young infants or on the slit lamp in older children. Fluorescein should be used to determine the fitting of rigid and silicone elastomer lenses. For lenses that are not centring very well or that often ride up under the eyelid it may be necessary to increase the overall diameter of the lens to improve stability or to switch to a different type of contact lens.

15.7.3 Over-refraction

Retinoscopy should be performed at every aftercare visit to determine the over-refraction. Frequent changes to the power of the contact lens will be necessary in the first three months due to the rapid growth of the eye. As previously mentioned very young infants are deliberately over-corrected by +2.00D to focus on a near point. This over-correction is usually reduced to +1.00D by the age of 12 months or when the infant becomes mobile. The over-refraction is again reduced to plano by the time the infant reaches pre-school with a near addition incorporated into bifocals.

It also important to assess the quality of the retinoscopy reflex – this can indicate the presence of any media opacity.

15.7.4 Slit-Lamp Examination

Once the infant is old enough to sit at the slit lamp a detailed assessment of the cornea can be made paying particular attention to any contact lens induced changes. Fluorescein should also be instilled to check for any corneal staining.

15.7.5 Common Aftercare Problems

In addition to lens fitting and handling problems, other common problems include:

- **Red or sticky eye** – this can be due to numerous causes, including tight-fitting lens, infection, inflammation or allergic reaction. Parents/carers should be instructed to remove the lens immediately and seek urgent advice from a contact lens practitioner or ophthalmologist.
- **Neovascularization** – especially where thick hydrogel lenses have been used for continuous wear. Consider refitting with rigid or silicone hydrogel lenses and encourage daily wear from the beginning.
- **Papillary conjunctivitis** – eye rubbing is often a sign of ocular irritation due to an allergy to care solutions or protein deposition on lenses. The use of a separate cleaning solution with demonstration to the parents of mechanical rubbing of the lenses to dislodge protein and lipid build-up as well as a hydrogen peroxide system can be used to minimize this.
- **Glaucoma** – long term monitoring of eyes after congenital cataract surgery is essential as up to two thirds will develop glaucoma or become glaucoma suspects by 10 years after surgery [12]. Intraocular pressure can be measured on

babies and young children with a hand-held non-contact tonometer, e.g., Pulsair, or rebound technology tonometer e.g., iCare and this is advised at each visit. Any rapid or unexpected myopic shifts in refractive error should always be investigated to rule out glaucoma as well as any unexpected changes to the way the contact lens is fitting such as a rigid lens suddenly becoming too steep or looking smaller on the eye [15].

15.8 Summary

Contact lenses have the benefits of providing optical correction without the infant having to wear bulky spectacle frames which can be easily taken off by the infant. They are also most beneficial in unilateral aphakia and pseudophakia where there is a high degree of anisometropia. Appropriate timing of contact lens intervention and diligence from parents in terms of handling and caring for the contact lenses, can lead to the successful optical management of these patients.

Acknowledgement The authors would like to thank the Department of Ophthalmic Imaging at Manchester Royal Eye Hospital for the production of the illustrations used in this chapter.

References

1. Amaya LG, Speedwell L, Taylor D. Contact lenses for infant aphakia. Br J Ophthalmol. 1990;74:150–4.
2. Amos C, Lambert SR, Ward M. Rigid gas permeable correction of aphakia following congenital cataract removal during infancy. J Pediatr Ophthalmol Strabismus. 1992;26:290–5.
3. Birch EE, Cheng C, Stager Jr DR, Weakley Jr DR, Stager Sr DR. The critical period for surgical treatment of dense congenital bilateral cataracts. JAAPOS. 2009;13:67–71.
4. Bruce AS, Brennan NA. Corneal pathophysiology with contact lens wear. Surv Ophthalmol. 1990;35:25–58.
5. Celano M, Hartmann EE, Drews-Botsch CD. Parenting stress in the Infant Aphakia Treatment Study. J Pediatr Psychol. 2013;38(5):484–93.
6. Efron N, Morgan PB, Cameron ID, Brennan NA, Goodwin M. Oxygen permeability and water content of silicone hydrogel contact lens materials. Optom Vis Sci. 2007;84:328–37.
7. Ghormley N, Jones LW. Managing lipid deposition on silicone hydrogel lenses. Contact Lens Spectrum. 2006;21:21.
8. Inagaki Y. The rapid change in corneal curvature in the neonatal period and infancy. Arch Ophthalmol. 1986;104:1026–7.
9. Jones L, Dumbleton K. Soft contact lens fitting. In: Phillips AJ, Speedwell L, editors. Contact lenses. 5th ed. London: Butterworth-Heinemann; 2006. p. 230–5.
10. Lambert SR, Buckley EG, Drews-Botsch C, DuBois L, Hartmann E, Lynn M, Plager D, Wilson ME. The Infant Aphakia Treatment Study: design and clinical measures at enrollment. Arch Ophthalmol. 2010;128:21–7.
11. Lambert SR, Lynn MJ, DuBois LG, Cotsonis GA, Hartmann EE, Wilson ME. Axial elongation following cataract surgery during the first year of life in the Infant Aphakia Treatment Study. Invest Ophthalmol Vis Sci. 2012;53:7539–45.
12. Lambert SR, Purohit A, Superak HM, Lynn MJ, Beck AD. Long-term risk of glaucoma after congenital cataract surgery. Am J Ophthalmol. 2013;156:355–61.
13. Larsen JS. The sagittal growth of the eye: IV: ultrasonic measurement of the axial length of the eye from birth to puberty. Acta Ophthalmol. 1971;49:873–86.
14. Lloyd IC, Ashworth J, Biswas S, Abadi RV. Advances in the management of congenital and infantile cataract. Eye. 2007;21:1301–9.
15. Lindsay RG, Chi JT. Management of infantile aphakia. Clin Exp Optom. 2010;93:3–14.
16. Moore BD. Mensuration data in infant eyes with unilateral congenital cataracts. Am J Optom Physiol Opt. 1987;64:204–10.
17. Moore BD. Paediatric cataracts-diagnosis and treatment. Optom Vis Sci. 1994;71:168–73.
18. Russell B, Ward MA, Lynn M, DuBois L, Lambert S. The Infant Aphakia Treatment Study conact lens experience: one-year outcomes. Eye Contact Lens. 2012;38(4):234–9.
19. Sorsby A, Sheridan M. The eye at birth: measurement of the principal diameters in forty-eight cadavers. J Anat. 1960;94:192–5.
20. Tromans C. Paediatric contact lenses. In: Efron N, editor. Contact lenses. 2nd ed. Butterworth: Heinemen; 2010. p. 303–9.
21. Visser ES. The silicone rubber contact lens: clinical indications and fitting technique. Cont Lens Anterior Eye. 1997;20:S19–25.
22. Wilson HL, Tromans C, Ashworth J, Biswas S, Lloyd IC. The use of contact lenses to correct the residual refractive error in pseudophakic infants at Manchester Royal Eye Hospital. 2012, Presented at MREH 200 Conference 2014 and as a poster presentation at BIPOSA 2013.

Complications Following Congenital Cataract Surgery

16

David A. Plager

16.1 Introduction

Results of cataract surgery in infants have undergone sea-change improvement in the half century since Costenbader and Albert wrote in 1957 that "surgery for unilateral congenital cataract is strongly advised against" [1]. Such surgery is now considered routine and excellent visual results can be obtained in many cases, though significant controversies still exist regarding optimal timing, technique and methods of optical rehabilitation. In addition, complications can be numerous and significant and many of them are unique to the pediatric patient, especially infants. Complications can be categorized by their timing – intra-operative events, those that occur in the immediate post- operative period (within the first week) and those that develop over a longer period of time but are still directly related to the surgical process.

The soft, collapsible infant eye has much different physical characteristics than the more rigid eye of the older child or adult. In addition, the infant lens capsule and lens cortex behave much differently. These properties lead to somewhat different common complications.

D.A. Plager, MD
Department of Ophthalmology,
Eugene and Marilyn Glick Eye Institute,
Indiana University Medical Center,
Indianapolis, IN, USA

Section of Pediatric Ophthalmology and Adult Strabismus, Riley Hospital for Children,
Indianapolis, IN, USA
e-mail: dplager@iu.edu

16.2 Intraoperative Complications

16.2.1 Iris Prolapse

Iris prolapse is not usually an issue in infant cataract surgery if no IOL is to be implanted because the corneo/scleral openings are quite small. However the combination of the soft infant eye and larger wound needed for IOL insertion led to an iris prolapse rate of 21 % in the Infant Aphakia Treatment Study [2–6]. Making the entrance into the anterior chamber farther anterior and paying careful attention to the intracameral pressure during the surgery can help mitigate this potential complication.

16.2.2 Iris Damage

Damage to the iris can occur most commonly from uncontrolled iris prolapse or by direct damage to the iris with the lens cutting device (vitrector). Care must be exercised anytime the vitreous cutting instrument is in cut mode inside the eye as the very pliable infant iris can be easily aspirated into the cutting instrument tip if the two are brought into close proximity (Fig. 16.1).

I.C. Lloyd, S.R. Lambert (eds.), *Congenital Cataract*, DOI 10.1007/978-3-319-27848-3_16

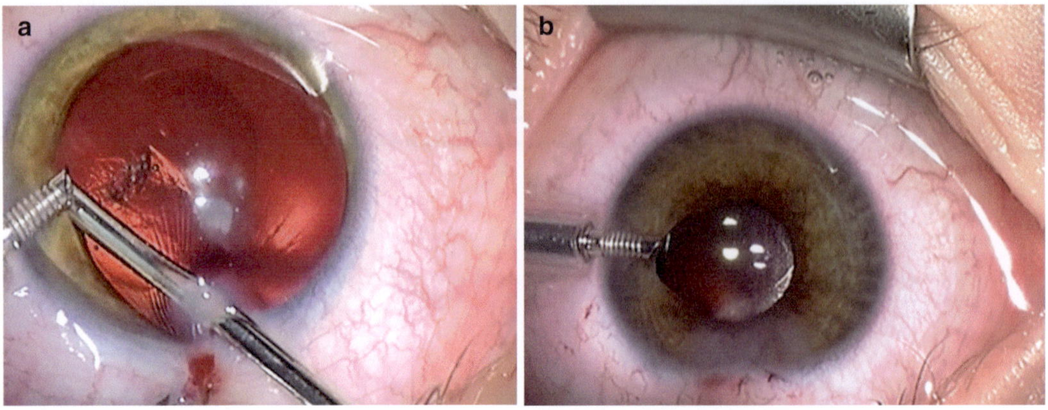

Fig. 16.1 (**a**) the vitrector has come too close to the iris while in cutting mode and the iris has been aspirated into the tip. (**b**) At conclusion of case with defect in iris apparent

16.2.3 Hyphema

Hyphema is a rare complication, occurring in <5 % of the IATS patients [3]. A persistent hyaloid vessel is commonly found in cases of PFV, but is only very rarely a cause of intraocular bleeding.

16.2.4 Ruptured Posterior Capsule

Because the posterior capsule left intact in very young children will opacify quickly and completely, it is common practice to perform a primary posterior capsulectomy in young children. When done in a controlled fashion with vitreous cutting instruments, this procedure is safe and effective. If the capsule ruptures prematurely and vitreous is allowed to escape uncontrolled into the anterior chamber or left incarcerated into the corneal wound, complications including CME, retinal detachment, pupillary block glaucoma and corectopia can ensue [7–9].

16.2.5 IOL Malposition

All efforts should be made to ensure that the IOL is secured in the capsular bag whenever possible. Although some IOL's can be placed in the ciliary sulcus, it is widely agreed that the safest long term resting place for an IOL is within the capsular bag (Fig. 16.2 and 16.3). Complications such as the UGH (uveitis-glaucoma hyphema) syndrome are more likely in cases where the IOL is malpositioned.

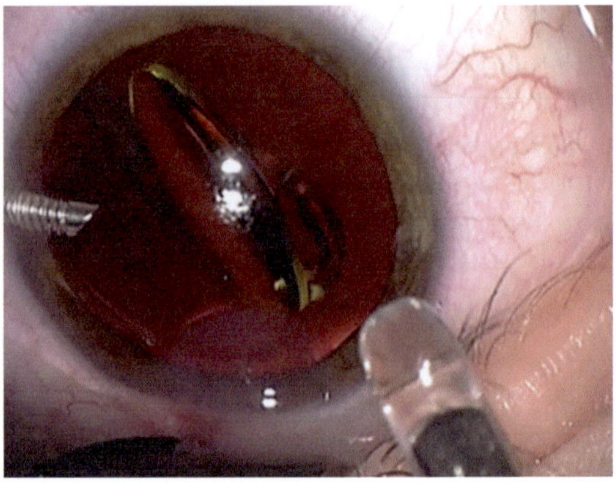

Fig. 16.2 IOL has been injected through an opening in the posterior capsule. This is one type of IOL malposition and a reason some surgeons favor doing a primary posterior capsulotomy after the IOL has been securely implanted in the capsular bag

16.3 Immediate Postoperative Complications

16.3.1 Wound Leak/Dehiscence

The infant sclera is soft and collapsible – all but the tiniest unsutured wounds tend to gape and become a source of wound leak, iris prolapse and

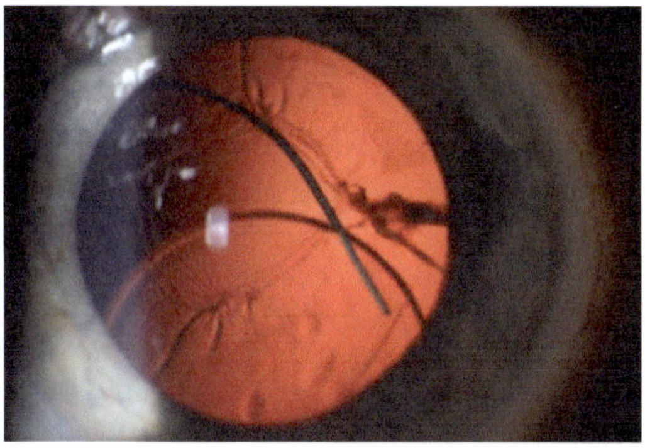

Fig. 16.3 A sulcus IOL that has become malpositioned over time

potentially endophthalmitis. Therefore it is highly recommended that most surgical wounds in young children be sutured closed. In addition to the challenging characteristics of the immature sclera, children cannot be relied on to keep their fingers away from the wounds during the early healing process. Using this philosophy, zero of 114 patients in the Infant Aphakia Treatment Study experienced a wound dehiscence (though one patient later developed a glaucoma-related wound dehiscence) [3].

16.3.2 Endophthalmitis

Endophthalmitis is perhaps the most feared complication of any intraocular surgery. Fortunately, the rate of endophthalmitis is very low in children – as it is in adults- but due to the relatively low number of patients involved, the rate in children is not as well established as it is in adult populations where it has ranged from 0.04–0.34 % in recent large studies [10–13].

Most cases in adults are due to gram-positive organisms such as *Staphylococcus epidermidis or Staph aureus,* but gram negative enterococci have also been implicated. Other important organisms found particularly in pediatric cases are *H influenza* and *pneumococci* [14, 15].

Interventions that may be appropriate to help reduce the incidence of endophthalmitis have become a controversial topic in recent years. Specifically, some surgeons have adopted the practice of mixing antibiotics into the intracameral irrigating solution and/or injecting antibiotic directly into the eye at the end of the cataract surgery [16]. For others, the scientific evidence supporting these measures and the cost/benefit ratio makes the idea of instituting them less attractive. In vitro studies have questioned the validity of mixing antibiotics into the irrigating solution and no in vivo studies have shown a statistical advantage to this measure [17].

A European study of injection of antibiotic directly into the eye at the conclusion of surgery provides the only Level 1 evidence supporting its adoption [10]. This study showed that intraocular injection of cefuroxime reduced the incidence of endophthalmitis to .07 % compared to .34 % in the control group not receiving the antibiotic. But the conclusion has been criticized because the endophthalmitis rate in the control group was much higher than other published large scale studies. The choice of cefuroxime has also been questioned because of its relatively poor efficacy against MRSA and gram negative organisms [17]. Other studies have not supported this salutary effect [18]. In addition, because the solutions need to be mixed by hand on a case by case basis (at least in the US), there exists the possibility of dilution error causing more harm than good. In addition to dilution errors leading to vision threatening complications such as macular infarction, serous detachment and cystoid macular edema, non-dose dependent idiosyncratic reactions to the injected antibiotic have been reported [19]. Shows just such a devastating reaction following injection of vancomycin post cataract surgery. Because this reaction may be delayed for days or even weeks, the second eye may be operated and sustain the same fate before the damage to the first eye is diagnosed.

Moxifloxacin has become a popular alternative antibiotic for intracameral injection because of its safety profile and the fact that it comes in a preservative-free solution that does not require reconstitution. However resistance rates to this antibiotic are rising with its increased use and the cost effectiveness for prophylactic treatment of a very rare entity has been questioned [20]. At one outpatient hospital that this author is aware of, the charge for a single dose of moxifloxacin injection is higher than the surgeon's Medicare fee for the cataract surgery.

16.3.3 Excessive Inflammation/Pupillary Membrane/Corectopia

Some degree of postoperative inflammation is expected after any cataract surgery, especially when an IOL is implanted, but the response is more intense in young children, particularly infants. If not controlled, this can lead to formation of inflammatory membranes causing pupil opacification and/or corectopia. Clearly aggressive use of steroids postoperatively is indicated in children. The route of administration- whether just topically or supplemented with intracameral or subconjunctival injection or orally- is not well settled [21, 22]. Interestingly, although the IATS was not designed to answer this question, the addition of subconjunctival steroid injection did not seem to reduce this complication- the number of babies that developed inflammatory pupillary membranes was 16 % in the eyes that had subconjunctival injection of steroid in addition to aggressive topical drops and only 13 % in the eyes that did not receive a subconjunctival injection in addition to the topical steroid [23].

16.3.4 Retinal Hemorrhages

Intraretinal hemorrhages are quite common after cataract surgery in infants, but these are invariably self-limited and non-sight threatening.

16.3.5 Vitreous Hemorrhage

Intraocular hemorrhage has been reported after surgery for congenital cataract especially in cases of PFV, but in this author's experience it is very rare. Even in cases where the persistent hyaloid vessel appears to be intact, any bleeding after transection of the vessel is usually mild and can be controlled by raising the infusion pressure in the eye for a short time.

16.4 Later Postoperative Complications

16.4.1 Lens Reproliferation into the Visual Axis

The most common complication of cataract surgery *with* IOL implantation in infants <*7 months* of age is lens reproliferation into the visual axis (VAO). It must be emphasized that this complication is common only if an IOL is placed and only in the very young, e.g., in the first 6 months of life. In the IATS, this occurred in 24 of 57 (42 %) of infants when an IOL was placed, but only 1 of 57 when the child was left aphakic [3, 4]. Similarly, in a separate study comparing children with and without IOL implant at various ages, up to 80 % of infants <6 months with an IOL developed VAO but only 12 % of the same age group when no IOL was implanted. Notably no children >8 months of age developed VAO even when an IOL was implanted [24].

16.4.2 Why Does This Occur Only in Infants and Mostly When an IOL Is Implanted?

The lens cells are still undergoing rapid proliferation in the first six months of life. When a lensectomy is performed at this young age, even when all visible cortical lens material has been aspirated from the capsular bag, more lens epithelial cell proliferation is yet to come. In most cases these re-proliferating cells will be sequestered out of the visual axis by forming a Sommerring ring (Fig. 16.4). If an IOL is placed in the capsular bag, the anterior and posterior capsule leaflets are prevented from fusing to sequester the proliferating lens cells and they are free to grow across the visual axis (Fig. 16.5). This is usually across the posterior surface of the IOL, but can be anterior to it. In either case, when they obscure the visual axis, a second procedure to aspirate the offending lens material becomes necessary (Fig. 16.6).

This reproliferation of lens cells could probably be prevented if the entire capsular bag was removed as part of the cataract surgery (this was a technique more commonly practiced before

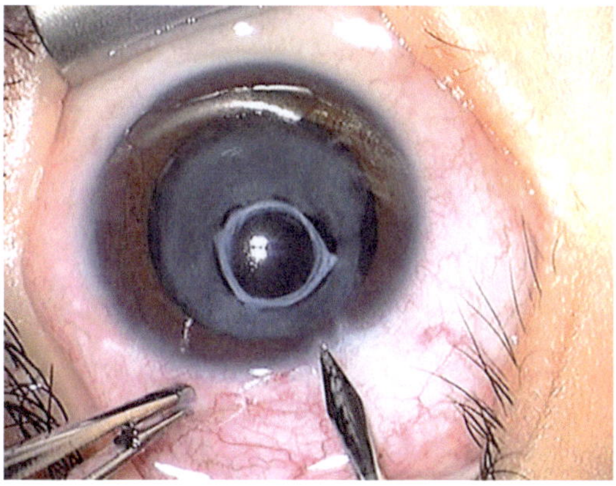

Fig. 16.4 A typical large Soemmerring ring that develops in the years following lensectomy done in the first few months of life when no IOL is placed in the capsular bag

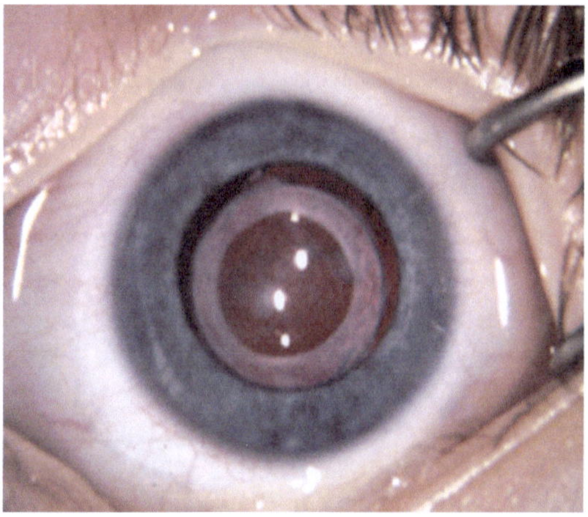

Fig. 16.5 Opacification of the visual axis that commonly occurs in infants in the months after lensectomy with posterior capsulectomy and anterior vitrectomy when an IOL is placed in the capsular bag

IOLs became widely used in children), but doing so destroys the most logical location for placement of an IOL either primarily or in later years as a second procedure.

16.4.3 Posterior Capsule Opacification

It is well known that the posterior capsule, if left intact, will opacify at some point in all children. In older children, it can take many years by which time the child will likely be cooperative enough to perform a standard YAG laser capsulotomy without need for anesthesia [25]. In young children, infants especially, the opacification of the intact posterior capsule may occur as rapidly as a few weeks. Therefore, it is standard practice to perform a primary posterior capsulectomy with anterior vitrectomy in all infants and most young children up to at least age 4 years.

16.4.4 Retinal Detachment

Retinal detachment is very rarely associated with pediatric cataract surgery, even when pars plana vitrectomy is used as part of the cataract procedure. Two of 114 infants in the IATS developed retinal detachment- one in the first month after uneventful lensectomy/vitrectomy and one following a pars plana vitrectomy to clear inflammatory debris from the visual axis [4]. Neither of these children had an IOL placed.

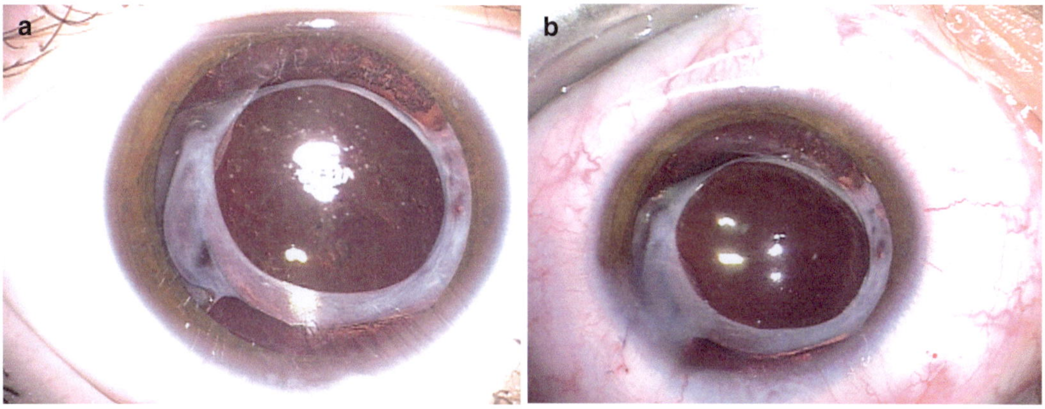

Fig. 16.6 (**a**) Opacification of the intact posterior capsule in an older child when the posterior capsule is left intact. (**b**) Posterior capsulectomy performed via pars plana in a child not cooperative enough for awake YAG laser capsulotomy

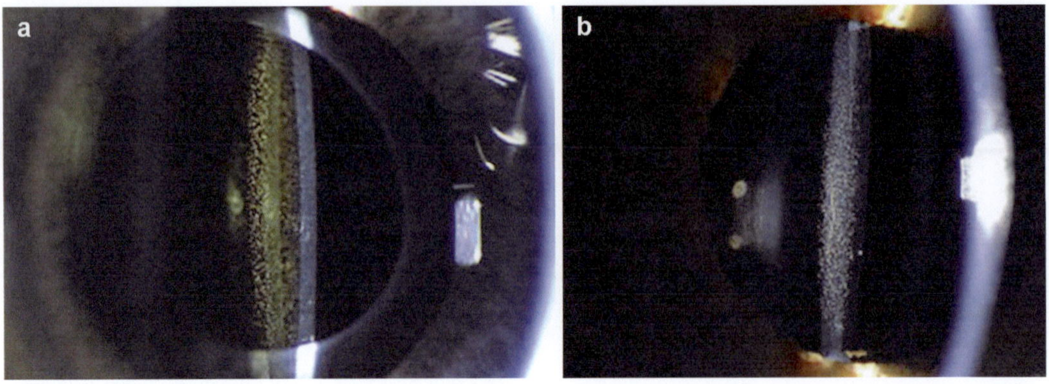

Fig. 16.7 Hydrophobic acrylic IOL glistenings

16.4.5 Cystoid Macular Edema

The incidence of CME is unknown in children but is not thought to be a visually significant issue. This is likely because the generally healthy vasculature of children is not prone to develop CME or it may be because of the difficulty of testing and/or documenting its presence in children. As a practical matter, CME typically elicits neither concern about its presence nor warrants an exhaustive search for it in children following cataract surgery.

16.4.6 IOL Glistenings

Glistenings are reflections of light seen in the slit beam of IOLs that are due to micro water vacuoles in the IOL matrix (Fig. 16.7). They can be found in modern IOL materials including PMMA, acrylic-both hydrophilic and hydrophobic and silicon. Long term studies to date have not shown an effect on visual acuity or contrast sensitivity [26].

16.5 Other

16.5.1 Glaucoma

Development of aphakic (and pseudophakic) glaucoma is an unfortunate reality when caring for children with cataracts. A detailed discussion on this topic can be found in Chap. 20, but in general, glaucoma is found almost exclusively in children with congenital (not acquired) cataracts who have undergone surgery at a young age. No effect, either deleterious or protective, of IOL implantation has been convincingly demonstrated. In the IATS, the rates of children diagnosed with glaucoma or as a glaucoma suspect were not different at 5 years of age between the groups who had an IOL implanted and those left aphakic.

It is more likely that the glaucoma is caused by or is at least strongly associated with some combination of abnormal anterior chamber anatomy found in eyes harboring congenital cataracts- mostly variants of PFV- and the young age at surgery. There are currently no known measures to reduce the incidence of glaucoma in this at-risk group. Vigilance in monitoring for development of glaucoma must be maintained for the life of the children who have undergone surgery for congenital cataracts.

16.5.2 Unpredicted Refractive Error

In general, the ability to predict the refractive error at maturity is inversely proportional to the age at which an IOL is implanted. In other words, the older the child, the less variability there will be in postoperative refractive change. At the other end, infants have extreme variability in the amount of refractive change they undergo between the time of IOL implantation and their visual maturity decades later. In the IATS, although all babies were implanted with an IOL designed to give them an immediate postoperative refraction between +6D and +8D, at 5 years of age the residual refractive errors ranged from +5D to −19D! [6]

References

1. Costenbader FD, Albert DG. Conservatism in the management of congenital cataract. AMA Arch Ophthalmol. 1957;58(3):426–30.
2. Lambert SR, Buckley EG, Drews-Botsch C, et al. The infant aphakia treatment study: design and clinical measures at enrollment. Arch Ophthalmol. 2010; 128(1):21–7.
3. Plager DA, Lynn MJ, Buckley EG, et al. Complications, adverse events, and additional intraocular surgery 1 year after cataract surgery in the infant Aphakia Treatment Study. Ophthalmology. 2011;118(12):2330–4.
4. Plager DA, Lynn MJ, Buckley EG, Wilson ME, Lambert SR, Infant Aphakia Treatment Study Group. Complications, in the first 5 years following cataract surgery in infants with and without intraocular lens implantation in the Infant Aphakia Treatment Study. Am J Ophthalmol. 2014;158:892–8.
5. Lambert SR, Buckley EG, Drews-Botsch C, et al. A randomized clinical trial comparing contact lens with intraocular lens correction of monocular aphakia during infancy: grating acuity and adverse events at age 1 year. Arch Ophthalmol. 2010;128(7):810–8.
6. Lambert SR, Lynn MJ, Hartmann EE, et al. Comparison of contact lens and intraocular lens correction of monocular aphakia during infancy: a randomized clinical trial of HOTV optotype acuity at age 4.5 years and clinical findings at age 5 years. JAMA Ophthalmol. 2014;132(6):676–82.
7. Kuhli-Hattenbach C, Luchtenberg M, Kohnen T, Hattenbach LO. Risk factors for complications after congenital cataract surgery without intraocular lens implantation in the first 18 months of life. Am J Ophthalmol. 2008;146(1):1–7.
8. Rabiah PK, Du H, Hahn EA. Frequency and predictors of retinal detachment after pediatric cataract surgery without primary intraocular lens implantation. J AAPOS. 2005;9(2):152–9.
9. Haargaard B, Andersen EW, Oudin A, et al. Risk of retinal detachmentafter pediatric cataract surgery. Invest Ophthalmol Vis Sci. 2014;55(5):2947–51.
10. Endophthalmitis Study Group, European Society of Cataract & Refractive Surgeons. Prophylaxis of postoperative endophthalmitis following cataract surgery: results of the ESCRS multicenter study and identification of risk factors. J Cataract Refract Surg. 2007; 33(6):978–88.
11. Eifrig CW, Flynn Jr HW, Scott IU, Newton J. Acute-onset postoperative endophthalmitis: review of incidence and visual outcomes (1995–2001). Ophthalmic Surg Lasers. 2002;33(5):373–8.
12. Taban M, Behrens A, Newcomb RL, et al. Acute endophthalmitis following cataract surgery: a systematic review of the literature. Arch Ophthalmol. 2005;123(5):613–20.
13. Packer M, Chang DF, Dewey SH, ASCRS Cataract Clinical Committee, et al. Prevention, diagnosis, and management of acute postoperative bacterial endophthalmitis. J Cataract Refract Surg. 2011;37(9): 1699–714.
14. Good WV, Hing S, Irvine AR, et al. Postoperative endophthalmitis in children following cataract surgery. J Pediatr Ophthalmol Strabismus. 1990;27(6):283–5.
15. Wheeler DT, Stager DR, Weakley Jr DR. Endophthalmitis following pediatric intraocular surgery for congenital cataracts and congenital glaucoma. J Pediatr Ophthalmol Strabismus. 1992;29(3):139–41.
16. Gills JP. Filters and antibiotics in irrigating solution for cataract surgery. J Cataract Refract Surg. 1991; 17(3):385.
17. Schimel AM, Alfonso EC, Flynn Jr HW. Endophthalmitis prophylaxis for cataract surgery: are intracameral antibiotics necessary? JAMA Ophthalmol. 2014;132(11):1269–70.
18. Sharma S, Sahu SK, Dhillon V, Das S, Rath S. Reevaluating intracameral cefuroxime as a prophylaxis against endophthalmitis after cataract surgery in India. J Cataract Refract Surg. 2015;41(2):393–9.
19. Alfonso EC, Flynn Jr HW. Controversies in endophthalmitis prevention: the risk for emerging resistance to vancomycin. Arch Ophthalmol. 1995;113(11):1369–70.
20. Schimel AM, Miller D, Flynn Jr HW. Endophthalmitis isolates and antibiotic susceptibilities: a 10-year review of culture-proven cases. Am J Ophthalmol. 2013;156(1):50–2, e1.
21. Cleary CA, Lanigan B, O'Keeffe M. Intracameral triamcinolone acetonide after pediatric cataract surgery. J Cataract Refract Surg. 2010;36(10):1676–81.
22. Dixit NV, Shah SK, Vasavada V, et al. Outcomes of cataract surgery and intraocular lens implantation with and without intracameral triamcinolone in pediatric eyes. J Cataract Refract Surg. 2010;36(9): 1494–8.
23. Lambert SR, Plager DA, Buckley EG, Wilson ME, DuBois L, Drews-Botsch CD, Hartmann EE, Lynn MJ, Infant Aphakia Treatment Study Group. The Infant Aphakia Treatment Study: further on intra- and postoperative complications in the intraocular lens group. J AAPOS. 2015;19(2):101–3.
24. Plager DA, Yang S, Neely DE, Sprunger DT, Sondhi N. Complications in the first year following cataract surgery with and without IOL in infants and older children. J AAPOS. 2002;6(1):9–14.
25. Plager DA, Lipsky SN, Snyder SK, et al. Capsular management and refractive error in pediatric intraocular lenses. Ophthalmology. 1997;104:600–7.
26. Henriksen BS, Kinard K, Olson RJ. Effect of intraocular lens glistening size on visual quality. J Cataract Refract Surg. 2015;41(6):1190–8.

Glaucoma Following Cataract Surgery in Aphakic or Pseudophakic Children

17

John Grigg and Cecilia Fenerty

17.1 Introduction

Glaucoma is a common, lifelong, potentially sight threatening complication for children undergoing cataract surgery. The World Glaucoma Association has defined childhood glaucoma as *intraocular pressure related damage to the eye*, to reflect the impact of raised pressure upon a range of ocular structures in the paediatric eye [1]. These changes have the potential to severely impact on the vision of a child, therefore glaucoma monitoring is essential in the management of children following cataract surgery.

J. Grigg, M.B.,B.S (QLD), MD (Syd) FRANZCO FRACS (✉)
Associate Professor, Head Discipline of Ophthalmology, Discipline of Ophthalmology, Save Sight Institute, Sydney Medical School, University of Sydney, 8 Macquarie Street, Sydney, NSW 2001, Australia

Consultant Ophthalmologist Sydney Eye Hospital, Honorary Visiting Medical Officer The Children's Hospital at Westmead, Eye Genetics Research Group Children's Medical Research Institute, The Children's Hospital at Westmead, & Save Sight Institute Sydney, Westmead, NSW, Australia
e-mail: john.grigg@sydney.edu.au

C. Fenerty, MD, FRCOphth
Manchester Royal Eye Hospital, Manchester, UK

Manchester University, Manchester, UK
e-mail: cecilia@fenerty.com

17.2 Childhood Cataract

Cataract aetiology includes: Congenital idiopathic cataract, congenital cataract associated with ocular anomalies/systemic disease (e.g. aniridia, congenital rubella syndrome etc.) and acquired cataract.

There are usually no pre-existent ocular features of glaucoma in congenital idiopathic cataract and gonioscopic findings are normal. Glaucoma arising in this group of children is therefore directly related to the surgical removal of the cataract and may occur in eyes rendered aphakic or pseudophakic [2–6].

Cases of congenital cataract associated with other ocular anomalies or systemic syndromes, may have a predisposition to glaucoma independent of cataract surgery. However the underlying ocular condition still defines the glaucoma, and influences the management.

17.3 Glaucoma

The Childhood Glaucoma Research Network has defined the diagnostic criteria for glaucoma in children [7] by the presence of two or more of the following:

- Intraocular pressure: IOP greater than 21 mmHg;
- Optic Disc features: Narrowing of the optic disc neuroretinal rim, progressive increase in the cup:disc ratio, cup:disc ratio asymmetry of

I.C. Lloyd, S.R. Lambert (eds.), *Congenital Cataract*, DOI 10.1007/978-3-319-27848-3_17

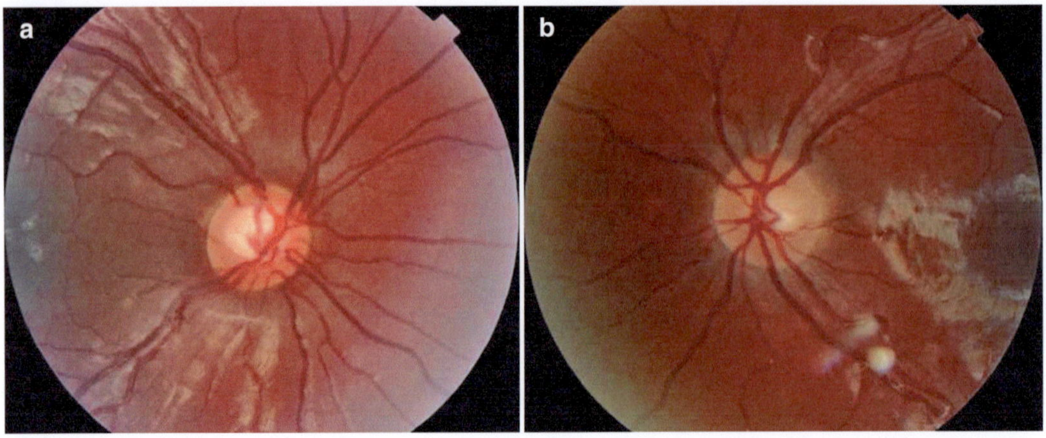

Fig. 17.1 Optic disc asymmetry with thinning of the neuroretinal rim in the right optic disc in comparison to the left optic disc

≥0.2 (assuming that the discs are of similar size); (Fig. 17.1)

- Cornea features: Haab's striae, enlarged corneal diameter (≥11 mm in newborn, > 12 mmHg in a child under 1 year of age, > 13 mHg at any age);
- Refractive error: progressive myopia or myopic shift coupled with an increase in ocular dimensions out of keeping with normal growth;
- Visual fields: Reproducible visual fields defect consistent with the glaucomatous optic disc findings with no other observable reason for the field defect.

17.3.1 Suspected Glaucoma

Glaucoma may be suspected when the constellation of features is incomplete, e.g. the presence of increasing ocular dimensions in the absence of raised IOP, or the presence of raised IOP without any other features of glaucoma. These children require close monitoring over time before a diagnosis of glaucoma can be made or excluded.

17.4 Incidence and Onset

A recent multicenter prospective study reported the incidence of glaucoma following cataract surgery to be 10% in the first year of monitoring, with cases arising in both aphakic and pseudophakic eyes [2, 3]. A retrospective review of 165 cases in the UK reported an annual incidence of glaucoma following cataract surgery to be 5.25 per 100 surgeries [8], whilst another from Australia reported an incidence of 3.9 per 100 person years [9]. Glaucoma is therefore a frequent complication of cataract surgery and the risk is life-long [2, 3, 8–13].

17.5 Mechanisms of Glaucoma

In the majority of cases there are no pre-operative gonioscopy features to indicate the pathogenesis of glaucoma [13] and removing the lens has a direct role in the development of glaucoma [14]. The two main mechanisms of glaucoma are:

- Open angle (>180° is open)
- Closed angle (<180° is open), associated with either
  - acute pupil block, or
  - progressive peripheral anterior synechiae (PAS) formation.

17.6 Pathogenesis of Open Angle Glaucoma Following Paediatric Cataract Surgery

Open angle glaucoma is the commonest mechanism, and may present at any time following surgery. The pathogenesis is poorly understood but may include the following:

- Trabecular meshwork (TM) dysfunction from inflammation and cellular obstruction
- Insult to developing angle structures from interaction with lens epithelial cells or vitreous leading to reduced outflow facility and or developmental arrest [15]
- Corticosteroid-induced mechanism [16, 17]
- TM collapse from lack of ciliary body traction
- Postoperative inflammation with damage to the trabecular meshwork, which may then progress to angle closure

Risk factors include:

- Age at time of cataract surgery – early surgery carries a higher risk of glaucoma [4, 10, 12, 18–22]
- Microcornea [2, 3, 8, 18, 23]
- Chronic Uveitis
- Family history of glaucoma following cataract surgery [12]

17.7 Pathogenesis of Closed Angle Glaucoma Following Paediatric Cataract Surgery

Angle closure mechanisms may occur either acutely with pupil block, or with progressive formation of PAS secondary to post-operative inflammation. It generally presents early following surgery.

Risk factors include:

- Microcornea [2, 3, 8, 18, 23]
- Poor pupil dilatation
- Retained lens matter
- Secondary lens proliferation
- Sulcus intraocular lens implantation
- Uveitis with pupillary membrane formation.

17.8 Risk Factors for Developing Glaucoma Following Cataract Surgery

Risks due to pre-existing ocular features should be identified prior to cataract surgery, whilst risks directly related to the surgery may be mitigated with meticulous surgical technique and careful postoperative management.

Microcornea carries a significant risk of postoperative glaucoma [2, 3, 8, 12, 18, 23] both open and closed angle. In one study of 48 eyes with aphakic glaucoma 45 (94 %) were found to have microcornea [23].

Persistent foetal vasculature may carry additional risks of glaucoma although the evidence is conflicting [2, 3, 24].

Intra-ocular lens placement: The risk of developing glaucoma following intraocular lens implantation has generated much debate. An initial report that the presence of an intraocular lens was protective for the development of glaucoma [25] was also supported by a large multicenter meta-analysis [26]. However, selection bias potentially contributes to the lower rate of glaucoma in pseudophakic infants reported in these studies as lens implantation in infants less than 12 months old occurs in only a few selected cases. Three studies have reported that an intraocular lens is not protective for the development of glaucoma [2, 4, 5]. The recent 5 year outcome from the Infant Aphakia Treatment Study found no difference in glaucoma rates between the two groups [3]. Modern surgical techniques do not eliminate the early development of glaucoma following congenital cataract surgery with or without an intraocular lens implant [2]. These studies highlight the need for lifelong surveillance for glaucoma.

Hypotony is a sight threatening complication, which increases the risk of glaucoma. It is often associated with a shallow or flat anterior chamber, and if left untreated, may result in either PAS with angle closure glaucoma, or more seriously, aqueous misdirection. Per-operative steps to avoid hypotony include the use of an anterior chamber infusion and ensuring all surgical wounds are securely sutured to avoid aqueous leaks. Postoperative cycloplegia helps to maintain a deep anterior chamber and therefore minimizes the risk of PAS formation and aqueous misdirection.

Postoperative inflammation may directly damage the functionality of the trabecular meshwork, or may lead to PAS with angle closure, or an occlusive pupillary membrane leading to pupil block glaucoma. Inflammation may be minimized by meticulously removing all the lens material, avoiding unnecessary iris surgical trauma, using intra-cameral heparin [27, 28] and subconjunctival steroid at the end of the procedure. Postoperative frequent topical steroids (e.g. dexamethasone three to four times a day as a starting point) should be used, supplemented if necessary with further peri-ocular steroid injections.

17.9 Assessment and Monitoring for Glaucoma

The glaucoma risk is lifelong [2, 3, 10–13] so monitoring should continue indefinitely, and should be aimed at early detection before vision has been affected, and before the child becomes symptomatic.

17.9.1 History

The child's caregivers, may identify features of raised IOP including: photophobia, lacrimation, blepharospasm, intolerance of contact lens, visible enlargement of the globe, dull corneal reflex (sometimes described as a change in colour of the child's eye by the parents), poor sleep pattern, signs of distress, refusal to feed and failure to thrive. These symptoms and signs are related to enlargement of the globe and corneal oedema. Observation of the child in the clinic setting will also often elicit many of the above signs.

17.9.2 Examination

Examination to assess for the presence of glaucoma requires the clinician to be patient and to adjust the techniques used to the age of the child and their level of cooperation (Fig. 17.2). More than one visit may be necessary to obtain all the necessary information. Lowering the ambient lighting levels may assist when photophobia is an issue, and opportunistically examining an infant when they are feeding or sleeping may be helpful.

Modern equipment allows assessment in the outpatients for most children, however it may be necessary to perform an examination under anesthesia to fully determine the glaucoma status. Inhaled anaesthetic agents are associated with a reduction in IOP and measurements need to be taken as early as possible in the induction process with agreement from the anaesthetist. Ketamine does not affect the IOP as dramatically as inhaled anaesthesia but is less frequently used in current clinical practice.

Monitoring should be at intervals chosen according to the perceived risk of developing glaucoma and according to breadth and accuracy of the possible assessments at each visit. Assuming the ophthalmologist is confident that adequate assessment has been achieved, and there is no evidence of glaucoma, some experts have suggested the following monitoring review intervals: 1 week and then 1 month following cataract surgery and then 2–4 month review; thereafter high risk cases may be monitored at 2–4 monthly intervals and low risk 6–12 monthly intervals [29]. However, when development of glaucoma is suspected, or when full assessment has not been possible earlier review must be considered (Table 17.1).

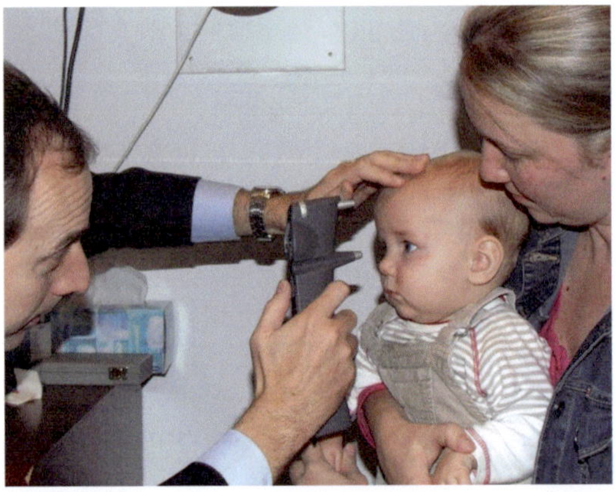

Fig. 17.2 iCare™ rebound tonometry (Icare Finland Oy Vantaa, Finland) allows regular and frequent clinic intra-ocular pressure measurements

Table 17.1 Examination features and techniques

Test	Features	Equipment	Notes
Visual Acuity	Sequential recordings assessing for change	Preferential Looking Cards for pre-verbal children,	
		Matching shapes (Kay Pictures) for toddlers,	
		Matching letters (HOTV, or Sheridan Gardner) pre-school age	
		Snellen charts with single or linear letters or LogMAR visual acuity charts for school aged children	
Intra-ocular pressure (IOP)	Sequential recordings: Accuracy may be affected by corneal thickness, off-axis measurements, corneal scarring, lid squeezing, breath holding, crying, and use of a speculum or fingers to hold the lids.	Goldmann applanation tonometry (GAT) GAT may be performed by Perkins tonometer	GAT is the reference standard for IOP measurement
		Other methods: iCare™ rebound tonometer Pneunotonometry Tonopen™	Non-GAT methods reasonably accurate when IOP within normal limits but may over-estimate compared to GAT at higher levels of IOP [30–40]
Corneal Assessment	Corneal Diameter	Calipers and ruler estimating to nearest 0.25 mm	Limbal-to-limbal measurement preferably in horizontal meridian. Progressive enlargement may indicate poor IOP control [41]
	Corneal edema	Direct observation	May indicate raised IOP
	Haab's Striae	Direct observation	
	Central corneal thickness (CCT)	Pachymetry	Often thicker following cataract surgery [42–48]. Changes in CCT may influence the accuracy of IOP measurements
Anterior chamber (AC) assessment	Anterior chamber depth	Redmond Smith method [49], anterior segment OCT, or UBM	
	Iris and pupillary profile	Direct observation	e.g. Bombé with pupil block, or peripheral tenting with PAS formation
	Inflammation	Direct observation	Inflammation should be graded during monitoring and treatment
	Angle	Gonioscopy	
	Additional features: e.g. pupillary membrane, Elschnig pearls, vitreous in the anterior chamber	Direct observation	

Table 17.1 (continued)

Test	Features	Equipment	Notes
Optic Disc Assessment	Size, shape, colour, neuroretinal rim configuration, Cup:disc ratio, Nerve fibre layer defects, congenital anomalies	Direct or indirect ophthalmoscopy, imaging e.g. photography, OCT, HRT, GDx	Baseline images should be obtained when possible with further images as and when changes occur.
Axial length measurement	Sequential recordings particularly up to age of 3 years of age	A-scan or B-scan ultrasound	Changes in axial length in excess of normal growth may indicate raised IOP [41, 50, 51]. Some reversal may be seen when the IOP is controlled.
Refraction	Sequential measurements	Retinoscopy or auto-refraction	Myopic shift, often with increased axial length, may be indicative of poorly controlled IOP; reversal of myopic shift may occur with improved IOP control
Visual Field Assessment	Sequential recordings	Confrontation visual field, or automated visual field testing	Use of automated perimetry to monitor visual field when ability of child allows

Other investigations that assist in assessment of glaucoma include: anterior segment OCT, ultra-sound biomicroscopy allowing imaging of the ciliary body and angle; B-scan ultrasound to image the posterior pole and exclude other pathology such as retinal detachment or supra-choroidal hemorrhage.

17.10 Management

Management of glaucoma or IOP rise following cataract surgery depends on the mechanism causing raised intra-ocular pressure:

17.10.1 Corticosteroid Induced IOP Rise

Topical corticosteroid therapy is the mainstay treatment for postoperative inflammation following cataract surgery. However steroid induced raised IOP is a significant risk in children. Children have been noted to have a higher frequency, worse severity and shorter time to peak corticosteroid response. Potency and mode of administration of corticosteroids plays a major role in the degree of corticosteroid response [16, 17]. It is important not to compromise the treatment of post-operative inflammation, and the addition of topical glaucoma medications may alleviate the raised IOP.

17.10.2 Pupil Block

Pupil block may occur in the post-operative period as a result of excessive post-operative inflammation and pupillary membrane formation, vitreous, remaining capsule or a proliferating lens fibers occluding aqueous flow through the pupil. Surgical intervention is then required to remove these and a peripheral iridectomy may also be performed as prophylaxis against recurrence of pupil block. Intra-cameral sodium heparin [27, 28] and intensive post-operative topical steroid may help reduce post-operative inflammation. Late pupil block may occur due to secondary lens

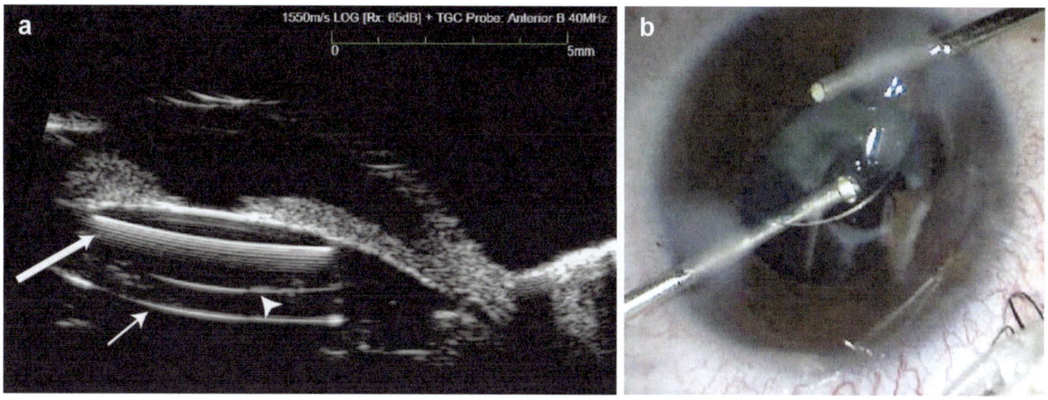

Fig. 17.3 (**a**) Ultrasound Biomicroscopy (UBM) of anterior segment of a pseudophakic eye with angle closure. The posterior chamber intraocular lens (IOL) located in the ciliary sulcus (*large arrow*). Anterior lens capsule (*arrow head*) and posterior capsule (*thin arrow*) with secondary lens proliferation (Soemmerring's ring) between the capsule leaflets. The combination of the secondary lens proliferation and sulcus IOL contribute to the angle closure. (**b**) Twenty three gauge cutter and infusion cannula removing secondary lens proliferation from under the sulcus placed IOL (same patient as **a**)

proliferation [52] or Soemmerring's ring formation (particularly in smaller eyes), which again is managed with surgical removal (Fig. 17.3).

17.10.3 Glaucoma Without Pupil Block

This is the most common presenting form of glaucoma following cataract surgery and in choosing the appropriate management consideration needs to be given to the following:

- The underlying cause and ocular characteristics of the glaucoma: Cataract surgery may be the sole cause of the glaucoma and the mechanism may be open angle, or closed angle with peripheral anterior synechiae formation. Alternatively there may be a pre-existent condition associated with glaucoma as the underlying cause e.g. aniridia
- The severity of the glaucoma including the level of IOP rise and the magnitude of the associated ocular changes including disc changes, corneal diameter and axial length. Mild to moderate intra-ocular pressure rise with early glaucomatous changes may respond well to topical medication. Advanced glaucoma usually warrants surgical intervention. If buphthalmos is present surgery is more challenging with a greater risk for complications including hypotony.
- The intolerance and allergy to topical medications: The dosage of topical medications is not titrated according to body mass, and children may suffer greater side effects from medications than do adults as a result of proportionally greater drug load, and their immature metabolism, blood–brain barrier and excretory systems. Local side effects from topical medication may reduce tolerance particularly when refractive correction is provided in the form of contact lenses. Preservative-free medication may be used in the presence of preservative intolerance or in the presence of a poor corneal surface, such as aniridia.
- Family and social factors: The effectiveness of any topical medication depends upon reliable instillation, with adherence to a regular dosing regimen and persistence in the long term. Parents and caregivers should be supported in learning the best method for instilling topical drops, which will vary according to the age and cooperation of the child. In determining a workable drop regimen, consideration must be given to social and family factors and constraints. Surgical treatment may reduce or eliminate the need for topical medications in the medium to long term. However, surgery often carries sig-

nificant risks, requires a commitment to a more intense topical drop regimen in immediate post-operative period and the need for more frequent hospital visits for post-operative assessment and monitoring in the short term.

Choice of treatment therefore needs to be tailored to the individual child and negotiated with the parents and caregivers with regular review as circumstances change.

17.11 Medical Therapy

In the absence of pupil block, topical medical therapy is the first line treatment for most children developing glaucoma following cataract surgery. The most efficacious drug classes should be used first-line with the lowest effective dose to minimize side effects and improve compliance. Availability and licensing of medication varies across different healthcare systems however currently available drug classes are listed below (Table 17.2):

17.12 Laser Treatment

Diode laser cyclophotocoagulation may be performed by the trans-scleral or endoscopic routes and both appear to have similar efficacy with 54 % qualified success and 43 % qualified success respectively [53, 54]. Retreatment rates as high as 66 % have been reported. This treatment is therefore usually performed as an adjunct to medical therapy or as a temporizing measure prior to surgery.

17.13 Surgical Treatment

When medication adequately controls IOP, or is not tolerated, or when there are continued signs of glaucoma progression, surgery is often required. Ultimately, the choice of surgical procedure will be dependent upon the clinical features of each case combined with the surgical experience of the clinician. However it is important to note that the first operation chosen for the child is often their best chance for long-term success.

Table 17.2 Medical treatment for glaucoma

Drug class	Use	Main side effects limiting tolerability	Notes
Beta-blockers	1st line	Bronchoconstriction Apnea Bradycardia.	Respiratory side effects may arise even in those children without pre-existing asthma
Prostaglandin analogues	1st line	Lash growth Hyperemia	Limited efficacy in some children
Carbonic anhydrase inhibitors[a]	Usually 2nd line	Local stinging, burning, itching hyperaemia Systemic side effects: Lethargy Loss of appetite Gastrointestinal disturbance Metabolic acidosis	Allergy to sulphonamide-type medications is a contra-indication due to cross-reactivity.
Adrenergic agonists	Limited	Somnolence Coma Respiratory depression	Should not be used in children under the age of 6 years or less than 20 kg
Miotics	Not usually 1st line	Sweating Salivation Miosis Bradycardia.	May be effective in cases of aphakic glaucoma

[a]Carbonic anhydrase inhibitors are also available as systemic treatment although side effects and intolerance limit their use in children to the short-term, often only as a temporizing measure prior to surgery. The appropriate dosage is calculated based on the body weight of the child and the minimum effective dosage should be used

- Angle Surgery (Goniotomy or Trabeculotomy)– Published data of angle surgery for glaucoma following cataract surgery is limited and mainly confined to eyes rendered aphakic. Absolute success rates may be as low as 15 %, with qualified success rates up to 57 % [13, 18, 55].
- Trabeculectomy – Success of enhanced trabeculectomy is particularly poor for aphakic cases and cases less than 1 year of age [56, 57]. An absolute success rate of 36.8 % has been reported for aphakic and pseudophakic glaucoma at 3 years [58]. Post-operative management of trabeculectomy requires intensive follow-up, sometimes combined with multiple interventions such as suture adjustment/removal and application of additional antimetabolite. Some older children may be able to tolerate these interventions at slit-lamp examination with topical anaesthesia, however most children will require general anaesthesia. These considerations therefore affect the selection of suitable cases for trabeculectomy. This procedure should be avoided when contact lens refractive correction is required because of an increased risk of blebitis and endophthalmitis [3, 58, 59].
- Glaucoma Drainage Devices (GDDs): have become the preferred primary procedure in the management of glaucoma following cataract surgery [60] partly due to the following benefits: children may still wear contact lens refractive correction if required after postoperative recovery; postoperative management is not as interventional as trabeculectomy in terms of follow up, suture manipulation or post-operative anti-metabolite application; success rates and possibly complication rates are more favorable in aphakic cases than with trabeculectomy [59, 61].

Drainage implants are available as valved devices (the Ahmed device being the most commonly used) and non-valved devices (the Baerveldt and Molteno devices being the most commonly used) [60]. All these implants are available in a range of plate sizes, and whilst the larger sizes offer some benefit in terms of achieving a lower IOP this needs to be balanced against the risk of inducing hypotony (Fig. 17.4).

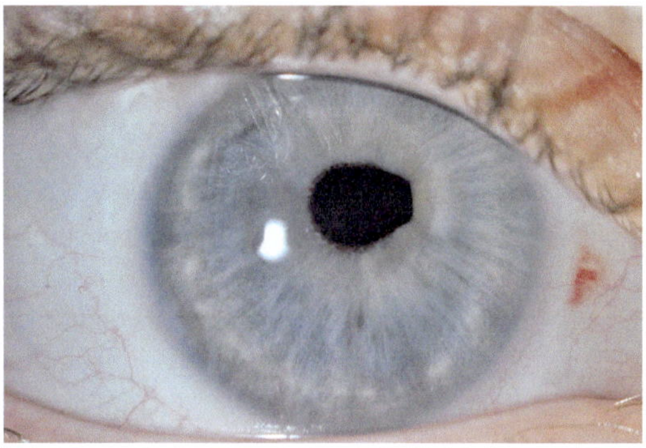

Fig. 17.4 Glaucoma drainage device sited in the superior-temporal quadrant of the eye in a case of aphakic glaucoma

17.13.1 Success Rates

One series reported a success rate of 90 % at 1 year with the use of GDDs in cases of glaucoma arising following cataract surgery, although at 10 years success dropped to 55 % [62]. Reported qualified success rates with Ahmed valve implantation in aphakic cases has been reported as high as 68 % [63] and low intraocular pressure levels may be achieved [64]. In a series of mixed pseudophakic and aphakic cases an 11 year success rate of 85 % has been reported with the Molteno tube implant [65]. When drainage implantation alone does not achieve adequate IOP control, supplementation with topical medical therapy is appropriate, although in some cases a second GDD may be warranted.

17.13.2 Complications

Although GDD surgery offers benefits over other procedures they also carry the risk of significant complications, in particular that of hypotony or from the tube itself [59, 60, 65–71].

Hypotony is a serious sight threatening complication which may be associated with a shallow or flat anterior chamber, maculopathy, choroidal effusion, serous retinal detachment, and suprachoroidal haemorrhage. If left untreated it may lead to further complications of aqueous misdirection or ultimately to phthisis. Buphthalmic eyes with low scleral rigidity are particularly at risk [62, 72–74]. The use of a per-operative anterior chamber infusion assists in maintaining a consistent IOP throughout the procedure, and the use of a 25 or 27 G needle to fashion a long tunnel for the tube ensures a snug fit reducing postoperative leakage around the tube [60]. Additional surgical techniques have evolved to mitigate the risk of hypotony in non-valved devices: Devices may be implanted as a two stage procedure [75], or with the use of an absorbable extra-luminal tie [76] with or without an additional intraluminal stent [77]. Valved devices have a variable risk of hypotony depending on other patient factors.

Tube-related complications include:

- Erosion through the conjunctiva – This is a significant risk which may lead to infection and endophthalmitis ultimately resulting in the need to remove the drainage device. The risk of erosion may be minimized by making a very long scleral tunnel for the tube starting several millimeters posterior to the limbus, or covering the tube with a patch e.g. donor sclera, corneal or pericardium or autografts such as fascia lata, or temporalis fascia [60].
- Occlusion of the tube tip by capsular remnants, fibrin, or vitreous etc. Care should be taken to site the tube away from the iris and capsule and careful vitrectomy should be performed for eyes rendered aphakic, particularly if the tube is being sited through the pars plana. Aggressive management of post-operative inflammation avoids occlusion of the tube with fibrin and inflammatory debris.
- 'Tube touch complications' may be as a consequence of poor placement of the tube or as a result of migration of the tube occurring either because the plate has not been secured properly at the time of surgery, or due to changes in the dimensions of the eye with reduction in IOP. Corneal touch and endothelial damage can be avoided by siting the tube just anterior to the iris plane or using a pars plana insertion. Iris touch with chaffing, persistent uveitis and corectopia can be avoided by ensuring the insertion of the tube is not too close to the iris root.
- Tube migration – Securing the plate with non-absorbable sutures helps to ensure the plate does not migrate towards the limbus as healing and encapsulation occurs, however changes in globe size associated with changes in IOP may result in migration of the intra-ocular portion of the tube.
- Regardless of where the tube is sited the intra-ocular portion should be long enough to visualize the tip of the tube. This assists in assessing for occlusion by iris, vitreous or capsular remnants, and provides a 'margin of error' for tube movement.
- Ocular motility disturbances may arise following drainage device implantation, particularly when recti muscles have been isolated for placement of the device plate.

Post-operative management: frequent topical steroid and antibiotic are used. In addition, some surgeons use cycloplegia to maintain a deep anterior chamber and systemic anti-inflammatory drugs or immunosuppressants to reduce inflammation particularly of the sclera and episcleral tissues.

17.14 Visual Prognosis

Early detection of glaucoma and successful control of raised intraocular pressure is key to preventing permanent visual loss in children undergoing cataract surgery. However, poor visual outcome for these children may also be as a result of amblyopia. Whilst the cataract itself may have resulted in visual deprivation amblyopia, raised intraocular pressure and the resulting corneal oedema may contribute further. Eyes undergoing cataract surgery require refractive correction to optimise the visual outcome, however changes in intraocular pressure may also result in significant changes in refractive error due to changes in corneal curvature and axial length. These changes may occur rapidly and reversibly with the onset and subsequent treatment of raised intraocular pressure, and refraction therefore needs to be tested frequently and correction provided as necessary, particularly when any deterioration in visual acuity is noted.

Ocular motility disturbances and strabismus impeding binocularity also arise in children undergoing cataract surgery, but this is also a potential complication when glaucoma is treated with drainage implants.

Whilst detection and adequate management of glaucoma is of utmost importance, attention still needs to be given to the assessment of refractive errors, amblyopia and strabismus, management of which should be maintained as far as possible throughout any glaucoma treatment schedule to maximize visual outcome.

References

1. Beck A, Chen T, Freedman S. Definition, Classification, Differential Diagnosis. In: Weinreb R, Grajewski A, Papadopoulos A, Grigg J, Freedman S, editors. Childhood Glaucoma: World Glaucoma Association, Consensus Series - 9. Amersterdam, The Netherlands: Kugler Pubications; 2013. Ch 1 p. 3.
2. Beck AD, Freedman SF, Lynn MJ, Bothun E, Neely DE, Lambert SR, et al. Glaucoma-related adverse events in the Infant Aphakia Treatment Study: 1-year results. Arch Ophthalmol. 2012;130(3):300–5.
3. Freedman SF, Lynn MJ, Beck AD, Bothun ED, Orge FH, Lambert SR, et al. Glaucoma-related adverse events in the first 5 years after unilateral cataract removal in the Infant Aphakia Treatment Study. JAMA Ophthalmol. 2015;133(8):907–14.
4. Trivedi RH, Wilson Jr ME, Golub RL. Incidence and risk factors for glaucoma after pediatric cataract surgery with and without intraocular lens implantation. J AAPOS. 2006;10(2):117–23.
5. Wong IB, Sukthankar VD, Cortina-Borja M, Nischal KK. Incidence of early-onset glaucoma after infant cataract extraction with and without intraocular lens implantation. Br J Ophthalmol. 2009;93(9):1200–3.
6. Urban B, Bakunowicz-Lazarczyk A. Aphakic glaucoma after congenital cataract surgery with and without intraocular lens implantation. Klin Oczna. 2010;112(4–6):105–7.
7. Beck A, Chen T, Freedman S. Definition, Classification, Differential Diagnosis. In: Weinreb R, Grajewski A, Papadopoulos A, Grigg J, Freedman S, editors. Childhood Glaucoma: World Glaucoma Association, Consensus Series - 9. Amersterdam, The Netherlands: Kugler Pubications; 2013. Ch 1 p. 5–6.
8. Chak M, Rahi JS, British Congenital Cataract Interest Group. Incidence of and factors associated with glaucoma after surgery for congenital cataract: findings from the British Congenital Cataract Study. Ophthalmology. 2008;115(6):1013–8.e2.
9. Ruddle JB, Staffieri SE, Crowston JG, Sherwin JC, Mackey DA. Incidence and predictors of glaucoma following surgery for congenital cataract in the first year of life in Victoria, Australia. Clin Experiment Ophthalmol. 2013;41(7):653–61.
10. Rabiah PK. Frequency and predictors of glaucoma after pediatric cataract surgery. Am J Ophthalmol. 2004;137(1):30–7.
11. Simon JW, Mehta N, Simmons ST, Catalano RA, Lininger LL. Glaucoma after pediatric lensectomy/vitrectomy. Ophthalmology. 1991;98(5):670–4.
12. Swamy BN, Billson F, Martin F, Donaldson C, Hing S, Jamieson R, et al. Secondary glaucoma after paediatric cataract surgery. Br J Ophthalmol. 2007;91(12):1627–30.
13. Walton DS. Pediatric aphakic glaucoma: a study of 65 patients. Trans Am Ophthalmol Soc. 1995;93:403–13; discussion 13–20.
14. Levin AV. Aphakic glaucoma: a never-ending story? Br J Ophthalmol. 2007;91(12):1574–5.
15. Michael I, Shmoish M, Walton DS, Levenberg S. Interactions between trabecular meshwork cells and lens epithelial cells: a possible mechanism in infantile aphakic glaucoma. Invest Ophthalmol Vis Sci. 2008;49(9):3981–7.
16. Lam D, Fan D, Ng J, Yu C, Wong C, Cheung A. Ocular hypertensive and anti-inflammatory responses to different dosages of topical dexamethasone in children: a randomized trial. Clin Experiment Ophthalmol. 2005; 33:252–8.
17. Jones RI, Rhee D. Corticosteroid-induced ocular hypertension and glaucoma: a brief review and update of the literature. Curr Opin Ophthalmol. 2006; 17(2):163–7.
18. Chen TC, Walton DS, Bhatia LS. Aphakic glaucoma after congenital cataract surgery. Arch Ophthalmol. 2004;122(12):1819–25.
19. Vishwanath M, Cheong-Leen R, Taylor D, Russell-Eggitt I, Rahi J. Is early surgery for congenital cataract a risk factor for glaucoma? Br J Ophthalmol. 2004;88(7):905–10.
20. Lambert SR, Lynn M, Drews-Botsch C, Loupe D, Plager DA, Medow NB, et al. A comparison of grating visual acuity, strabismus, and reoperation outcomes among children with aphakia and pseudophakia after unilateral cataract surgery during the first six months of life. J AAPOS. 2001;5(2):70–5.
21. Haargaard B, Ritz C, Oudin A, Wohlfahrt J, Thygesen J, Olsen T, et al. Risk of glaucoma after pediatric cataract surgery. Invest Ophthalmol Vis Sci. 2008;49(5):1791–6.
22. Koc F, Kargi S, Biglan AW, Chu CT, Davis JS. The aetiology in paediatric aphakic glaucoma. Eye (Lond). 2006;20(12):1360–5.

23. Wallace DK, Plager DA. Corneal diameter in childhood aphakic glaucoma. J Pediatr Ophthalmol Strabismus. 1996;33(5):230–4.
24. Johnson CP, Keech RV. Prevalence of glaucoma after surgery for PHPV and infantile cataracts. J Pediatr Ophthalmol Strabismus. 1996;33(1):14–7.
25. Ahmadieh H, Javadi MA. Intra-ocular lens implantation in children. Curr Opin Ophthalmol. 2001;12(1):30–4.
26. Mataftsi A, Haidich A-B, Kokkali S, Rabiah PK, Birch E, Stager Jr DR, et al. Postoperative glaucoma following infantile cataract surgery an individual patient data meta-analysis. JAMA Ophthalmol. 2014; 132(9):1059–67.
27. Vasavada VA, Praveen MR, Shah SK, Trivedi RH, Vasavada AR. Anti-inflammatory effect of low-molecular-weight heparin in pediatric cataract surgery: a randomized clinical trial. Am J Ophthalmol. 2012;154(2):252–8.e4.
28. Dada T, Dada VK, Sharma N, Vajpayee RB. Primary posterior capsulorhexis with optic capture and intracameral heparin in paediatric cataract surgery. Clin Experiment Ophthalmol. 2000;28(5):361–3.
29. Fenerty C, Freeman N, Grigg J. Glaucoma Following Cataract Surgery. In: Weinreb R, Grajewski A, Papadopoulos M, Grigg J, Freedman S, editors. Childhood Glaucoma World Glaucoma Association Consensus Series -9. Amsterdam: Kugler; 2013. Ch 10 p. 233-7.
30. Flemmons MS, Hsiao YC, Dzau J, Asrani S, Jones S, Freedman SF. Icare rebound tonometry in children with known and suspected glaucoma. J AAPOS. 2011;15(2):153–7.
31. Dahlmann-Noor AH, Puertas R, Tabasa-Lim S, El-Karmouty A, Kadhim M, Wride NK, et al. Comparison of handheld rebound tonometry with Goldmann applanation tonometry in children with glaucoma: a cohort study. BMJ open. 2013;3(4):1–6.
32. Poostchi A, Mitchell R, Nicholas S, Purdie G, Wells A. The iCare rebound tonometer: comparisons with Goldmann tonometry, and influence of central corneal thickness. Clin Experiment Ophthalmol. 2009;37(7):687–91.
33. Martinez-de-la-Casa JM, Garcia-Feijoo J, Saenz-Frances F, Vizzeri G, Fernandez-Vidal A, Mendez-Hernandez C, et al. Comparison of rebound tonometer and Goldmann handheld applanation tonometer in congenital glaucoma. J Glaucoma. 2009;18(1):49–52.
34. Lambert SR, Melia M, Buffenn AN, Chiang MF, Simpson JL, Yang MB. Rebound tonometry in children: a report by the American Academy of Ophthalmology. Ophthalmology. 2013;120(4):e21–7.
35. Radtke ND, Cohan BE. Intraocular pressure measurement in the newborn. Am J Ophthalmol. 1974; 78(3):501–4.
36. Sihota R, Tuli D, Dada T, Gupta V, Sachdeva MM. Distribution and determinants of intraocular pressure in a normal pediatric population. J Pediatr Ophthalmol Strabismus. 2006;43(1):14–8.
37. Levy J, Lifshitz T, Rosen S, Tessler Z, Biedner BZ. Is the tono-pen accurate for measuring intraocular pressure in young children with congenital glaucoma? J AAPOS. 2005;9(4):321–5.
38. Garcia-Resua C, Gonzalez-Meijome JM, Gilino J, Yebra-Pimentel E. Accuracy of the new ICare rebound tonometer vs. other portable tonometers in healthy eyes. Optom Vis Sci. 2006;83(2):102–7.
39. Bradfield YS, Kaminski BM, Repka MX, Melia M; Pediatric Eye Disease Investigator Group; Davitt BV, et al. Comparison of Tono-Pen and Goldmann applanation tonometers for measurement of intraocular pressure in healthy children. J AAPOS. 2012; 16(3):242–8.
40. Eisenberg DL, Sherman BG, McKeown CA, Schuman JS. Tonometry in adults and children. A manometric evaluation of pneumatonometry, applanation, and TonoPen in vitro and in vivo. Ophthalmology. 1998;105(7):1173–81.
41. Sampaolesi R. Corneal diameter and axial length in congenital glaucoma. Can J Ophthalmol. 1988;23(1):42–4.
42. Simon JW, O'Malley MR, Gandham SB, Ghaiy R, Zobal-Ratner J, Simmons ST. Central corneal thickness and glaucoma in aphakic and pseudophakic children. J AAPOS. 2005;9(4):326–9.
43. Simsek T, Mutluay AH, Elgin U, Gursel R, Batman A. Glaucoma and increased central corneal thickness in aphakic and pseudophakic patients after congenital cataract surgery. Br J Ophthalmol. 2006;90(9):1103–6.
44. Tai TY, Mills MD, Beck AD, Joos KM, Ying GS, Liu C, et al. Central corneal thickness and corneal diameter in patients with childhood glaucoma. J Glaucoma. 2006;15(6):524–8.
45. Lim Z, Muir KW, Duncan L, Freedman SF. Acquired central corneal thickness increase following removal of childhood cataracts. Am J Ophthalmol. 2011; 151(3):434–41.e1.
46. Resende GM, Lupinacci AP, Arieta CE, Costa VP. Central corneal thickness and intraocular pressure in children undergoing congenital cataract surgery: a prospective, longitudinal study. Br J Ophthalmol. 2012;96(9):1190–4.
47. Ventura MC, Ventura BV, Ventura CV, Ventura LO, Nose W. Congenital cataract surgery with intracameral triamcinolone: pre- and postoperative central corneal thickness and intraocular pressure. J AAPOS. 2012;16(5):441–4.
48. Filous A, Osmera J, Hlozanek M, Mahelkova G. Central corneal thickness in microphthalmic eyes with or without history of congenital cataract surgery. Eur J Ophthalmol. 2011;21(4):374–8.
49. Smith RJ. A new method of estimating the depth of the anterior chamber. Br J Ophthalmol. 1979;63(4):215–20.
50. Sampaolesi R, Caruso R. Ocular echometry in the diagnosis of congenital glaucoma. Arch Ophthalmol. 1982;100(4):574–7.
51. Law SK, Bui D, Caprioli J. Serial axial length measurements in congenital glaucoma. Am J Ophthalmol. 2001;132(6):926–8.

52. Kappelhof JP, Vrensen GFJM, de Jong PTVM, Pameyer J, Willekens BLJC. The ring of Soemmerring in man: an ultrastructural study. Graefes Arch Clin Exp Ophthalmol. 1987;225(1):77–83.
53. Kirwan JF, Shah P, Khaw PT. Diode laser cyclophotocoagulation: role in the management of refractory pediatric glaucomas. Ophthalmology. 2002;109(2): 316–23.
54. Neely DE, Plager DA. Endocyclophotocoagulation for management of difficult pediatric glaucomas. J AAPOS. 2001;5(4):221–9.
55. Bothun ED, Guo Y, Christiansen SP, Summers CG, Anderson JS, Wright MM, et al. Outcome of angle surgery in children with aphakic glaucoma. J AAPOS. 2010;14(3):235–9.
56. Azuara-Blanco A, Wilson RP, Spaeth GL, Schmidt CM, Augsburger JJ. Filtration procedures supplemented with mitomycin C in the management of childhood glaucoma. Br J Ophthalmol. 1999;83(2):151–6.
57. Beck AD, Wilson WR, Lynch MG, Lynn MJ, Noe R. Trabeculectomy with adjunctive mitomycin C in pediatric glaucoma. Am J Ophthalmol. 1998;126(5):648–57.
58. Mandal AK, Bagga H, Nutheti R, Gothwal VK, Nanda AK. Trabeculectomy with or without mitomycin-C for paediatric glaucoma in aphakia and pseudophakia following congenital cataract surgery. Eye (Lond). 2003;17(1):53–62.
59. Beck AD, Freedman S, Kammer J, Jin J. Aqueous shunt devices compared with trabeculectomy with mitomycin-C for children in the first two years of life. Am J Ophthalmol. 2003;136(6):994–1000.
60. Papadopoulos M, Edmunds B, Chiang M, Mandal A, Grajewski A, Khaw PT. Glaucoma surgery in children. In: Weinreb RN, Grajewski AL, Papadopoulos M, Grigg J, Freedman S, editors. Childhood glaucoma. World Glaucoma Association consensus series – 9. Amsterdam: Kugler Publications; 2013. p. 118.
61. Pakravan M, Homayoon N, Shahin Y, Ali Reza BR. Trabeculectomy with mitomycin C versus Ahmed glaucoma implant with mitomycin C for treatment of pediatric aphakic glaucoma. J Glaucoma. 2007;16(7):631–6.
62. O'Malley Schotthoefer E, Yanovitch TL, Freedman SF. Aqueous drainage device surgery in refractory pediatric glaucomas: I. Long-term outcomes. J AAPOS. 2008;12(1):33–9.
63. Kirwan C, O'Keefe M, Lanigan B, Mahmood U. Ahmed valve drainage implant surgery in the management of paediatric aphakic glaucoma. Br J Ophthalmol. 2005;89(7):855–8.
64. Chen TC, Bhatia LS, Walton DS. Ahmed valve surgery for refractory pediatric glaucoma: a report of 52 eyes. J Pediatr Ophthalmol Strabismus. 2005;42(5):274–83; quiz 304–5.
65. Cunliffe IA, Molteno AC. Long-term follow-up of Molteno drains used in the treatment of glaucoma presenting in childhood. Eye (Lond). 1998;12(Pt 3a): 379–85.
66. Fellenbaum PS, Sidoti PA, Heuer DK, Minckler DS, Baerveldt G, Lee PP. Experience with the baerveldt implant in young patients with complicated glaucomas. J Glaucoma. 1995;4(2):91–7.
67. Al-Mobarak F, Khan AO. Two-year survival of Ahmed valve implantation in the first 2 years of life with and without intraoperative mitomycin-C. Ophthalmology. 2009;116(10):1862–5.
68. Hill RA, Heuer DK, Baerveldt G, Minckler DS, Martone JF. Molteno implantation for glaucoma in young patients. Ophthalmology. 1991;98(7):1042–6.
69. Eid TE, Katz LJ, Spaeth GL, Augsburger JJ. Long-term effects of tube-shunt procedures on management of refractory childhood glaucoma. Ophthalmology. 1997;104(6):1011–6.
70. Djodeyre MR, Peralta Calvo J, Abelairas GJ. Clinical evaluation and risk factors of time to failure of Ahmed Glaucoma Valve implant in pediatric patients. Ophthalmology. 2001;108(3):614–20.
71. Al-Torbak AA, Al-Shahwan S, Al-Jadaan I, Al-Hommadi A, Edward DP. Endophthalmitis associated with the Ahmed glaucoma valve implant. Br J Ophthalmol. 2005;89(4):454–8.
72. Coleman AL, Smyth RJ, Wilson MR, Tam M. Initial clinical experience with the Ahmed Glaucoma Valve implant in pediatric patients. Arch Ophthalmol. 1997;115(2):186–91.
73. Englert JA, Freedman SF, Cox TA. The Ahmed valve in refractory pediatric glaucoma. Am J Ophthalmol. 1999;127(1):34–42.
74. Morales J, Al Shahwan S, Al Odhayb S, Al Jadaan I, Edward DP. Current surgical options for the management of pediatric glaucoma. J Ophthalmol. 2013; 2013:763735.
75. Molteno AC, Ancker E, Van Biljon G. Surgical technique for advanced juvenile glaucoma. Arch Ophthalmol. 1984;102(1):51–7.
76. Molteno AC, Polkinghorne PJ, Bowbyes JA. The vicryl tie technique for inserting a draining implant in the treatment of secondary glaucoma. Aust N Z J Ophthalmol. 1986;14(4):343–54.
77. Sherwood MB, Smith MF. Prevention of early hypotony associated with Molteno implants by a new occluding stent technique. Ophthalmology. 1993; 100(1):85–90.

Part V

Outcomes

18 Visual Outcomes

Scott R. Lambert

18.1 Historical Background

In 1957 Costenbader and Albert [8] published an article entitled "Conservatism in the management of congenital cataract" in which they divided children with congenital cataracts into five groups: (Group 1) bilateral minimal involvement; (Group 2) unilateral cataract; (Group 3) bilateral moderate lamellar involvement; (Group 4) bilateral dense nuclear involvement with clear cortex; and (Group 5) bilateral extensive involvement. They recommended that cataract surgery be deferred until after the first year of life for children in all of these groups with the exception of children with bilateral total cataracts (Group 5). In fact, for children with unilateral cataracts (Group 2) they made the following recommendation:

> …we would unequivocally advise against surgery…unless the cataract is becoming hypermature. The appearance of the eye is usually not improved; function has not been helped, and the eye has been jeopardized if surgery is performed.

Much has changed since then in the management of congenial cataracts due to a better understanding of neurodevelopment, the widespread adoption of newborn red reflex screening, improved surgical techniques and the availability of high plus contact lenses with excellent oxygen permeability and foldable intraocular lenses (IOLs). Whereas congenital cataracts were once thought to consign a child to a life of visual impairment, cataracts are now considered to be one of the most avoidable causes of childhood visual impairment [19]. In fact, cataract surgery is now considered to be the treatment of choice for all children with visually significant cataracts (e.g. all but Group 1 in Costenbader's classification).

18.2 Factors Affecting Visual Outcome

18.2.1 Age at Surgery

Congenital cataracts differ from cataracts in older children and adults because they interfere with the development of central visual pathways. Therefore, early surgery is essential to achieve a good visual outcome. Both basic science research and clinical studies have helped us to understand the critical relationship between the age of congenital cataract surgery and the visual outcome.

18.2.1.1 Latent and Critical Periods

Animal Models

In the 1960s Hubel and Wiesel [16] introduced the concept of a "latent period" and a "critical period" for the development of central visual

S.R. Lambert, MD
Department of Ophthalmology, Stanford University School of Medicine, Stanford, CA, USA
e-mail: slamber@emory.edu

I.C. Lloyd, S.R. Lambert (eds.), *Congenital Cataract*, DOI 10.1007/978-3-319-27848-3_18

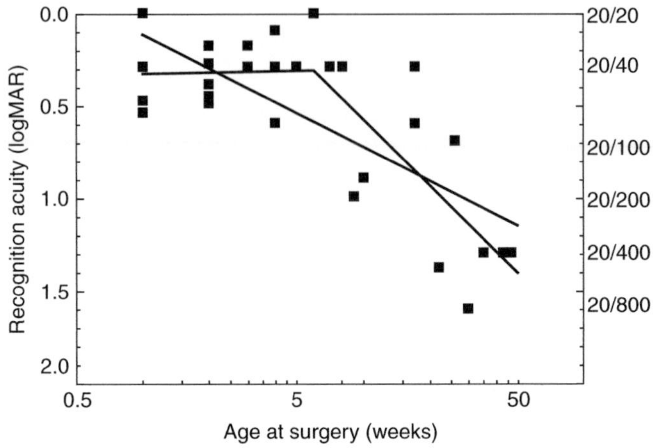

Fig. 18.1 Recognition acuity versus age at surgery for children treated for a dense unilateral congenital cataract showing a better fit with a bilinear than a linear model (Used with permission from Birch and Stager [6])

pathways. In kittens, they noted that the latent period extended from birth to age 4 weeks during which time unilateral eyelid suturing had no long-term effect on visual acuity in the deprived eye. However, after the latent period until age 3 months, there was a critical period during which visual deprivation resulted in irreversible vision loss in the deprived eye that was associated with a reduction in the size of the neurons in the lateral geniculate nucleus subserving the deprived eye. Furthermore, they noted that bilateral visual deprivation during the critical period resulted in a reduction in binocularly driven neurons in the visual cortex [37]. Latent and critical periods are species specific and they differ for unilateral and bilateral visual deprivation [9]. In humans, the latent period has been reported to extend to at least 6 weeks of age for unilateral visual deprivation [11]. While there is less consensus regarding the latent period for bilateral visual deprivation, it may extend to 8–10 weeks of age. It is generally accepted that the critical period extends to age 7 years [6]. As a result, visual outcomes in children with congenital cataracts vary widely depending on the age that cataract surgery is performed.

Unilateral Cataract Surgery

The optimal age for cataract surgery in a child with a unilateral congenital cataract is generally believed to be between 4 and 6 weeks of age. Birch and Stager [6] evaluated the relationship between the age at cataract surgery and the visual outcomes for 45 children who were diagnosed with dense unilateral congenital cataracts as newborns. Only children with good to excellent compliance with contact lens, spectacle and occlusion therapy were included in the study. The model that best fit their data was a bilinear model (Fig. 18.1). They found no relationship between age and the visual outcome for infants undergoing cataract surgery ≤6 weeks of age. However, after age 6 weeks, there was a linear decline in visual outcomes related to the age at cataract surgery. Their model suggests that there is a latent period until age 6 weeks for children with a dense unilateral cataract. More recently, Hartmann and coworkers [13] evaluated the relationship between age at surgery and the visual outcome among children enrolled in the Infant Aphakia Treatment Study [20]. They found that age at cataract surgery was only weakly associated with visual acuity (Fig. 18.2). While median visual acuity was better among patients who had cataract surgery between ages 4 and 6 weeks, the association between age at cataract surgery and the visual outcome was less robust than the data reported by Birch and Stager [6]. These studies differ in that Hartmann and coworkers analyzed the visual outcome for all of the children enrolled in the Infant Aphakia Treatment Study whereas Birch and coworkers only analyzed the visual outcome for children who were compliant with optical and occlusion therapy. In addition, Birch and coworkers only analyzed data from patients who were confirmed to have a dense unilateral cataract as a newborn whereas Hartmann did not include this as an inclusion criterion.

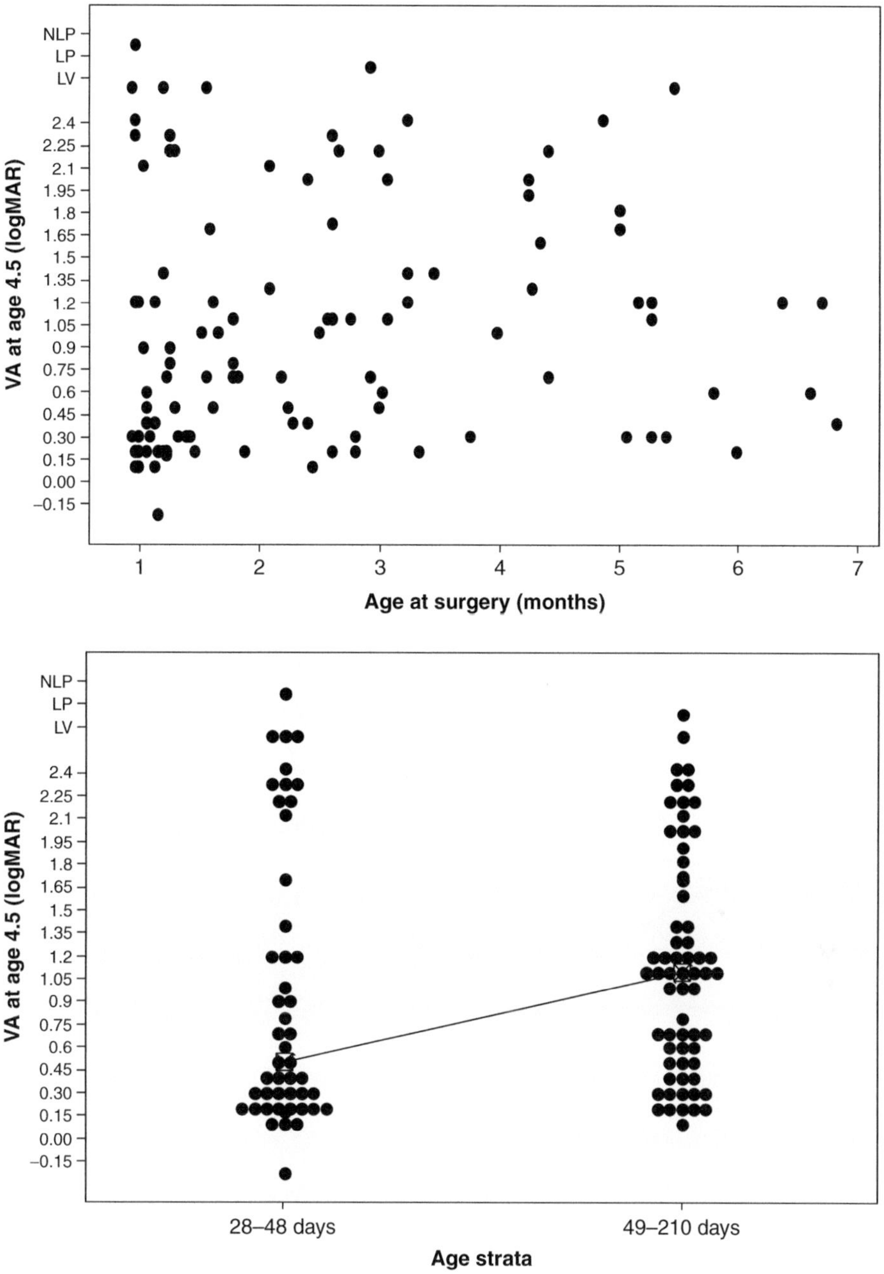

Fig. 18.2 Visual outcome data for 112 children treated for a dense unilateral congenital cataract in the Infant Aphakia Treatment Study: (**a**) Scatterplot of recognition visual acuity at 4.5 years of age versus age at cataract surgery; (**b**) Plot comparing recognition visual acuity at 4.5 years of age versus age at cataract surgery (Used with permission from Hartmann et al. [13])

Bilateral Cataract Surgery

It is generally believed that bilateral congenital cataracts should be removed by 8 weeks of age to achieve the best visual outcomes. Lambert and coworkers [22] evaluated the long-term visual outcomes for 43 children with dense bilateral congenital cataracts and found a linear relationship between the age of cataract surgery and the

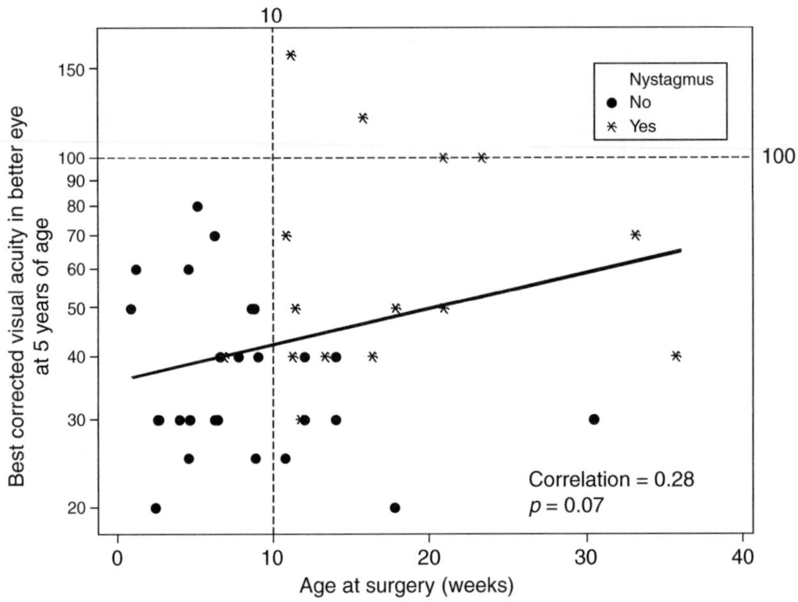

Fig. 18.3 Best corrected visual acuity (BCVA) at 5 years of age in the better seeing eye versus age at surgery for 43 children treated for dense bilateral congenital cataracts. Symbols indicate the status of nystagmus at the initial exam. *Dotted lines* indicate BCVA of 20/80 and age of 10 weeks (Used with permission from Lambert et al. [22])

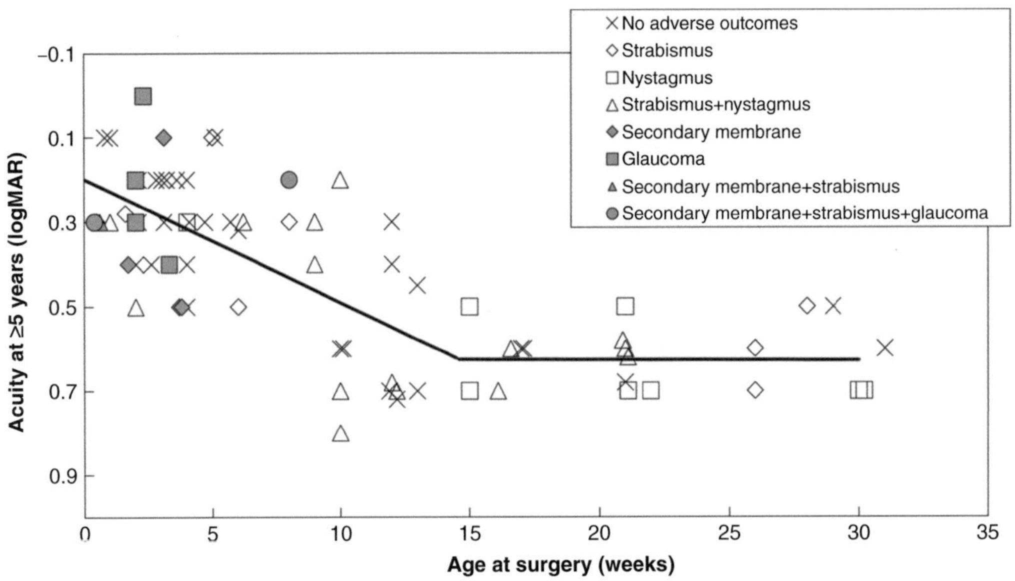

Fig. 18.4 Long-term visual outcome data for 37 children treated for dense bilateral congenital cataracts along with the best-fit linear model of the critical period (Used with permission from Birch et al. *JAAPOS*. 2009;13:67–71)

visual acuity in the better seeing eye (correlation coefficient=0.28) (Fig. 18.3). They noted that delaying cataract surgery to 10 week of age or later increased the likely of a poor visual outcome (20/100 or worse). In contrast, Birch and coworkers [4] reported a bilinear relationship between the age of surgery and the visual outcome in 37 infants with dense bilateral congenital cataracts. Between birth and 14 weeks of age they noted a progressively worse visual outcome the older a child was at the time of cataract surgery (visual acuity decreased by 1 line with each 3 week delay in surgery). However, after age 14 weeks until 31 weeks, the visual outcome was independent of age at the time of cataract surgery (Fig. 18.4). These two studies suggest that unlike

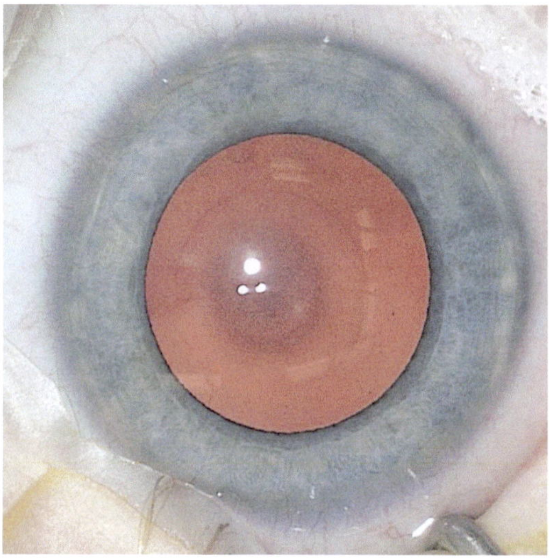

Fig. 18.5 Lamellar cataract in a 2-year-old child

children with unilateral congenital cataracts, children with dense bilateral congenital cataracts do not have a well-defined latent period. However, other considerations such as the increased risk of glaucoma associated with very early cataract surgery and comorbidities should dictate the timing of cataract surgery.

18.2.2 Cataract Morphology

The type of cataract has been reported to be a predictor of the visual outcome [34]. However, confounding variables make it difficult to ascertain the relative contribution of the type of cataract on the visual outcome. Certainly the density of lens opacities and the age of onset are important considerations. For example, eyes with partial cataracts that are acquired after birth (e.g. posterior lentiglobus and lamellar cataracts) are usually associated with better visual outcomes (Fig. 18.5) than cataracts associated with dense congenital opacities such as nuclear cataracts (Fig. 18.6) [30]. Cataracts arising from persistent fetal vasculature (PFV) have been reported to have a worse visual prognosis, but eyes with PFV vary greatly in their severity and some subtypes may be associated with good visual outcomes [31]. While personal photographs may allow the age of

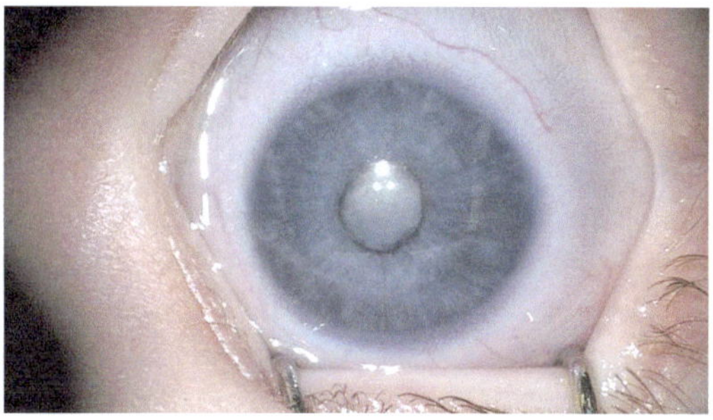

Fig. 18.6 Dense nuclear cataract in a newborn

onset of cataracts to be ascertained in some instances [35], it is still difficult to ascertain the rate that cataracts progress using photographs alone.

18.2.3 Amblyopia Therapy

Occlusion therapy is critical for the successful visual rehabilitation of children with a unilateral congenital cataract after cataract surgery. Selected children with bilateral congenital cataracts also require occlusion therapy after cataract surgery. Little is known about the best patching regimen to optimize visual acuity and binocular vision following unilateral congenital cataract surgery. Lambert and coworkers [23] reviewed the medical records of 9 children who underwent unilateral congenital cataract surgery when 6 weeks of age or younger. All of these children were compliant with patching therapy until 12 months of age and optical correction until 6 years of age. At age 12 months, the fellow eyes were patched a mean of 6.7 h/day. However, by 6 years of age, patching had declined to a mean of 1.7 h/day. Furthermore, 4 of the 9 children abandoned patching therapy entirely between the ages of 3 and 6 years. Nevertheless, visual acuity only worsened in one child after the cessation of patching therapy suggesting that visual acuity was not adversely affected by early termination of patching therapy provided the correct optical correction was being worn by the child.

Patching regimens for children with unilateral aphakia, unlike patching regimens for children with anisometropic and strabismic amblyopia

[15, 25, 36], are not evidence based. However in recent years, there has been a trend to reduce the number of hours that patients are patched each day to potentiate the development of binocular vision in these children [18, 21]. Patching a child for longer than 6 h each day probably does not improve the visual outcome and may contribute to the loss of binocularity and contribute to the development of strabismus. This is illustrated by two case studies from my clinical practice. Both of these children underwent unilateral congenital cataract surgery during early infancy and both achieved 20/20 visual acuity in their aphakic eyes. However, Patient 1 had the fellow eye patched nearly full-time for 2 ½ years and now has no stereopsis and has required two strabismus surgeries to achieve satisfactory ocular alignment. In contrast, the fellow eye of Patient 2 was never patched for more than 6 h a day and patching was tapered beginning at age 14 months. These cases illustrate that good visual outcomes can be achieved with part-time patching. In addition, part-time patching may facilitate the development of binocular vision. Based on the excellent visual and stereopsis outcome achieved with the patching regimen for Patient 2, I now advise parents to only patch their child's fellow eye for one-half of their waking hours until age 14 months. I then advise them to gradually reduce the frequency of patching until age 7 years when I recommend patching therapy be discontinued.

Patient 1

A child with a dense nuclear cataract in his left eye underwent a lensectomy at age 3 weeks. Immediately after cataract surgery, he was treated with an extended wear contact lens and patching therapy of his fellow eye for one-half of his waking hours. At age 8 months, his patching therapy was increased to 9 ½ h/day and then increased to 11 h/day at age 18 months. This patching regimen was then maintained for the next 2 ½ years. At age 4 years, his patching therapy was gradually tapered (age 4 years: 10 h/3 days a week; 4 ½ years: 6–7 h/day; 5 years: 4 h/3 days; and 6 years: 4 h/2 days a week) and then discontinued at age 7 ½ years. At age 10 months he underwent a left medial rectus recession to correct an esotropia.

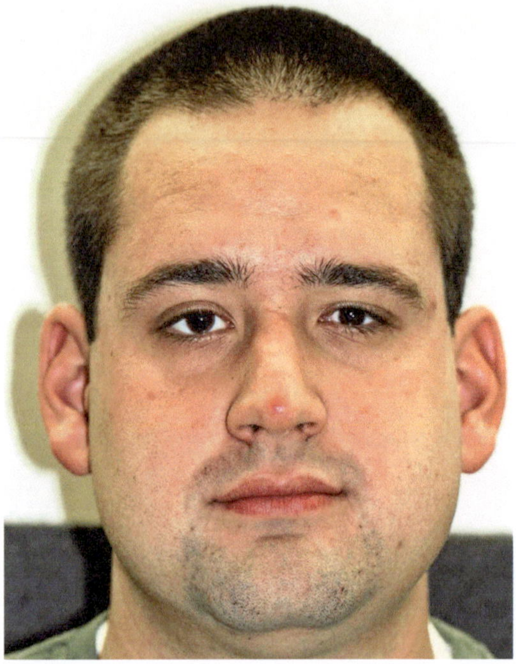

Fig. 18.7 A dense cataract was diagnosed in the left eye of this patient as a newborn. At age 3 weeks, a lensectomy was performed and he wore an aphakic contact lens until age 21 years when an intraocular lens was implanted in the sulcus. He received nearly full-time patching therapy of his right eye until age 4 years. He is now 30 years old and has visual acuity of 20/15 in his right eye and 20/20 in his left eye. He has undergone two strabismus surgeries and continues to have a dissociated vertical deviation and a small angle exotropia. He has no stereopsis

At age 17 years, his left medial rectus muscle was advanced to correct a consecutive exotropia. At age 21 years, an intraocular lens was implanted in the left eye. At age 30 years (Fig. 18.7), his best corrected visual acuity was 20/15 in the right eye and 20/20-2 in his left eye. He reports using his left eye for reading at night since he only has low myopia in this eye, but high myopia in his right eye. He has never had measurable stereopsis and his exotropia has recurred.

Patient 2

A child with a dense nuclear cataract in her left eye underwent a lensectomy at age 6 weeks. One week after cataract surgery, she started wearing an extended wear contact lens on her aphakic eye and began patching her fellow eye 1 h/day. Patching was gradually increased by 1 h/day/month of life

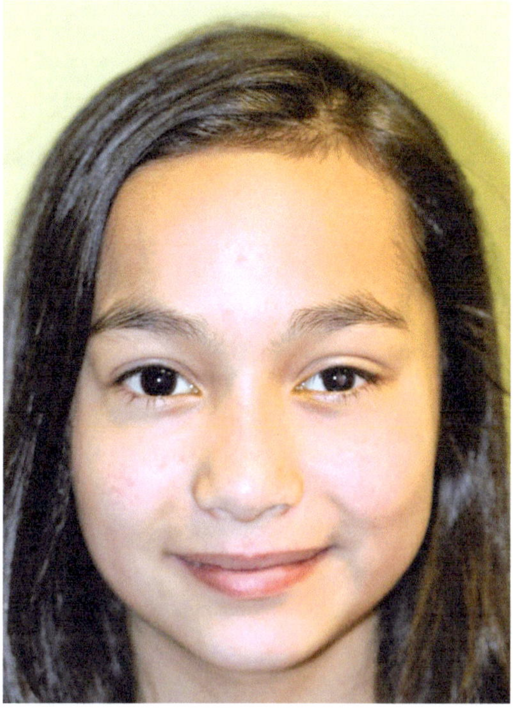

Fig. 18.8 Twelve year old patient who was diagnosed with a dense cataract in the left eye as a newborn. At age 6 weeks, a lensectomy was performed on her left eye. Postoperatively, her left eye was corrected optically with a contact lens and she underwent part-time patching therapy of her right eye until age 7 years. She continues to wear an aphakic contact lens on her left eye. She is orthophoric and has 120 s/arc of stereopsis. Her best corrected visual acuity is 20/20 in both eyes

until she was being patched 6 h/day. Patching was maintained at this level until age 14 months, when patching was reduced to 5 h/day. Patching was then slowly tapered (age 2 ½ years: 3–4 h/day; 3 years: 2 h/day; 4 years: 4 h every other day; and 5 years: 4 h/day twice a week) and then discontinued at age 7 ½ years. At age 12 years (Fig. 18.8), her best corrected visual acuity was 20/20 in both eyes. She was orthophoric and had 120 s/arc of stereopsis using the Randot stereoacuity test.

18.2.4 Nystagmus

Nystagmus occurs commonly in children with bilateral congenital cataracts. If cataracts are left untreated, nystagmus usually develops between the ages of 10 and 12 weeks. Lambert and coworkers [22] reported that in children with bilateral congenital cataracts, preoperative nystagmus was a better predictor of a poor visual outcome than age at cataract surgery (Fig. 18.3). Only 38 % of children with preoperative nystagmus developed a best corrected visual acuity of 20/40 or better compared to 74 % of children with no preoperative nystagmus. Children with preoperative nystagmus underwent cataract surgery at a mean age of 18 weeks compared to 8 weeks for children undergoing cataract surgery without nystagmus. Young and coworkers [38] also found that nystagmus was a predictor of a worse visual outcome in children with bilateral congenital cataracts. However, they reported that most children developed nystagmus after cataract surgery, rather than before cataract surgery. While nystagmus can develop after cataract surgery, this is unusual. It is likely that the nystagmus was present preoperatively, but not documented since this was a retrospective chart review.

18.2.5 Type of Optical Correction

The type of optical correction worn probably does not affect the visual outcome in children with congenital cataracts provided the optical correction is worn on a consistent basis. However, compliance may be better with certain types of optical corrections than others. The Infant Aphakia Treatment Study found that children with a unilateral congenital cataract had similar visual outcomes at age 4 ½ years if an eye underwent primary IOL implantation or was left aphakic and corrected with a contact lens (Fig. 18.9) [17]. Birch and coworkers [3] also reported similar visual outcomes in children with dense unilateral cataracts after cataract extraction with or without IOL implantation when patients had good-to-excellent contact lens compliance. However, they reported worse visual outcomes in eyes left aphakic and treated with contact lenses when contact lens compliance was moderate-to-poor. Another case series reported similar visual outcomes in 15 children who underwent bilateral congenital cataract surgery coupled with primary IOL implantation

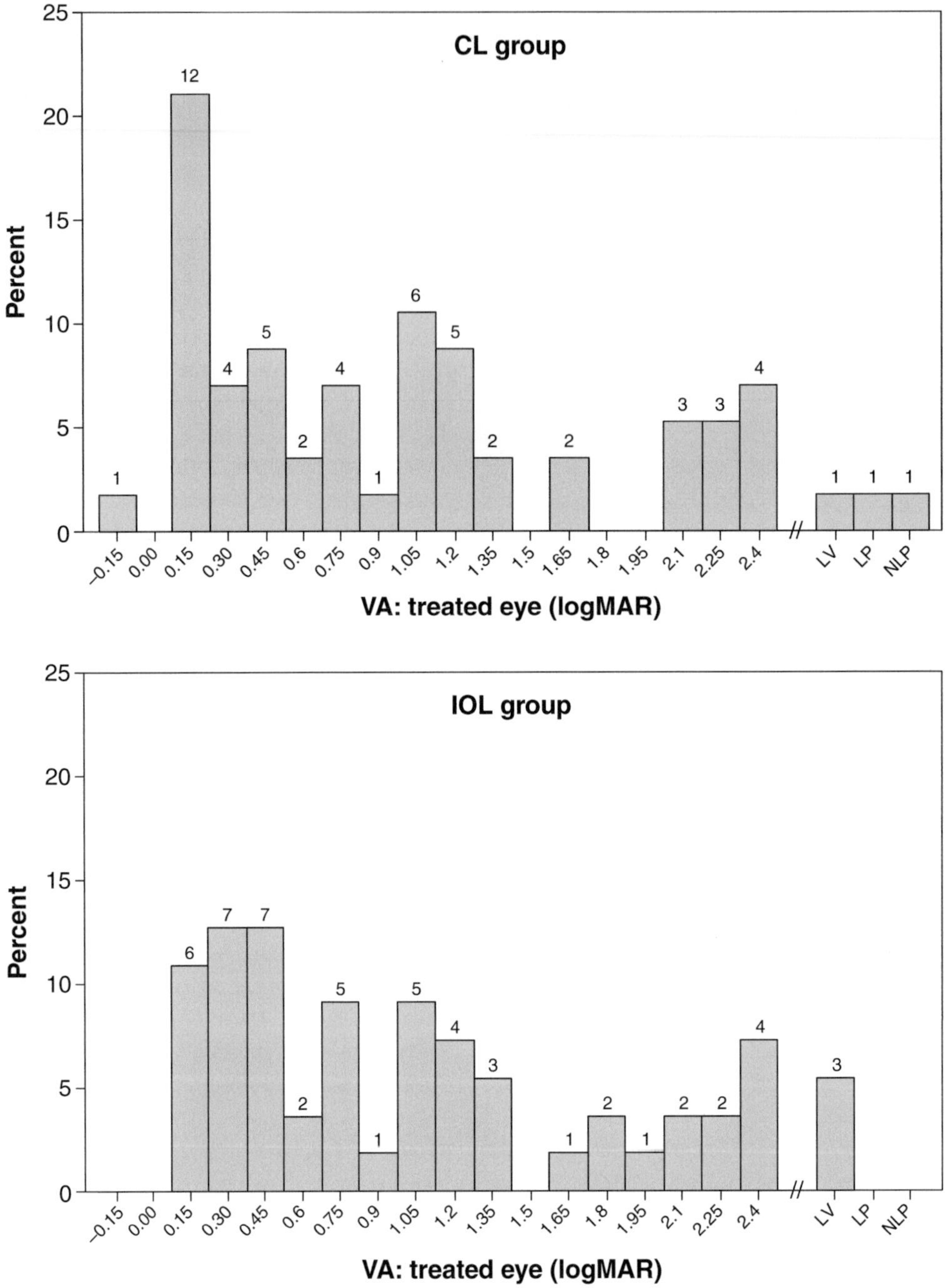

Fig. 18.9 Histogram of recognition visual acuity at age 4.5 years by treatment group (*CL* contact lens, *IOL* intraocular lens) for 112 children treated for a dense unilateral congenital cataract in the Infant Aphakia Treatment Study. The median visual acuities were 0.90 logMAR (20/159) for both groups. *LP* indicates light perception, *LV* low vision (Teller Acuity Card), *NLP* no light perception (Used with permission from The Infant Aphakia Treatment Study Group [17])

compared to 18 children who underwent bilateral lensectomies and were initially optically corrected with contact lenses and only later underwent secondary IOL implantation [28]. Therefore the type of optical correction does not appear to be a major factor in determining the visual outcome if

Table 18.1 Visual outcomes in children with bilateral congenital Cataracts

Country	# of patients	Mean age at surgery (months)	VA ≥20/30 (%)	VA 20/40-20/100 (%)	VA ≤ 20/200 (%)
Sweden [26]	13	1	31	61	8
USA [22]	43	3	28	72	0
India [12]	32	NA	NA[a]	41	59
Tanzania [7]	94	NA	NA[a]	62	13
Bangladesh [32]	408	87	13	29	58

[a]Visual acuity only recorded as 20/20-20/60. No data is given for the percent of patients with VA ≥20/30

there is good to excellent compliance with the optical correction.

18.2.6 Co-morbidities

18.2.6.1 Visual Outcomes

Bilateral Congenital Cataracts

Pattern of Visual Recovery

Maurer and coworkers [29] evaluated the pattern of visual recovery following unilateral and bilateral congenital cataract surgery in children treated with aphakic contact lenses. They noted on average a 0.40 octave improvement in monocular acuity in the treated eye 1 hour after contact lens correction and another 0.60 octave improvement 1 month later. The pattern of improvement was similar for unilateral and bilateral cataracts and was not related to age at the time of cataract surgery. They hypothesized that patterned visual input alone supports some visual improvement independent of any competitive interaction with the fellow eye.

Visual Acuity

In a recent multi-center series from the U.S.A., 28 % of children who underwent bilateral congenital cataract surgery at a mean age of 11.5 weeks were able to see 20/30 or better in their better seeing eye after long-term follow-up (Fig. 18.3) [22]. Furthermore, none of these children had a visual outcome worse than 20/100. Similar visual results have been reported in a series from Sweden (Table 18.1) [26]. In contrast a recent series from India reported that only 22 % of children with bilateral cataracts were able to see 20/60 or better in their better seeing eye after cataract surgery and 59 % had a visual outcome worse than 20/200 [12]. One of the likely causes for the worse visual outcomes in India was that cataract surgery was often delayed until later in childhood; only 18 of the 46 (38 %) children in the study underwent cataract surgery before 6 months of age. There was even a greater delay in cataract surgery in a series reported from Tanzania. Cataract surgery was performed at a mean age of nearly 4 years. However, since only 25 % of these children had preoperative nystagmus, it is likely that some of these children had acquired cataracts [7].

It is likely that a higher percentage of the patients from Bangladesh had congenital cataracts since 50 % of these patients were noted to have nystagmus postoperatively. The poor visual outcomes in the series likely reflects the mean 5+ year delay between the time cataracts were first noted by the parents until cataract surgery was performed [32]. Even though most of these children likely them had congenital cataracts, only 12 % of them underwent cataract surgery during the first year of life.

While immediate sequential bilateral cataract surgery has been hypothesized to reduce interocular differences in visual outcomes in children with congenital cataracts, there is no empirical data to support a better visual outcome using this surgical approach [10].

Visuospatial Deficits

Project Prakash evaluated the visual recovery of children in India after having congenital cataracts removed surgically at older ages. Ostrovsky and

Table 18.2 Visual outcomes in children with a unilateral congenital cataract

Country author/year	# of patients	Mean age at surgery (weeks)	VA ≥20/30 (%)	VA 20/40-20/100 (%)	VA ≤ 20/200 (%)
Sweden [27]	30	15	3	16	81
Czech Republic [2]	41	12	5	93	2[a]
England [1]	62	5	6	67	27
U.S.A. [17]	114	10	17	34	49

[a]Patients were only included in this series who were compliant with optical and patching therapy

coworkers [33] reported that these children had difficulty separating overlapping static images and identifying the correct spatial relationship of overlapping images. However, they were more successful in distinguishing objects in motion from the background. These children also had difficulty recognizing objects that they had previously handled by sight. However, after 1 week, their ability to integrate visual and tactile inputs improved [14]. LeGrand and coworkers [24] also noted long-term deficits in recognizing subtle differences in facial features in children who had undergone bilateral congenital cataract surgery independent of their visual acuity or the length of time they were visual deprived prior to cataract surgery.

18.2.6.2 Unilateral Congenital Cataracts

Visual Acuity

Less than 20 % of patients who undergo unilateral congenital cataract surgery have an excellent visual outcome in the treated eye (Table 18.2). While normal visual acuity can be achieved in these eyes, this requires early cataract surgery, and excellent compliance wearing the correct optical correction and patching therapy. The Infant Aphakia Treatment Study reported that nearly 50 % of the children enrolled in this randomized clinical trial had a poor visual outcome in their treated eye. While Autrata and coworkers [2] reported a poor visual outcome in only a small percentage of patients in their series, they excluded from their series children who were not compliant with optical correction and patching therapy.

Reading Performance

Birch and coworkers [5] found no difference in the monocular reading performance between treated and fellow eyes of children who had undergone unilateral congenital cataract who had excellent visual outcomes and age matched normal eyes. However, monocular reading performance was subnormal in treated eyes with reduced visual acuity.

Conclusions

About 30 % of children with bilateral congenital cataracts and about 20 % of children with a unilateral congenital cataract who are diagnosed and treated during infancy develop excellent visual acuity. However, about 50 % of patients with a unilateral congenital cataract versus ≤10 % of children with bilateral congenital cataracts have a poor visual outcome in high income countries. Visual outcomes are worse in low income countries because treatment is more commonly delayed. Earlier diagnosis and treatment and refinements in patching regimens should allow a higher percentage of children with unilateral congenital cataracts to develop excellent visual outcomes in the future.

References

1. Allen RJ, Speedwell L, Russell-Eggitt I. Long-term visual outcome after extraction of unilateral congenital cataracts. Eye (Lond). 2010;24(7):1263–7. doi:eye2009295 [pii]. 10.1038/eye.2009.295.
2. Autrata R, Rehurek J, Vodickova K. Visual results after primary intraocular lens implantation or contact lens correction for aphakia in the first year of age. Ophthalmologica. 2005;219(2):72–9. doi:OPH2005219002072 [pii]. 10.1159/000083264.
3. Birch EE, Cheng C, Stager Jr DR, Felius J. Visual acuity development after the implantation of unilateral intraocular lenses in infants and young children. J AAPOS.

2005;9(6):527–32. doi:S1091-8531(05)00228-4 [pii]. 10.1016/j.jaapos.2005.07.008.
4. Birch EE, Cheng C, Stager DR, Jr., Weakley DR, Jr., Stager DR, Sr. The critical period for surgical treatment of dense congenital bilateral cataracts. J AAPOS. 2009;13(1):67–71.
5. Birch EE, Cheng C, Vu C, Stager Jr DR. Oral reading after treatment of dense congenital unilateral cataract. J AAPOS. 2010;14(3):227–31. doi:S1091-8531(10)00236-3 [pii]. 10.1016/j.jaapos.2010.04.007.
6. Birch EE, Stager DR. The critical period for surgical treatment of dense congenital unilateral cataract. Invest Ophthalmol Vis Sci. 1996;37(8):1532–8.
7. Bowman RJ, Kabiru J, Negretti G, Wood ML. Outcomes of bilateral cataract surgery in Tanzanian children. Ophthalmology. 2007;114(12):2287–92. doi:S0161-6420(07)00127-3 [pii]. 10.1016/j.ophtha.2007.01.030.
8. Costenbader FD, Albert DG. Conservatism in the management of congenital cataract. AMA Arch Ophthalmol. 1957;58(3):426–30.
9. Crawford ML, Blake R, Cool SJ, von Noorden GK. Physiological consequences of unilateral and bilateral eye closure in macaque monkeys: some further observations. Brain Res. 1975;84(1):150–4.
10. Dave H, Phoenix V, Becker ER, Lambert SR. Simultaneous vs sequential bilateral cataract surgery for infants with congenital cataracts: Visual outcomes, adverse events, and economic costs. Arch Ophthalmol. 2010;128(8):1050–4. doi:128/8/1050 [pii]. 10.1001/archophthalmol.2010.136.
11. Elston JS, Timms C. Clinical evidence for the onset of the sensitive period in infancy. Br J Ophthalmol. 1992;76(6):327–8.
12. Gogate PM, Sahasrabudhe M, Shah M, Patil S, Kulkarni AN, Trivedi R, Bhasa D, Tamboli R, Mane R. Long term outcomes of bilateral congenital and developmental cataracts operated in Maharashtra, India. Miraj pediatric cataract study III. Indian J Ophthalmol. 2014;62(2):186–95. doi:10.4103/0301-4738.128630.
13. Hartmann EE, Lynn MJ, Lambert SR, Infant Aphakia Treatment Study G. Baseline characteristics of the infant aphakia treatment study population: predicting recognition acuity at 4.5 years of age. Invest Ophthalmol Vis Sci. 2015;56(1):388–95. doi:10.1167/iovs.14-15464.
14. Held R, Ostrovsky Y, de Gelder B, Gandhi T, Ganesh S, Mathur U, Sinha P. The newly sighted fail to match seen with felt. Nat Neurosci. 2011;14(5):551–3. doi:10.1038/nn.2795.
15. Holmes JM, Kraker RT, Beck RW, Birch EE, Cotter SA, Everett DF, Hertle RW, Quinn GE, Repka MX, Scheiman MM, Wallace DK. A randomized trial of prescribed patching regimens for treatment of severe amblyopia in children. Ophthalmology. 2003;110(11): 2075–87.
16. Hubel DH, Wiesel TN. The period of susceptibility to the physiological effects of unilateral eye closure in kittens. J Physiol. 1970;206(2):419–36.
17. Infant Aphakia Treatment Study G, Lambert SR, Lynn MJ, Hartmann EE, DuBois L, Drews-Botsch C, Freedman SF, Plager DA, Buckley EG, Wilson ME. Comparison of contact lens and intraocular lens correction of monocular aphakia during infancy: a randomized clinical trial of HOTV optotype acuity at age 4.5 years and clinical findings at age 5 years. JAMA Ophthalmol 2014;132(6):676–82. doi:10.1001/jamaophthalmol.2014.531
18. Jeffrey BG, Birch EE, Stager DR, Jr., Stager DR, Sr., Weakley DR, Jr. Early binocular visual experience may improve binocular sensory outcomes in children after surgery for congenital unilateral cataract. J AAPOS. 2001;5:209–16.
19. Kong L, Fry M, Al-Samarraie M, Gilbert C, Steinkuller PG. An update on progress and the changing epidemiology of causes of childhood blindness worldwide. J AAPOS. 2012;16(6):501–7. doi:10.1016/j.jaapos.2012.09.004.
20. Lambert SR, Buckley EG, Drews-Botsch C, DuBois L, Hartmann E, Lynn MJ, Plager DA, Wilson ME. The infant aphakia treatment study: design and clinical measures at enrollment. Arch Ophthalmol. 2010;128(1):21–7. doi:128/1/21 [pii]. 10.1001/archophthalmol.2009.350.
21. Lambert SR, DuBois L, Cotsonis G, Hartmann EE, Drews-Botsch C. Factors Associated with a Good Visual Acuity Outcome and Stereopsis in the Infant Aphakia Treatment Study Eye. 2016;30:1221–1228.
22. Lambert SR, Lynn MJ, Reeves R, Plager DA, Buckley EG, Wilson ME. Is there a latent period for the surgical treatment of children with dense bilateral congenital cataracts? J AAPOS. 2006;10(1):30–6. doi:S1091-8531(05)00297-1 [pii]. 10.1016/j.jaapos.2005.10.002.
23. Lambert SR, Plager DA, Lynn MJ, Wilson ME. Visual outcome following the reduction or cessation of patching therapy after early unilateral cataract surgery. Arch Ophthalmol. 2008;126(8):1071–4. doi:126/8/1071 [pii]. 10.1001/archopht.126.8.1071 [doi].
24. Le Grand R, Mondloch CJ, Maurer D, Brent HP. Neuroperception. Early visual experience and face processing. Nature. 2001;410(6831):890. doi:10.1038/35073749.
25. Lloyd IC, Dowler JG, Kriss A, Speedwell L, Thompson DA, Russell-Eggitt I, Taylor D. Modulation of amblyopia therapy following early surgery for unilateral congenital cataracts. Br J Ophthalmol. 1995;79(9):802–6.
26. Lundvall A, Kugelberg U. Outcome after treatment of congenital bilateral cataract. Acta Ophthalmol Scand. 2002;80(6):593–7. doi:aos800607 [pii].
27. Lundvall A, Kugelberg U. Outcome after treatment of congenital unilateral cataract. Acta Ophthalmol Scand. 2002;80(6):588–92. doi:aos800606 [pii].
28. Magli A, Forte R, Rombetto L. Long-term outcome of primary versus secondary intraocular lens implantation after simultaneous removal of bilateral congenital cataract. Graefes Arch Clin Exp Ophthalmol. 2013;251(1): 309–14. doi:10.1007/s00417-012-1979-7.
29. Maurer D, Lewis TL, Brent HP, Levin AV. Rapid improvement in the acuity of infants after visual input. Science. 1999;286(5437):108–10.

30. Mistr SK, Trivedi RH, Wilson ME. Preoperative considerations and outcomes of primary intraocular lens implantation in children with posterior polar and posterior lentiglobus cataract. J AAPOS. 2008;12(1):58–61. doi:S1091-8531(07)00418-1 [pii]. 10.1016/j.jaapos.2007.08.003.
31. Morrison DG, Wilson ME, Trivedi RH, Lambert SR, Lynn MJ. Infant Aphakia Treatment Study: effects of persistent fetal vasculature on outcome at 1 year of age. J AAPOS. 2011;15(5):427–31. doi:10.1016/j.jaapos.2011.06.004. S1091-8531(11)00476-9 [pii].
32. Negretti GS, Ayoub T, Ahmed S, Deb R, Majumder U, Jewel J, Muhit M, Gilbert CE, Bowman RJ. Cataract surgery outcomes in Bangladeshi children. Ophthalmology. 2015. doi:10.1016/j.ophtha.2015.01.013.
33. Ostrovsky Y, Meyers E, Ganesh S, Mathur U, Sinha P. Visual parsing after recovery from blindness. Psychol Sci. 2009;20(12):1484–91. doi:10.1111/j.1467-9280.2009.02471.x.
34. Parks MM, Johnson DA, Reed GW. Long-term visual results and complications in children with aphakia. A function of cataract type. Ophthalmology. 1993; 100(6):826–40; discussion 840–21.
35. Sawhney GK, Hutchinson AK, Lambert SR. The value of serial personal photographs in timing the onset of unilateral cataracts in children. J AAPOS. 2009; 13(5):459–62. doi:10.1016/j.jaapos.2009.08.007. doi:S1091-8531(09)00272-9 [pii].
36. Wallace DK, Pediatric Eye Disease Investigator G, Edwards AR, Cotter SA, Beck RW, Arnold RW, Astle WF, Barnhardt CN, Birch EE, Donahue SP, Everett DF, Felius J, Holmes JM, Kraker RT, Melia M, Repka MX, Sala NA, Silbert DI, Weise KK. A randomized trial to evaluate 2 hours of daily patching for strabismic and anisometropic amblyopia in children. Ophthalmology 2006;113(6):904–12. doi:10.1016/j.ophtha.2006.01.069
37. Wiesel TN, Hubel DH. Comparison of the effects of unilateral and bilateral eye closure on cortical unit responses in kittens. J Neurophysiol. 1965;28(6): 1029–40.
38. Young MP, Heidary G, VanderVeen DK. Relationship between the timing of cataract surgery and development of nystagmus in patients with bilateral infantile cataracts. J AAPOS. 2012;16(6):554–7. doi:10.1016/j.jaapos.2012.08.008.

19 Strabismus in Children with Cataracts

Erick D. Bothun

The presence of a pediatric cataract in a visually immature child may interfere with the development of binocularity and the maintenance of orthophoria [1–12]. A number of factors related to pediatric lens anomaly have been suggested to interrupt motor and sensory ocular alignment. These include suppression by the cataract, associated ocular anomalies, aggressive occlusive regimens and the presence of anisometropia and aniseikonia. Approximately 50 % of children with cataract will develop strabismus [9]. It can occur with varying severity of bilateral and unilateral lens opacities but appears more common in the latter. Younger age at the onset of cataract and denser opacity correlates to a higher risk of strabismus. Thus presence of strabismus is seen as indicator that pediatric cataract had an early onset, is long standing, and/or is associated with amblyopia. To the contrary, patients with older age, partial cataract and better preoperative visual acuity are more likely to be orthophoric. Timely management of visually significant lens opacities is important for ocular alignment outcomes. Despite appropriate management of cataract, strabismus may develop after cataract surgery, irrespective of refractive and amblyopia rehabilitation.

E.D. Bothun, MD
Department of Ophthalmology, Mayo Clinic, 200 First Street South West, Rochester, MN 55905, USA
e-mail: bothu003@umn.edu

19.1 Introduction

The association between pediatric cataract surgery and strabismus is well documented. In 1977, Hiles and Sheridan [9] reported strabismus in 50 % of 350 consecutive children treated for pediatric cataract. They reported that children with bilateral cataracts had the same frequency of strabismus as those with a unilateral cataract (49 % verses 45 %). In 1984, France and Frank [13] also reported strabismus in 71 % of such children at the completion of rehabilitative care. Despite improvements in surgical and optical care in recent decades, the rates of strabismus have remained unchanged. Watts and colleagues [8] later documented strabismus developing in 42 % of bilateral and 50 % of monocular cataract patients in 2003. Utilizing only the literature since 1980, Wilson and colleagues [14] documented strabismus in 78 % of patients following cataract surgery. The incidence of strabismus after the treatment of unilateral congenital cataracts has been well documented and range from 34 to 100 % [1–12]. In the randomized clinical trial, The Infant Aphakia Treatment Study (IATS), 70 % of infants develop strabismus by 12 months after unilateral cataract surgery [15] (Fig. 19.1).

19.2 Cataract Morphology

There are conflicting reports on the association between the etiology and morphology of pediatric cataracts and strabismus. Such a relationship may

I.C. Lloyd, S.R. Lambert (eds.), *Congenital Cataract*, DOI 10.1007/978-3-319-27848-3_19

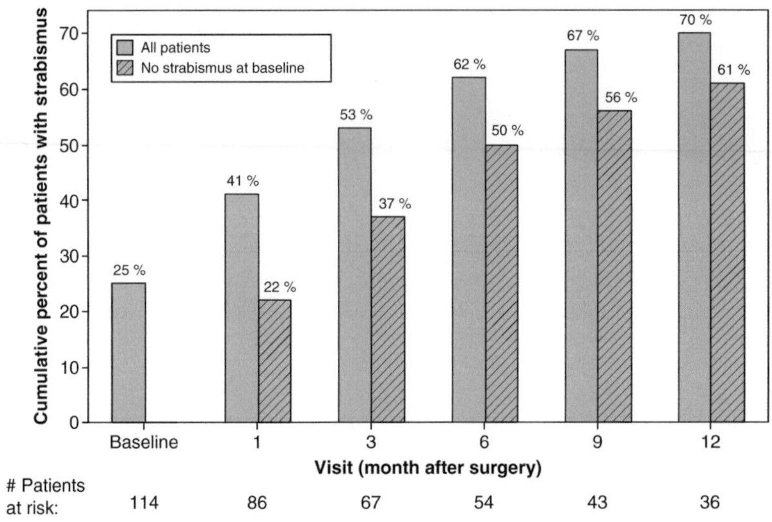

Fig. 19.1 Life-table estimates of the cumulative percent of patients developing strabismus over time [15]

be masked by the myriad of associated ocular, syndromic, and neurologic anomalies that are also risk factors for strabismus the same child. Hiles [9] did not detect an increased risk of strabismus with severity or type of cataract or with other ocular and systemic findings. No difference in strabismus prevalence was found when Weisberg and colleagues [16] looked at different cataract types. However, Gregg and Parks [17] reported a strong correlation between cataract morphology and the rate of strabismus. Strabismus was found in 21 % of lamellar cataracts, 48 % of posterior lentiglobus, 65 % of nuclear cataracts, and 100 % of patients with persistent fetal vasculature. Hosal et al. [6] showed better binocular functioning in patients with traumatic cataract and posterior lenticonus and lower levels in congenital and complicated cataracts. France and Frank [13] reported children with acquired cataracts had less strabismus that those with congenital cataract (61 verses 86 %). The lower rate of strabismus with acquired and traumatic pediatric cataracts is likely linked to the development of normal binocular fusion prior to ocular trauma and a more rapid surgical treatment.

19.3 Types of Strabismus

Although reports vary, esotropia is the most common type of strabismus in children with cataracts. Studies have reported esotropia in 50–76 % of children with cataracts (Lambert [1] 50 %, Spanou et al. [3] 76.5 %, Parks and Hiles [11] 66 %, Cheng et al. [5] 59 %). In both the historic studies by Hiles and Cheng and the recent IATS, the percentage of patients with esotropia outnumbered those with exotropia by a ratio of 2:1. In IATS, esotropia (2–70 prism diopters) was present in 50 % and exotropia (3–50 prism diopters) was present in 27 % of children at age 5. Horizontal deviations were typically constant and present at distance and near. Exotropia may be more common with acquired cataracts or in strabismus with delayed onset after prior treatment of cataract (Hiles). Small, vertical deviations, inferior oblique overaction and pattern deviations have been reported but appear uncommon.

19.3.1 Time Course of the Development of Strabismus

The longitudinal development of strabismus has been documented even after timely and successful cataract surgical intervention. In the studies by Hiles [9], France [13], Wilson [14] and Bothun [15], strabismus developed after the cataract surgery at least half of all cases. Wilson's literature review showed that the presence of strabismus grew from 33 % of patients preoperatively to

78 % with postoperative follow up. In the prospective study of monocular cataracts in the IATS, strabismus prevalence in this study rose from 24 % preoperatively to 70 % at 12 months postoperative to 81 % through age 5 [18]. Although many factors may contribute to the detection and development of strabismus, this report shows that ocular alignment is not stable even 1 year after cataract surgery.

19.3.2 Spontaneous Resolution Rate of Strabismus

Despite excellent vision outcomes, it is unusual to have strabismus resolve simply by removing the cataract and rehabilitating the vision. Awner et al. [10] reported that two of 21 children in his retrospective series regained orthophoria through cataract surgery only. Five of the 27 with strabismus at baseline in the Infant Aphakia Treatment Study regained and maintained orthotropia to 12 months postoperatively [15]. Similarly 19 of 82 patients in the Hiles [9] series became orthophoric once the cataract was removed. Lastly, the development or course of strabismus in the IATS did not correlate to the occurrence of adverse events or need for additional intraocular surgeries in children after initial removal of infantile cataract.

19.3.3 Relationship Between Binocularity and Strabismus

Suppression from a cataract early in infancy may disrupt both vision and binocular development. Thus timely cataract surgery before the critical window in developing sensory fusion closes may minimize strabismus. In the study of France, surgery in the first 2 weeks of life for congenital cataract was associated with lower rates of strabismus. In the Infant Aphakia Treatment Study, orthotropia was found in 27 % of children who underwent early cataract surgery (between 28 and 48 days of life) compared to 13 % who had surgery at an older age (p = 0.085) [18].

Unfortunately maintaining orthophoria after infantile cataract surgery does not guarantee meaningful stereopsis. Despite rare reports of high grade stereopsis after infantile cataract surgery, most children do not demonstrated stereopsis after rehabilitation for unilateral congenital cataract surgery. In addition to the sensory interruption by the cataract or refractive error, full time patching regimens for amblyopia have been implicated as a potential compounding factor poor stereopsis. The hope for better stereopsis was ignited in the 1990s when retrospective studies of part time patching protocols showed improved motor and sensory fusion [4, 7, 19, 20]. With guarded patching in the first 6 months of life, Wright and colleagues [4] obtained sensory fusion in 3 of 13 patients, one with Randot Stereo Acuity of 250 s of arc. After comparable patching regimen in the IATS, gross stereopsis was measured on one or more of three tests in 25.5 % of children at age 4.5 years [21]. Detectable stereopsis is close to three times more likely (18 verses 46 %) in children with orthotropia vs. those with strabismus (P = 0.005). In Hartmann's report, the highest levels of measured stereopsis were detected by Frisby Stereotest (2 with 170 s of arc).

19.3.4 Relationship Between the Type of Optical Correction and Strabismus

Some reports have suggested that primary intraocular lens (IOL) placement might lower the frequency of strabismus and improve stereopsis. Lambert and colleagues [1] described rates of strabismus of 75 % using IOLs and 92 % using contact lenses in a small series of infants after unilateral cataract surgery. Autrata et al. [2] reported a similar finding with 55 % developing strabismus after IOL vs 83 % using CL. Greenwald and Glaser [22] reported better stereopsis in patients implanted with an IOL. Yet a consistent limitation to these retrospective, small series was that the decision to place an IOL was not randomized. Eyes with higher risk characteristics, such as younger age and associated structural defects, have been less likely to receive IOL at the time.

The recently completed IATS study showed randomized infants undergoing monocular cataract surgery to aphakia treatment with contact lens vs IOL [23–25]. After 5 years of age, the development of strabismus was similar whether the child received contact lens or primary IOL implantation for the correction of unilateral aphakia (86 % verses 77 %, p = 0.33) [18].

19.3.5 Timing of Strabismus Surgery

The strabismus associated with pediatric cataract can be monitored as optical rehabilitation and amblyopia treatment ensues. A common approach is to maximize the vision outcome prior to strabismus surgery. This provides time to further assess the stability or frequency of manifest strabismus patterns and console the family on chronic management options. As most motility disorders in pediatric aphakic or pseudophakic patients are constant deviations, extraocular muscle surgery is typically warranted. The timing of strabismus surgery is elective and may be delayed until an exam under anesthesia is warranted or just prior to school to avoid negative psychosocial impact. Hiles [9] reported an alignment success of less than 10 prism diopters in 80 % of patients undergoing strabismus surgery after prior lensectomy. Most were unilateral recess and respect procedures, typically performed after cataract surgery. Weisber [16], Hiles [9], and Merino et al. [26] also reported success rates between 75 and 83 % in older children.

Conclusions

Despite significant advancement in visual outcomes, strabismus rates remain high and stereopsis values remain low for children with pediatric cataracts. Strabismus is all frequent with both bilateral and unilateral cataracts, developing at any point in the rehabilitative care of a child and irrespective of optical choice in aphakia management. Although timely surgical intervention, effective optical correction and a controlled patching regimen may reduce the prevalence, we have yet to find the key to maximize binocular outcomes.

References

1. Lambert SR, Lynn M, Drews-Botsch C, et al. A comparison of grating visual acuity, strabismus, and reoperation outcomes among infants with aphakia and pseudophakia after unilateral cataract surgery during the first six months of life. J AAPOS. 2001;5:70–5.
2. Autrata R, Rehurek J, Vodickova K. Visual results after primary intraocular lens implantation or contract lens correction for aphakia in the first year of age. Ophthalmologica. 2005;219:72–9.
3. Spanou N, Alexopoulos L, Manta G, et al. Strabismus in pediatric lens disorders. J Pediatr Ophthalmol Strabismus. 2011;48:163–6.
4. Wright KW, Matsumoto E, Edelman PM. Binocular fusion and stereopsis associated with early surgery for monocular congenital cataracts. Arch Ophthalmol. 1992;110:1607–9.
5. Cheng KP, Hiles DA, Biglan AW, et al. Visual results after early surgical treatment of unilateral congenital cataract. Ophthalmology. 1991;98:903–10.
6. Hosal BM, Biglan AW, Elhan AH. High levels of binocular function are achievable after removal of monocular cataracts in infants before 8 years of age. Ophthalmology. 2000;107:1647–55.
7. Brown SM, Archer SA, Del Monte MA. Stereopsis and binocular vision after surgery for unilateral infantile cataract. J AAPOS. 1999;3(2):109–13.
8. Watts P, Abdolell M, Levin AV. Complications in infants undergoing surgery for congenital cataract in the first 12 weeks of life: is early surgery better? J AAPOS. 2003;7:81–5.
9. Hiles DA, Sheridan SJ. Strabismus associated with infantile cataracts. Int Ophthalmol Clin. 1977;17(4):193–202.
10. Awner S, Buckley EG, DeVaro JM, et al. Unilateral pseudophakia in children under 4 years. J Pediatr Ophthalmol Strabismus. 1996;33:230–6.
11. Parks MM, Hiles DA. Management of infantile cataracts. Am J Ophthalmol. 1967;63:10–9.
12. Deweese MW. A survey of the surgical management of congenital cataracts. Am J Ophthalmol. 1962;53: 853–8.
13. France TD, Frank JW. The association of strabismus and aphakia in infants. J Pediatr Ophthalmol Strabismus. 1984;21:223–6.
14. Wilson Jr ME, Trivedi RH, Hoxie JP, et al. Treatment outcomes of congenital monocular cataracts: the effects of surgical timing and patching compliance. J Pediatr Ophthalmol Strabismus. 2003;40:323–9.
15. Bothun ED, Cleveland J, Lynn MJ, et al. Infant Aphakic Treatment Study. One-year strabismus outcomes in the Infant Aphakia Treatment Study. Ophthalmology. 2013;120(6):1227–31.
16. Weisberg OL, Sprunger DT, Plager DA, et al. Strabismus in pediatric pseudophakia. Ophthalmology. 2005;112:1625–8.
17. Gregg FM, Parks MM. Stereopsis after congenital monocular cataract extraction. Am J Ophthalmol. 1992;114:314–7.

18. Bothun ED, Lynn MJ, Christiansen SP, Neely DE, Vanderveen DK, Kruger SJ, Lambert SR; Infant Aphakia Treatment Study. Sensorimotor outcomes by age 5 years after monocular cataract surgery in the Infant Aphakia Treatment Study (IATS). JAAPOS. 2016;20(1):49–53.
19. Birch EE, Swanson WH, Stager DR, et al. Outcome after very early treatment of dense congenital unilateral cataract. Invest Ophthalmol Vis Sci. 1993;34(13):3687–99.
20. Fawcett SL, Wang Y, Birch EE. The critical period for susceptibility of human stereopsis. Invest Ophthalmol Vis Sci. 2005;46:521–5.
21. Hartman EE, Stout AU, Lynn MJ, et al. Infant Aphakia Treatment Study. Stereopsis results at 4.5 years of age in the infant aphakia treatment study. Am J Ophthalmol. 2015;159:64–70.
22. Greenwald MJ, Glaser SR. Visual outcomes after surgery for unilateral cataract in children more than two years old; posterior chamber intraocular lens implantation verses contact lens correction of aphakia. J AAPOS. 1998;2:168–76.
23. Infant Aphakia Treatment Study Group. The Infant Aphakia Treatment Study: design and clinical measures at enrollment. Arch Ophthalmol. 2010;128:21–7.
24. Infant Aphakia Treatment Study Group, Lambert SR, Lynn MJ, Hartmann EE, et al. Comparison of contact lens and intraocular lens correction of monocular aphakia during infancy: a randomized clinical trial of HOTV optotype acuity at age 4.5 years and clinical findings at age 5 years. JAMA Ophthalmol. 2014;132(6):676–82.
25. Plager DA, Lynn MJ, Buckley EG, et al. Infant Aphakia Treatment Study Group. Complications in the first 5 years following cataract surgery in infants with and without intraocular lens implantation in the Infant Aphakia Treatment Study. Am J Ophthalmol. 2014;158(5):892–8.
26. Merino P, Gomez-de-Liano P, Gil MR, et al. Strabismus and congenital cataract. Arch Soc Esp Oftalmol. 2007;82:623–8.

20 Nystagmus in the Child with Congenital Cataract

Jay Self and Ian Christopher Lloyd

20.1 Human Eye Movements – A Brief Overview

Eye movements have evolved to subserve the specific visual requirements of particular organisms. For example, afoveate animals such as the mouse (that lack a fovea) require eye movements primarily to stabilize the eyes in space during head movement. To achieve this, two distinct mechanisms evolved to stabilize images on the retina during such head perturbations. The first comprises the Vestibulo-Ocular Reflexes (VOR), which depend on the ability of the labyrinthine mechanoreceptors to sense head accelerations. The second consists of visually mediated reflexes (Optokinetic and Smooth-Pursuit tracking), which depend on the ability of the brain to determine the speed of image drift on the retina. Together, these reflexes stabilize the angle of gaze and eyes remain pointed at the object of regard whenever the head is moving [5].

With the evolution of the fovea, it became necessary to change the line of sight independently of head movements. Eye movement subsystems evolved both to bring eccentric targets onto the fovea (foveation) and keep it there [5]. Saccades are fast foveating eye movements that bring the object of interest onto the fovea. This function was described elegantly as early as the late nineteenth century by the American Ophthalmologist William James who wrote;

> The peripheral retina is like a Sentinel and when an object of regard falls upon it, it shouts 'hark, who goes there' and calls the fovea to the spot [6].

However, it is necessary to hold the position of even stationary objects on the fovea and for this purpose a gaze-holding system evolved. This constantly maintains the object of regard on the fovea and prevents the gaze from drifting off target.

With the evolution of frontal vision and binocularity came a requirement to place the object of interest on the fovea of both eyes simultaneously. Vergence movements are binocular movements which achieve this aim by moving the eyes simultaneously in opposite directions such as adduction of one eye and abduction of the other.

Thus, for foveate primates such as humans, the ocular motor system consists of several subsystems that generate different types of eye movements in response to different stimuli [7]. The development of, and the necessary hierarchical ordering of, these systems are sensitive to disruption in early infancy. Such disruption is thought to be the cause of a variety of oculomotor disturbances including nystagmus [8].

J. Self, BM, FRCOphth, PhD (✉)
University of Southampton, Southampton, UK
e-mail: J.E.Self@soton.ac.uk

I.C. Lloyd, MB, FRCS, FRCOphth
Department of Clinical and Academic Ophthalmology, Great Ormond Street Hospital for Children, London WC1N 7EH, UK

Paediatric Ophthalmology, Manchester Royal Eye Hospital, University of Manchester, Manchester, UK
e-mail: IanChristopher.Lloyd@gosh.nhs.uk

I.C. Lloyd, S.R. Lambert (eds.), *Congenital Cataract*, DOI 10.1007/978-3-319-27848-3_20

20.2 What Is Nystagmus?

Nystagmus is a disorder of eye movement which can be defined as "a repetitive, to-and-fro movement of the eyes that is initiated by slow phases" [7].

The word nystagmus is derived from a Greek word 'nustagmos' meaning nodding of the head or drowsiness. The word is thought to have evolved due to a comparison with slow downward drift and sudden upward jerk of the head during drowsiness [9].

In humans, there are three main control mechanisms for maintaining steady gaze; the fixation movements, the vestibulo-ocular reflex; and the gaze-holding system. Failure of any of these control systems will bring about a disruption of steady fixation. Two types of abnormal fixation can result; nystagmus and saccadic intrusions/oscillations. The difference between them lies in the initial movement that takes the line of sight away from the object of regard. The initial anomalous movement in saccadic intrusions/oscillations is a fast saccadic movement. In the case of nystagmus, it is a slow drift or 'slow phase' away from the target such that the corrective movement (which is a fast saccade in the case of jerk nystagmus) is a normal compensatory movement.

It has been suggested that that nystagmus results from an anomaly within the gaze-holding pathways or the tissues comprising the brainstem mechanism that generates the tonic innervation needed to maintain lateral gaze (neural integrator).

20.3 Types of Nystagmus

It is important to remember that 'Nystagmus' is purely a descriptive term. It occurs in a bewildering number of clinical scenarios. For example, it can be a normal finding on extreme eccentric gaze (end-point nystagmus), it can occur as a seemingly isolated phenomenon or it can be the first sign of a devastating visual or neurological condition [1, 2]. Consequently, with such complexity and ambiguity surrounding the significance of its presence, physicians have attempted to understand nystagmus by classification since its earliest descriptions. For this reason, over 40 different named types of nystagmus are described in the literature and the nomenclature is exceptionally inconsistent, with some classification systems relying on eye movement behaviour (gaze-evoked nystagmus), some using direction (downbeat nystagmus), some using age of onset (early onset nystagmus) and other purely using eponymous description (for example, Bruns' nystagmus) [4, 10]. These different ways of defining nystagmus have been designed for, and are therefore biased in favour of, use by different groups of researchers/clinicians.

In 2001 the National Eye Institute sponsored a workshop by the Committee for the Classification of Eye Movement Abnormalities and Strabismus (CEMAS). The remit was 'to produce a new classification system for eye movement anomalies including nystagmus' which was based on up-to-date clinical and scientific information and designed to be used as a resource for scientists, clinicians and educators' [3]. This system also has limitations but for clarity and consistency, we will use it (with reference to older nomenclature when prudent) in this chapter.

We will focus on the two commonest types of nystagmus seen in the pediatric cataract clinic; Fusion Maldevelopment Nystagmus Syndrome, FMNS (previously Manifest Latent Nystagmus MLN) and Infantile Nystagmus Syndrome (previously Congenital Idiopathic Nystagmus, CIN and also some forms of sensory deficit nystagmus, SDN). We will also discuss eye movements called 'Saccadic Intrusions' which are non-nystagmus eye movements, often observed in children with cataract.

20.4 Fusion Maldevelopment Nystagmus Syndrome, FMNS (Previously Manifest Latent Nystagmus MLN)

FMNS describes a nystagmus which is of infantile onset, usually associated with strabismus, with linear or decelerating slow-phases on eye movement recordings (see Fig. 20.1), beating in the direction of the fixing eye and which may include a high-frequency, low amplitude pendular nystagmus. It is often associated with strabismus and amblyopia and thought to occur due to early

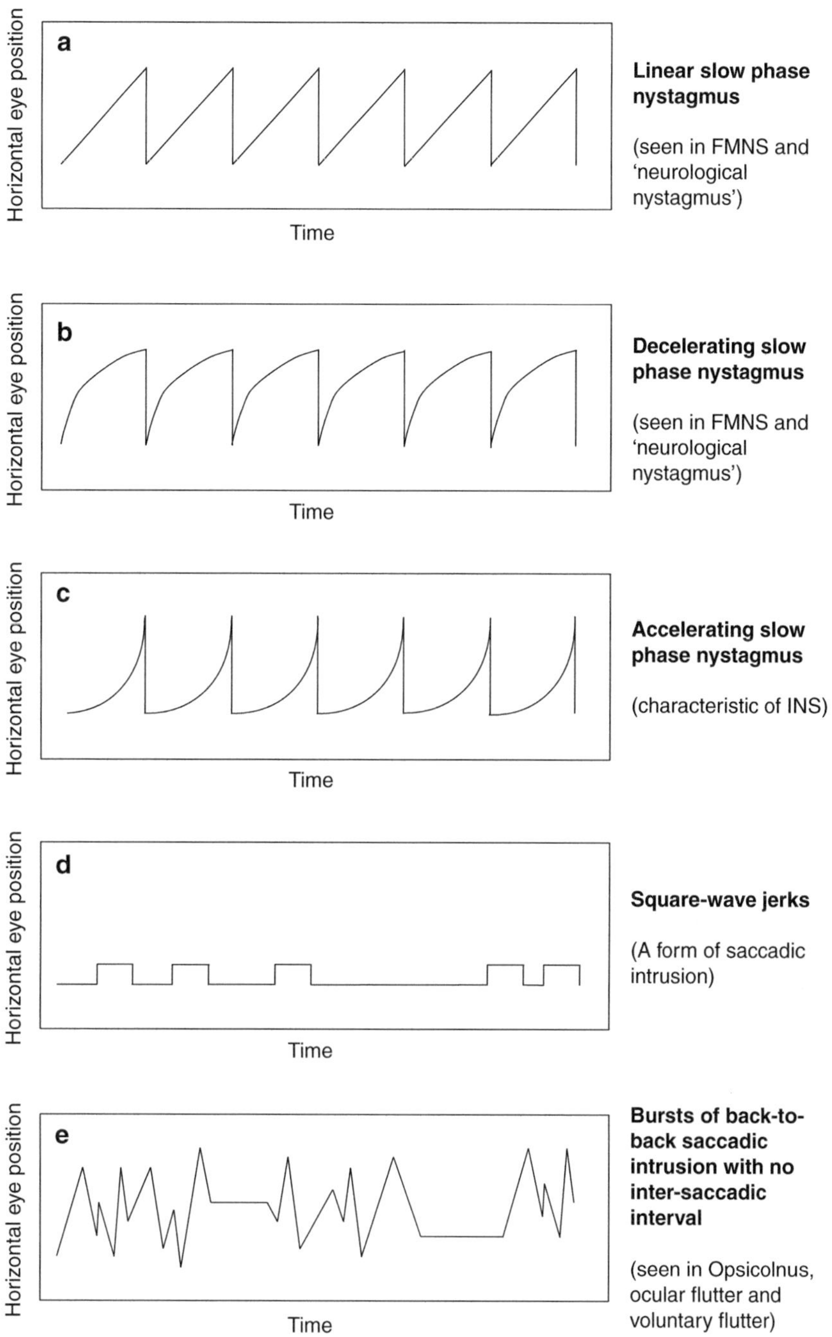

Fig. 20.1 Waveforms seen on eye movement recordings in children

interruption of binocular development from any cause [11–13]. MLN (prior to its renaming as FMNS) was subdivided into four groups in a continuum termed Latent Manifest Latent Nystagmus (LMLN) according to the ocular movements seen during binocular viewing [14]. Type 1 LMLN describes ocular stability during binocular viewing; also termed Latent Nystagmus (LN). In the authors' experience, LN is very rare in the context of childhood cataract. The generic term FMNS will be used for all previous MLN categories according to the above description.

FMNS is common in childhood cataract especially where there are significant interocular differences in visual acuity (such as typically seen in unilateral cataract). In some cases, it can be associated with a head posture or even cross-fixation, in order to hold the fixing (better) eye in adduction. This is thought to reduce the nystagmus intensity by holding gaze in the opposite direction to that of the nystagmus fast phases, a phenomenon seen in many forms of nystagmus (Alexanders law) [15].

20.5 Infantile Nystagmus Syndrome (Previously Including Congenital Idiopathic Nystagmus, CIN and Some Forms of Sensory Deficit Nystagmus, SDN)

The criteria for diagnosis of Infantile Nystagmus Syndrome (INS) include; infantile onset (usually identified between 3 and 6 months) and diagnostic accelerating slow phases on eye movement recordings (see Fig. 20.1) [3]. Typically, it is predominantly horizontal, increases with fixation attempt, stays horizontal in up and down-gaze, decreases with convergence and is associated with null zones. OKN can be either absent, or in some cases described as 'reverse' and squints and refractive errors are common. Some diagnostic confusion can occur here as the presence of INS does not point to a specific etiology and patients with sensory deficits such as albinism, achromatopsia and even congenital cataract may fall into this category if they meet the other diagnostic criteria (particularly accelerating waveforms on eye movement recordings).

20.6 Saccadic Intrusions

Saccadic intrusions are fast eye movements taking the fovea away from the object of regard. According to the CEMAS classification [3], the group of eye movements collectively named 'saccadic intrusions and oscillations' comprises 12 different subtypes including: square wave jerks, opsoclonus and psychogenic (voluntary) flutter. However, the term saccadic intrusion has been used in much of the paediatric cataract literature to describe any involuntary, conjugate, horizontal fast eye movement of less than 1° in amplitude [16]. The term will therefore be used in this context in this chapter (see Fig. 20.1).

20.7 What Type of Oculomotor Instabilities Do Children with Cataract Have?

Studies have found a variety of oculomotor instabilities in children with cataract. The most commonly reported is FMNS but INS, undefined multiplanar nystagmus and saccadic intrusions have also been reported in a number of studies [16–18].

Interestingly, saccadic intrusions can be recorded in normal infants, whenever they are in a reduced state of arousal and bursts of monophasic square-wave intrusions have also been recorded in healthy infants aged between 2 and 7 weeks of age [16, 19, 20]. They are also known to occur more commonly in amblyopia.

It has been observed that saccadic intrusions are a common physiological finding in younger children dependent upon their state of arousal and perhaps reflecting a failure to attend to, or actively engage in, fixation [16]. Therefore, the significance of their presence in children with cataract is difficult to interpret although features separating them from those seen in healthy infants appears to be their increased amplitude and occurrence in short bursts [16].

Early publications describing nystagmus associated with childhood cataract were typically limited to noting the presence or absence of nystagmus and did not differentiate between FMNS and INS or any other type of nystagmus [21, 22].

In the small number of studies that have used eye movement recordings to differentiate between FMNS and INS in children with cataract, the patient cohorts have differed substantially as have the criteria used for diagnosis of FMNS or INS. Unsurprisingly the reported relative frequency of FMNS to INS [16, 18] has varied between series. Interestingly, it has in some cases, also varied between the two eyes of individual patients and between pre and postoperative measurements in individual patients [16]. There is some evidence that the type and risk of nystagmus does not appear to vary with laterality of the cataract [16]. It is also evident that the characteristics of the nystagmus seen in children with cataract can evolve over time as they do in 'pure' FMNS or INS seen in other contexts.

In 2012, Birch et al studied 41 children with dense cataracts from a variety of aetiologies. They found that by 5 years of age, 29 (71 %) had nystagmus. Of these, 18 had a predominantly INS phenotype and 11 had a predominantly FMNS phenotype. They found that risk factors for nystagmus included: infantile onset of cataract (<12 months of age) and duration of cataract of longer than 6 weeks but interestingly *NOT* congenital onset (cataract observed in the 1st week of life) or laterality (unilateral vs bilateral). Furthermore, they found that congenital onset and unilaterality WERE associated with a significant risk of inter-ocular asymmetry of nystagmus [18]. Strabismus was also strongly associated with the presence of nystagmus.

Much debate still exists over the anatomical substrates for FMNS and INS and the observations of their coexistence in many patients with congenital cataract suggests that each is a consequence of a unique combination of timing, duration, laterality and the nature of sensory deprivation [18].

In summary, it seems that there are overlapping oculomotor disturbances at play in children with cataract, each perhaps with different but overlapping sensitive periods. However, early interruption of binocular vision appears to be a common causative insult. There are quite significant differences in the reported prevalence of nystagmus and in the characteristics of the nystagmus noted, between studies using eye movement recordings and others using cruder clinical assessment. This may explain why series describing children assessed using eye movement recordings report no difference in the incidence of fixation instabilities between bilateral and unilateral cataract cases [16, 18] whereas clinical reviews have described nystagmus as 'rare' in unilateral cataract [23].

20.8 How Common Is Nystagmus in Children with Cataract and Is It a Useful Prognostic Indicator for Cataract Surgery?

The reported prevalence of nystagmus and ocular oscillations in children with cataract varies between 38 and 100 % [16, 17, 24–27]. This makes judging the prognostic value of the presence of nystagmus difficult. However, the reported series and the types of patients included within them, varied widely in parameters including laterality, morphology of cataract, age of intervention, age of examination, stage of examination (pre-op or post-op), eye movement examination technique (observation or recordings) and discrepancy between types of ocular oscillations (i.e. saccadic intrusions vs nystagmus) [16, 17, 24, 25]. However, it is generally agreed that untreated dense bilateral cataracts in early infancy are associated with nystagmus or roving eye movements which develop by the age of 13 weeks [26, 27].

Robb and Peterson reported the visual results of 51 patients with congenital cataract following surgery and included a clinical observation of the presence of 'nystagmus'. A precise description of the abnormal eye movements observed is not provided but clinically defined 'nystagmus' was associated with the following: density of the cataract, signs of other ocular developmental anomalies (such as poor pupillary dilation and reduced corneal diameter) as well as poor acuity outcome [21]. Bradford et al studied 33 patients with dense bilateral congenital cataract and found that 'clinically observed nystagmus' was not a prognostically significant determinant of visual outcome either as a pre *or* post op finding [22] (although interestingly they similarly also found that in this series age at surgery was *not* a significant factor in determining visual outcome).

However, in a later study Lambert et al found that in 43 children undergoing surgery for dense bilateral congenital cataracts, the presence of preoperative nystagmus was a more powerful predictor of visual outcome than age at surgery [28].

Interestingly, other clinical studies have reported good visual outcomes in children with nystagmus but this appears to be largely confined to when the nystagmus is described as 'mild' [26, 29].

As described above, early studies provided qualitative judgement of eye movements and did not include eye movement recordings or assessment of the waveforms or beat direction of the oscillations [16]. In 2006, Abadi et al addressed some of these issues by studying 33 neonates, infants and children with infantile cataract without other associated ocular or systemic abnormalities [16]. The cataracts were graded according to morphology, density and position. Eye movement recordings were taken before and after surgery where possible. The authors found that those children with denser cataract, representing more severe form deprivation had a high probability of developing nystagmus.

In summary, most published work supports the premise that pre and post-operative nystagmus is associated with poorer final visual acuity outcomes. However, it remains unclear whether nystagmus is separate from other types of oculomotor instability such as saccadic intrusions or part of a spectrum of fixation instability. Similarly it is unclear whether the nystagmus subtype is important or whether the association with poorer vision is because nystagmus *per se* reduces acuity. Furthermore, given that the critical periods for visual acuity and oculomotor stability are generally considered to be distinct (but perhaps overlapping), it is possible that risk factors such as the timing, depth and duration of form deprivation operate independently on the development of acuity and ocular stability.

We would thus recommend that clinicians include careful assessment of the presence or absence of nystagmus and some details of its type (see section below) in their pre-operative assessment of children with cataract but advise that its presence does not necessarily preclude a good outcome from surgery.

20.9 Can Cataract Surgery Affect or Alter Nystagmus/Fixation Instability?

Felius et al described the oculomotor recordings, taken at 4.5 years old from 83 children who had undergone surgery at less than 7 months of age for unilateral cataract as part of the IATS study [17]. Preoperative measurements were not reported but nystagmus was identified in 38 % of subjects and 'saccadic oscillations' in 31 %. Although it is not possible to comment on the effect of surgery here it is notable that there was no difference between children who had contact lens or an intraocular lens for correction of aphakia.

Very little data is available for the effect of cataract surgery on fixation instability in childhood cataract. Abadi et al described change from INS waveform to the more benign FMNS in some infants after successful surgery [16]. Clinical descriptive series have also reported a reduction in the intensity of nystagmus or even apparent disappearance of nystagmus following surgery [26, 30]. This seems to be more common when the nystagmus is deemed 'mild' preoperatively [26] and in cases where the duration of visual deprivation is least [30].

20.10 What Details Should the Paediatric Cataract Surgeon Record About Nystagmus and Fixation Instability?

Careful pre-operative history and examination should identify clinical indicators linked to outcome and nystagmus development as well as a meaningful pre-operative baseline assessment of fixation enabling post-operative comparison. Atypical nystagmus warranting further investigation should be identified and eye movement studies considered where these are available and deemed clinically useful (Figs. 20.2 and 20.3). A typical assessment might document:

- Presence or absence of fixation instability/ nystagmus prior to surgery
- Onset and duration
- Direction of fast phase of nystagmus, assessment of frequency, laterality, effect of gaze, effect of monocular occlusion and a gross description of the waveform if possible - such as jerk or pendular nystagmus or apparent saccadic dysfunction (fast movements).
- Age appropriate examination of OKN, VOR, Saccades and Smooth pursuit eye movements
- A short video recording of the eyes in primary position and with either eye occluded is useful.

20.11 How to Manage Nystagmus Associated with Paediatric Cataract?

Nystagmus in children with paediatric cataract is most commonly of an FMNS type. These cases typically have a preferred fixing eye and the nystagmus (which is predominantly horizontal) beats towards this eye when viewing binocularly

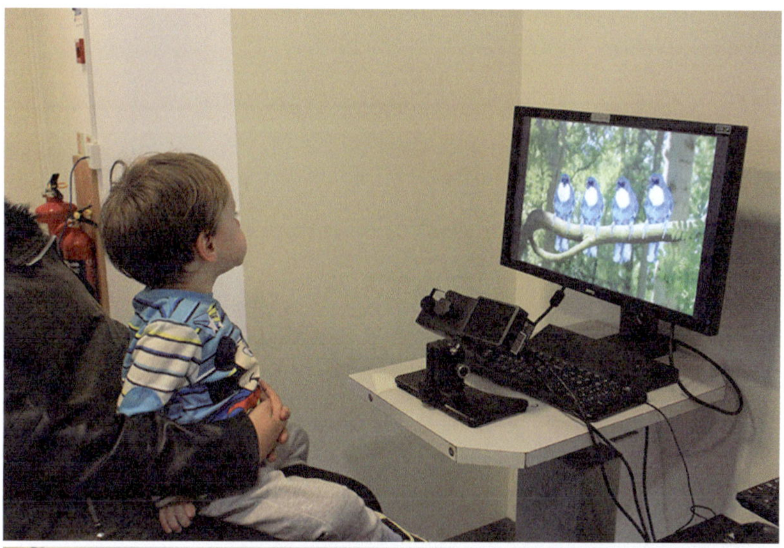

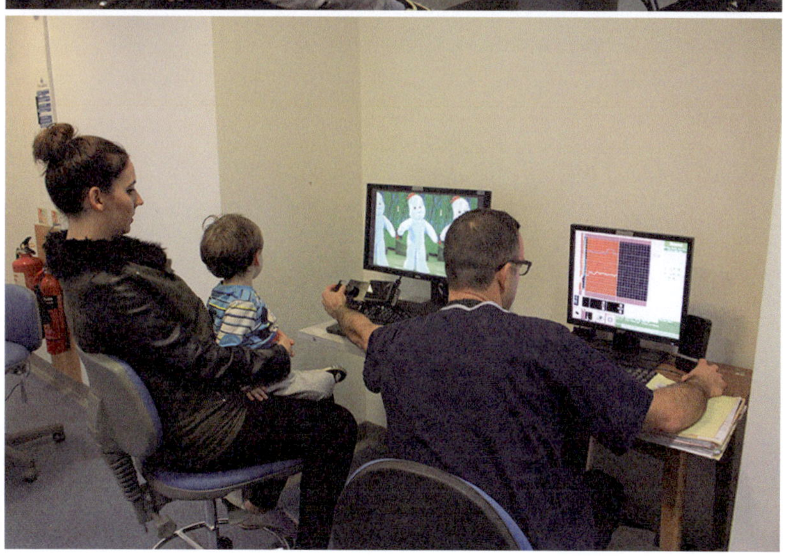

Figs. 20.2 and 20.3 A young child undergoing eye movement recording

and may change direction when the eye is occluded. The frequency (intensity) of the nystagmus tends to reduce with gaze away from the fixing eye (opposite to the fast phase of the nystagmus) due to Alexander's law [4]. This can be accompanied by esotropia or even cross fixation. In these cases surgical management of the strabismus and head posture can be helpful to improve cosmesis and comfort.

As nystagmus can develop well after the age at which surgery is considered and because it can occur in both eyes of patients with unilateral cataract, parents must be counselled about it at the pre-operative clinic visits.

At present there are no proven treatments for reducing nystagmus associated with childhood cataract although various medications and surgeries have been employed in childhood nystagmus in other contexts [31–37]. Treatment relies upon supportive measures and surgery where indicated for associated strabismus and abnormal head positions.

20.12 Summary

The available literature in this area suggests that the period of maturation of visual modalities, and hence plasticity/vulnerability, is made up of separate and specific sensory and motor control systems which develop at different rates [16]. The link between ocular instabilities and childhood cataract appears to be complex and thus it is important to:

1. Consider pre-operative nystagmus as a poor prognostic indicator in children with cataracts but be aware that this should be considered with other risk factors for poor visual outcome including patient age, density of cataract etc.
2. Be aware that even with optimum clinical care, postoperative nystagmus (even when not present pre-operatively), is a common finding.
3. Identify uncommon eye movement anomalies in children with cataract in order to identify patients with other pathologies (given that patients with neurological and metabolic disorders can often present to the pediatric cataract clinic).

References

1. Casteels I, et al. Nystagmus in infancy. Br J Ophthalmol. 1992;76(7):434–7.
2. Self J, Lotery A. The molecular genetics of congenital idiopathic nystagmus. Semin Ophthalmol. 2006;21(2): 87–90.
3. Workshop C. Classification of eye movement abnormalities and strabismus (CEMAS) workshop report. 2001: National Eye Institute Sponsored Workshop.
4. Heimann E. Einseitiger nystagmus. Klin Monatsbl J Augenheilkd. 1902;49:99–105.
5. Walls GL. The evolutionary history of eye movements.Vision Res. Pergamon Press, Printed in Great Britain. 1962;2:69–80.
6. Daroff RB. A personal introduction to eye movements. Ann NY Acad Sci. 2002;956:1–6.
7. Leigh RJ, Zee DS. The neurology of eye movements, vol. 3. New York: Oxford University Press; 1999.
8. Brodsky MC, Dell'Osso LF. A unifying neurologic mechanism for infantile nystagmus. JAMA Ophthalmol. 2014;132(6):761–8.
9. Oxford University Press. AskOxford.com, online dictionary. 2006.
10. Abel LA. Infantile nystagmus: current concepts in diagnosis and management. Clin Exp Optom. 2006; 89(2):57–65.
11. Richards M, et al. Duration of binocular decorrelation predicts the severity of latent (fusion maldevelopment) nystagmus in strabismic macaque monkeys. Invest Ophthalmol Vis Sci. 2008;49(5):1872–8.
12. Abadi RV, Bjerre A. Motor and sensory characteristics of infantile nystagmus. Br J Ophthalmol. 2002; 86(10):1152–60.
13. Dell'Osso LF. Congenital, latent and manifest latent nystagmus – similarities, differences and relation to strabismus. Jpn J Ophthalmol. 1985;29(4):351–68.
14. Abadi RV, Dickinson CM. Waveform characteristics in congenital nystagmus. Doc Ophthalmol. 1986; 64(2):153–67.
15. Baloh RW. Robert Bárány and the controversy surrounding his discovery of the caloric reaction. Neurology. 2002;58(7):1094–9.
16. Abadi RV, Forster JE, Lloyd IC. Ocular motor outcomes after bilateral and unilateral infantile cataracts. Vision Res. 2006;46(6–7):940–52.
17. Felius J, et al. Nystagmus and related fixation instabilities following extraction of unilateral infantile cataract in the Infant Aphakia Treatment Study (IATS). Invest Ophthalmol Vis Sci. 2014;55(8):5332–7.
18. Birch EE, et al. Fixation control and eye alignment in children treated for dense congenital or developmental cataracts, in J AAPOS. 2012;16:156–60. Inc: United States.
19. Hainline L, et al. Characteristics of saccades in human infants. Vision Res. 1984;24(12):1771–80.
20. Hainline L. Conjugate eye movements in infants in early visual development: normal and abnormal. Oxford: Oxford University Press; 1993. p. 47–79.

21. Robb RM, Petersen RA. Outcome of treatment for bilateral congenital cataracts. Trans Am Ophthalmol Soc. 1992;90:183–94; discussion 194–200.
22. Bradford GM, Keech RV, Scott WE. Factors affecting visual outcome after surgery for bilateral congenital cataracts. Am J Ophthalmol. 1994;117(1):58–64.
23. Ma F, Wang Q, Wang L. Advances in the management of the surgical complications for congenital cataract. Front Med. 2012;6(4):360–5.
24. Parks MM, Johnson DA, Reed GW. Long-term visual results and complications in children with aphakia. A function of cataract type. Ophthalmology. 1993; 100(6):826–40; discussion 840–1.
25. Rahi JS, Dezateux C. Congenital and infantile cataract in the United Kingdom: underlying or associated factors. British Congenital Cataract Interest Group. Invest Ophthalmol Vis Sci. 2000;41(8):2108–14.
26. Rabiah PK, et al. Results of surgery for bilateral cataract associated with sensory nystagmus in children. Am J Ophthalmol. 2002;134(4):586–91.
27. Tomkins O, et al. Outcomes of pediatric cataract surgery at a tertiary care center in rural southern Ethiopia. Arch Ophthalmol. 2011;129(10):1293–7.
28. Lambert SR, et al. Is there a latent period for the surgical treatment of children with dense bilateral congenital cataracts? J AAPOS. 2006;10(1):30–6.
29. Wright KW, Christensen LE, Noguchi BA. Results of late surgery for presumed congenital cataracts. Am J Ophthalmol. 1992;114(4):409–15.
30. Yagasaki T, et al. Changes in nystagmus after simultaneous surgery for bilateral congenital cataracts. Jpn J Ophthalmol. 1993;37(3):330–8.
31. Verbuch-Heller L, et al. A double-blind controlled study of gabapentin and baclofen as treatment for acquired nystagmus. Ann Neurol. 1997;41(6): 818–25.
32. Shery T, et al. The effects of gabapentin and memantine in acquired and congenital nystagmus – A retrospective study. Br J Ophthalmol. 2006;90(7):839–43.
33. McLean R, et al. Congenital nystagmus: randomized, controlled, double-masked trial of memantine/gabapentin. Ann Neurol. 2007;61(2):130–8.
34. Kumar A, et al. Improvement in visual acuity following surgery for correction of head posture in infantile nystagmus syndrome. J Pediatr Ophthalmol Strabismus. 2011;48:1–6.
35. Dell'osso LF, et al. Effects of topical brinzolamide on infantile nystagmus syndrome waveforms: eyedrops for nystagmus. J Neuroophthalmol Off J North Am Neuro Ophthalmol Soc. 2011;31(3):228–33.
36. Hertle RW, Dell'Osso LF. Benefits of retroequatorial four horizontal muscle recession surgery in congenital idiopathic nystagmus in adults. J AAPOS. 2007;11(3): 313–4.
37. Self J, et al. Infantile nystagmus and late onset ataxia associated with a CACNA1A mutation in the intracellular loop between s4 and s5 of domain 3. Eye. 2009;23(12):2251–5.

21 Stereopsis Outcomes in Children Treated for Congenital Cataracts

Eileen E. Birch and Anna R. O'Connor

Our eyes look at the world from two distinct viewpoints, yet we perceive a single three-dimensional environment. To perform this task, we need three essential elements: simultaneous perception, fusion, and stereopsis. Simultaneous perception allows us to see the details in both monocular images and fusion combines the slightly dissimilar images into a single percept. Stereopsis extracts data from the pair of two-dimensional retinal images by matching corresponding points, and reconstructs the third dimension by computing residual retinal disparities.

Before 1980, there was scarcely any information about when and how the brain develops the capacity for stereopsis. Initial studies at MIT and Vanderbilt University in 1979 addressed the question of when an infant was first able to demonstrate the capacity for stereopsis. The first publications of forced-choice preferential-looking data in 1980 showing the onset of stereopsis occurred at 3–4 months of age [1, 2]. This finding was confirmed with a variety of additional psychophysical, electrophysiological, and eye movement studies in a number of independent laboratories (for review, see Birch and Wang) [3]. Infants with stereopsis are not only able to discriminate binocular disparity but also appear to experience the perception of depth. They preferentially look at and track horizontally disparate targets that give rise to the perception of depth in adults, but do not track vertically disparate targets that appear diplopic to adults [1, 4]. Also, infants reach to grasp horizontally disparate targets that appear close to them but do not reach to grasp horizontally disparate targets that are far away or vertically disparate targets [5].

Following the abrupt onset of stereopsis at 3 to 4 months of age, stereoacuity maturation proceeds rapidly during the next 3–6 months (Fig. 21.1 left) [4, 6–8]. There is some evidence that sensitivity to crossed disparities may develop earlier and/or more rapidly than sensitivity to uncrossed disparities [4]. Slower continued improvement in stereoacuity continues during the next several years (Fig. 21.1 right) [9–15].

21.1 Stereoacuity Testing of Infants and Children

Two classes of tests are used to assess stereoacuity, contour tests and random- dot tests. Contour tests have the disadvantage of providing cues that enable some children with nil stereoacuity to

E.E. Birch, PhD (✉)
Crystal Charity Ball Pediatric Vision Laboratory,
Retina Foundation of the Southwest,
9600 North Central Expressway, Suite 200, Dallas,
TX, USA

Department of Ophthalmology, University of Texas
Southwestern Medical Center, Dallas, TX, USA
e-mail: ebirch@retinafoundation.org

A.R. O'Connor, PhD
Orthoptics and Vision Science, School of Health
Science, University of Liverpool, Liverpool, UK

I.C. Lloyd, S.R. Lambert (eds.), *Congenital Cataract*, DOI 10.1007/978-3-319-27848-3_21

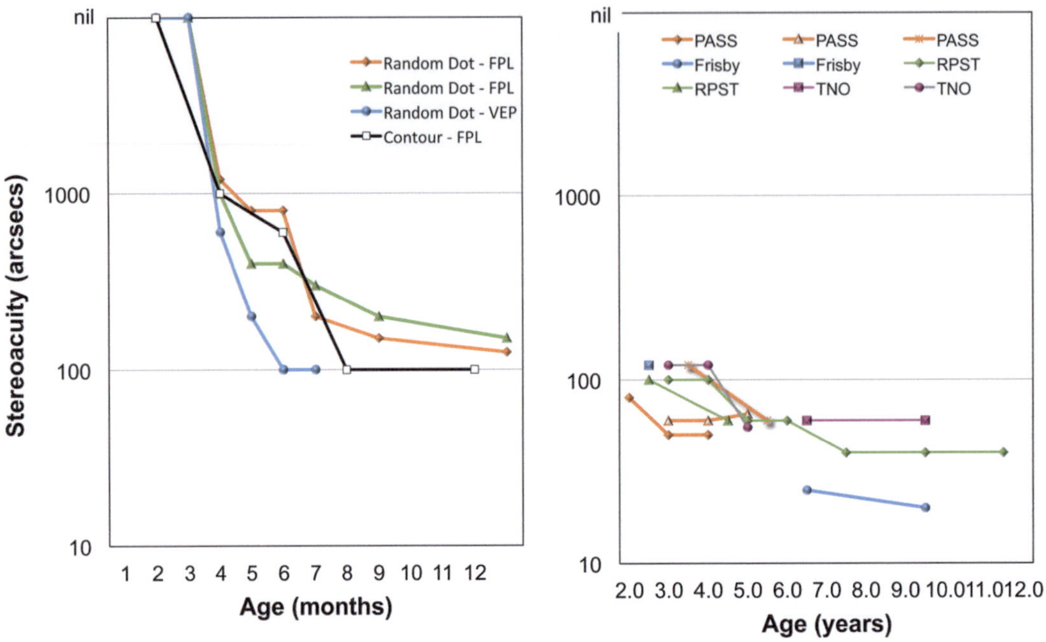

Fig. 21.1 Median random dot stereoacuity as a function of age for infants and children with normally developing vision

pass the initial 2–4 levels of the tests, typically disparities in the range >100 arcsecs [16, 17]. Large disparity contour targets be identified as different from the other targets on the basis of monocular or nonstereoscopic binocular cues [16, 17]. Most children treated for congenital cataracts will have nil or reduced stereoacuity, so it is especially important to use a random-dot format to distinguish true stereopsis from responses based on other cues in this clinical population. Random-dot tests contain no monocular or nonstereoscopic binocular cues; depth can only be appreciated via a global binocular evaluation of corresponding points and disparate points.

Most stereoacuity tests are conducted at a near viewing distance, usually at 40 cm. Because stereoacuity is sensitive to blur, it is important to optically correct for the viewing distance. It is always best to perform stereoacuity testing early in the examination, before the child's eyes are dissociated for visual acuity and ocular alignment assessments. For infants and pre-verbal children, forced-choice preferential looking tests can be performed using the PASS Stereotest ("Preschool Assessment of Stereopsis with a Smile" Stereotest; Vision Assessment Corporation, Elk Grove Village, IL, USA). The test set includes 6 vectographic random dot cards that the child can view while wearing polarized glasses. The test begins by holding the demo card with a two-dimensional smiley face side-by-side with the blank card. The child will look at and/or point to the card with the face. Once the child and tester are comfortable with the demo card, the test proceeds in the same way with the other four cards, holding them side-by-side, either to the left or the right of the blank card to determine whether the child consistently prefers to look at or point to the random dot smiley face. The four cards present four levels of stereoacuity: 440, 240, 120, and 60 arcsec. The smallest level of disparity that elicits consistent looking or pointing behavior provides an estimate of the child's stereoacuity. Normative data are summarized in Table 21.1 [9–15].

For children age 3 years and older, stereoacuity can be tested with matching and pointing tasks, and as they become more verbal, by asking them to name shapes or indicate locations. In this age range, the Randot® Preschool, TNO, and Frisby Stereoacuity tests have become widely

Table 21.1 Normative values for the most commonly used pediatric random dot stereoacuity tests

Age (y)	PASS [10]		PASS [9]		PASS [11]		Frisby [12]		Frisby [14]		RPST [13]		RPST [11]		TNO [12]		TNO [15]	
	Norm	Lower limit	Norm	Lower limit	Norm	Lower limit	Norm	Lower limit	Norm	Lower limit	Norm	Lower limit	Norm	Lower limit	Norm	Lower limit	Norm	Lower limit
0.5–0.9	300	480																
1	250	480																
2	80	240			120	480			120	480			100	400				
3	50	120	60	480							100	400					120	480
4	50	120	60	240	60	240					100	200	60	100			120	240
5			60	240							60	200					60	120
6							25	75			60	100			60	120		
7											40	60						
8																		
9							20	85			40	60			60	120		
10																		
11											40	60						
12																		

accepted standards for random-dot stereoacuity measurement. The Randot® Preschool Stereoacuity Test (Stereo Optical Co, Inc., Chicago, IL) was designed as a matching game in which the patient matches black-and-white pictures on the left side of a booklet with random-dot stereogram pictures on the right. The child wears polarizing glasses to view the stereograms. All of the stereogram pictures are age appropriate for children age 3 years and up (e.g., heart, car, duck, tree). Six levels of disparity are available in the standard set: 800, 400, 200, 100, 60, and 40 arcsecs. An optional supplemental book provides 30 and 20 arcsecs. The TNO (Lameris Ootech, Ede, Netherlands) stereoacuity test plates show discs with a missing sector and the child is asked to "point to where the piece of cake is missing." Plates V–VII are used for stereoacuity testing and present disparities of 480, 240, 120, 60, 30 and 15 arcsec. The Frisby Stereo Test (Stereotest Ltd, Sheffield, UK) presents "real depth" objects viewed with natural vision; no glasses are required. The test is comprised of 3 plastic plates of different thicknesses. Each plastic plate has four random-pattern squares printed on one side, but one of the squares has a central circle of pattern elements printed on the other side, so that it lies in a different depth plane relative to its surrounding square. The child must identify which of the four squares contains the circle. Using all three plates at varying viewing distances of 30–80 cm, it is possible to test stereoacuity in the range of 600 to 15 arcsecs. Normative data for each of these tests have been published (Table 21.1) but in some cases it is also important to ensure the normative values being used are for the correct version of the test, as variations may be present [18].

Despite the difficulties associated with interpretation of performance on the Titmus Fly, Titmus Animals, and the first 4 levels of the Titmus circles and Randot circles, results from these stereoacuity tests are commonly reported as outcomes for children treated for congenital cataracts. Passing the Titmus Fly test without stereopsis may be possible because the child knows it is a fly and expects the wings to be elevated, because the child has been repeatedly exposed to the same test with only two possible responses, or because the child alternates fixation and observes image jump in disparate portions of the test. Similarly, the location of the disparate circle in the first 4 levels of the Titmus and Randot circles and animal tests can be easily detected by ether monocular or nonstereoscopic binocular cues [16, 17]. Thus, we will include results obtained with these contour stereoacuity tests here with the caveat that stereoacuity values of 140 arcsecs or worse may be the result of artifact rather than evidence of true stereopsis.

Overall, the evidence regarding the prevalence of stereoacuity in children with congenital cataracts is necessarily limited by design characteristics of the currently available stereoacuity tests [19]. While high-grade stereoacuity is unlikely, children treated for congenital cataracts may have stereoacuity that simply is not measurable due to the limited range of disparities available. A second factor that may limit performance on current random dot stereoacuity tests is dot size; most random dot tests require visual acuity of 0.4 logMAR or better in order to be able to appreciate the dot texture sufficiently to extract disparity information. In addition, the clinical tests consist of relatively small images that are static; there is some evidence to suggest that larger, dynamic stimuli provide additional information that may allow children who appear to have nil stereoacuity on standardized tests to appreciate depth [20, 21].

21.2 Visual Deprivation and the Critical Period for Binocular Vision

The sudden post-natal onset of stereopsis exhibited by infants at 3 months of age corresponds to the start of a critical period, during which binocular function can be severely and permanently disrupted by abnormal visual experience. This maturational time course is consistent with a model of visual development that posits a precritical period, guided by genetically programmed molecular and neuronal signals, and a critical period during which environmental signals maintain and refine the neuronal circuitry for stereopsis. This model grew from Hubel and Wiesel's series of simple but elegant experiments in which they showed that closing one eye during early visual development permanently altered the structure of the columnar structure of the visual cortex, shifting the ocular dominance of cortical cells to the non-deprived eye [22, 23]. They hypothesized that visual experience guides the development of ocular dominance columns during a critical period shortly, but not immediately, after birth. During this period of experience-dependent maturation, neuronal connectivity and function is highly susceptible to disruption by visual deprivation.

However, this simple model of the critical period is incomplete. Cortical ocular dominance columns form very early, with at least a proto-map present prenatally [24, 25]. The development of neural circuitry in the primary visual cortex to support topographic maps and orientation selectivity is not dependent on visual experience, but is instead guided by molecular signaling and spontaneous neural activity. However, during the critical period, visual experience guides further refinement of the selective properties of striate neurons to harmonize inputs from the two eyes (Fig. 21.2). Prior to the critical period, striate neurons are commonly selective for different orientations when driven by the left versus the right eye [26, 27]. With normal visual experience during the critical period, striate neurons gradually shift their tuning to respond maximally to the same orientation regardless of which eye is viewing. Monocular or binocular visual deprivation during the critical period disrupts this developmental matching process and results in persistent mismatch and loss of binocular excitatory neurons [26, 27].

Classically, the critical period for ocular dominance plasticity has been considered to end at the onset of adolescence [28, 29]. More recent evidence suggests that sensitivity to visual deprivation actually diminishes very slowly and persists beyond adolescence, as does the potential for rehabilitation [30, 31] and is present even in adult striate cortex [32]. The diminishing potential for rehabilitation is reflected in studies that demonstrate a need for longer, more intense treatment and less stability of the gains in visual function obtained with treatment. It has been proposed that the increase in inhibitory cortical function that is a

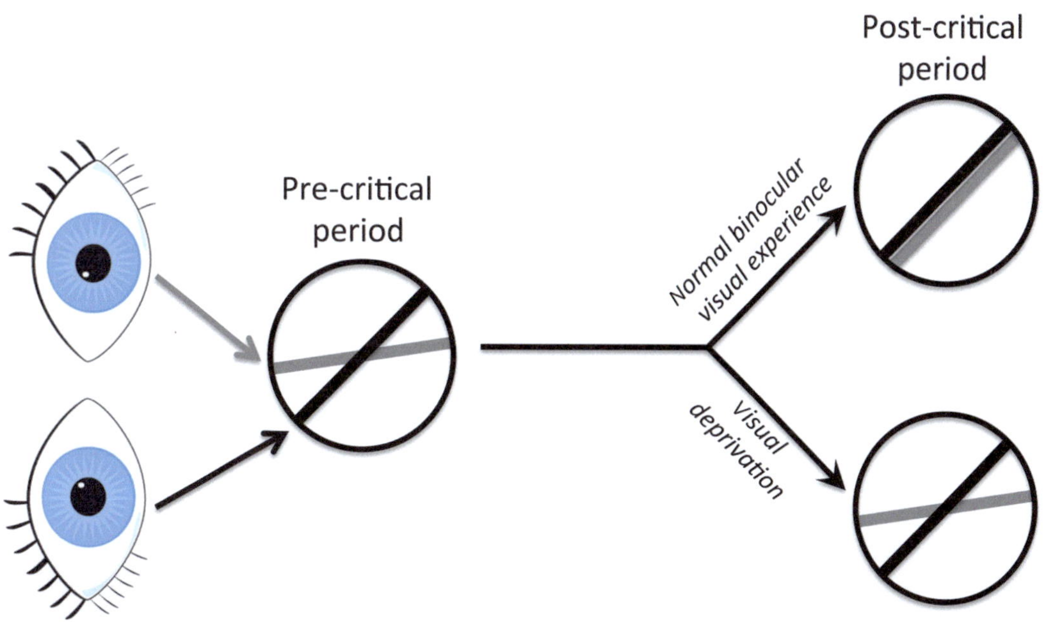

Fig. 21.2 Visual experience dependent refinement of orientation selectivity) harmonizes preferred orientation of the two eyes' inputs to binocular neurons in the striate cortex (V1) during the critical period. Visual deprivation during the critical period blocks binocular matching permanently

pronounced characteristic of the critical period [26] may also result in maturation of structural factors that restrict remodeling of circuits and promote closure of the critical period [33].

21.3 Stereoacuity Outcomes Following Congenital Cataract Extraction

The key role of surgery during the first weeks of life to minimize the effects of visual deprivation due to congenital cataract on visual acuity development is well established (for review, see Birch and O'Connor [34]). As good visual acuity is a prerequisite for high-grade stereoacuity, it is a reasonable assumption that for a good stereoacuity outcome, early surgery is essential. However, like visual acuity, stereoacuity outcome is dependent on multiple factors, not just the timing of cataract extraction. These factors include the laterality of the cataract, treatment modalities, and post-surgical complications.

Unilateral congenital cataract presents multiple barriers to the development of stereoacuity that may be present, both prior to cataract extraction and post-extraction. Prior to extraction, a unilateral cataract deprives the developing visual system of an important excitatory stimulus and also results in a severe imbalance in developing suppressive interocular interactions. Early surgery (≤8 weeks of age) is known to minimize the impact of deprivation and suppression on the development of visual acuity and appears to be of some benefit for stereoacuity development as well. Thus, children who are able to achieve visual acuity outcomes of 0.6 logMAR or better (20/80 or better) are much more likely to pass the various stereoacuity tests than those with visual acuity outcomes worse than 0.6 logMAR (20/100 or worse) (Table 21.2) [35–46].

In congenital unilateral cataract, optical correction after extraction is most commonly accomplished with a contact lens or intraocular lens (IOL). From the perspective of the development of stereoacuity, an IOL may provide improved optical quality, as it is consistently in place and may produce less aniseikonia. With these potential advantages, we might expect that use of IOLs for optical correction would result in higher rates of stereoacuity or better stereoacuity. However, while there is some variation in results depending on which stereoacuity test or combination of tests was used to assess outcome, overall stereoacuity outcomes with IOLs and contact lenses appear similar (Table 21.2) [35–39, 41–46, 48].

Post-extraction, the stimulus deprivation amblyopia that results from unilateral congenital cataract requires treatment, primarily by occlusion therapy, which may create a barrier to the development of binocular vision. The negative impact of occlusion therapy on binocular visual development appears to be greatest with intensive occlusion during the early months, where there is normally rapid stereoacuity development. The challenge is to ensure that occlusion therapy is sufficient to optimize visual acuity development of the formerly deprived eye but not at the expense of binocular vision. Progressive occlusion regimes are now widely used, with the number of hours of occlusion determined by the age of the child in the early months (typically 1 h of occlusion per month of life up to a maximum of 6 h per day or 50 % of waking hours). Several studies suggest that the reduced number of hours of occlusion during the first few months following cataract extraction are beneficial for the development of stereoacuity but, overall, the evidence is inconclusive (Table 21.2) [35, 37–40, 42, 45, 47].

Stereoacuity outcomes for children treated for bilateral congenital cataracts are generally similar to those for children treated for unilateral congenital cataracts. Children who have early surgery and better visual acuity outcomes are much more likely to demonstrate stereoacuity than children who have surgery >8 weeks of age [43, 44, 51–54] or those who have visual acuity outcomes of 20/100 or worse (Table 21.2) [41, 50–53].

21.4 Why Do Stereoacuity Outcomes Matter?

Due to significant visual deprivation during a critical period in visual development, high-grade stereoacuity may not be a realistic goal following

Table 21.2 Stereoacuity outcomes in children treated for congenital cataracts

	Titmus fly	Animals/circles	PRST/TNO/Frisby	Other or multiple tests
Unilateral				
VA ≤0.6 logMAR	10/14 (71 %) [37, 40, 46]	11/19 (58 %) [37, 38, 40, 41]		1/20 (5 %) [35]
VA >0.6 logMAR	1/15 (7 %) [37, 40, 46]	1/27 (4 %) [37, 40, 41]		0/42 (0 %) [35]
Surgery ≤8 weeks	14/32 (44 %) [37, 40, 45]	12/33 (36 %) [36–38, 41, 45]		28/121 (23 %) [35, 39, 42]
Surgery >8 weeks	3/10 (30 %) [37, 46]	2/41 (5 %) [36, 37, 41, 44]		10/99 (10 %) [35, 39, 43]
Intraocular lens	14/62 (23 %) [39, 46]	1/22 (5 %) [41]	7/59 (12 %) [39, 47]	12/21 (57 %) [43, 48]
Contact lens	16/66 (24 %) [37, 39, 45]	13/41 (32 %) [36–38, 45]	12/101 (12 %) [39, 47]	21/146 (14 %) [35, 42, 43, 48]
Intensive occlusion	5/10 (50 %) [40]	5/24 (21 %) [40, 47]		4/33 (12 %) [42, 49]
50 % or progressive occlusion	32/135 (23 %) [37, 39, 45]	10/27 (37 %) [37, 38, 45]		18/178 (10 %) [35, 39, 42]
Bilateral				
VA ≤0.6 logMAR		8/19 (42 %) [41, 50]		10/37 (27 %) [51–53]
VA >0.6 logMAR		1/36 (3 %) [41, 50]		0/14 (0 %) [51, 52]
Surgery ≤8 weeks		8/28 (29 %) [41, 51]		15/46 (33 %) [51–53]
Surgery >8 weeks		2/64 (3 %) [41, 44, 51]		3/89 (3 %) [43, 51, 52, 54]

congenital cataract extraction. Nonetheless, the achievement of subnormal stereoacuity may have real benefits to the child. Experimental data clearly establishes a relationship between accurate prehension and stereoacuity. Studies evaluating the kinematics of reaching and grasping (including speed, accuracy, grip aperture and changes over time) demonstrate that removal of disparity cues by occluding or defocusing one eye of a normal control observer significantly impacts performance [55–60]. When forced to rely on monocular cues alone, normal control observers, make more errors in velocity (young children tend to overshoot their targets and older children undershoot) and more errors in spatial path planning [56].

These experimental findings in normal controls with short-term simulated loss of stereoscopic cues are also evident in patients with reduced and nil stereoacuity, where stereodeficits are associated with poorer performance of functional skills, both in real world tasks and utilizing 3D displays [61]. These deficits are apparent even at a young age, where children with nil stereoacuity lag in achievement of sensorimotor developmental milestones during infancy, compared with infants who have stereopsis [62]. At an older age, when a child's motor capabilities are greater, the benefits of having stereoacuity extend to a range of motor skill tasks. Children with stereoacuity do a better job of threading beads, catching balls, and completing a battery of timed manual dexterity tasks (sorting, drawing, placing pegs, etc.) [63–65]. While motor skill tasks generally can be completed using only monocular cues, the presence of stereoacuity improves accuracy. The best (quickest/most accurate) motor responses are associated with high-grade stereoacuity, but those with reduced stereoacuity consistently perform better than those with nil stereoacuity.

As shown in Table 21.3, there is some variation in the impact of nil stereoacuity on task performance among different types of tasks [63–67]. Tasks with proprioceptive feedback are easier to complete using only monocular cues than those without [68], and increasing the task difficulty (e.g., by reducing the target size or increasing the complexity of the motion path required) results in larger deficits [64].

In the studies presented in Table 21.3, the studies of normal control observers with one eye occluded or defocused as a surrogate for nil stereoacuity facilitates the evaluation of disparity cues and allows for a within-subjects comparison of normal versus nil stereoacuity performance. However, this approach eliminates more than the binocular disparity cue; it removes other nonstereoscopic binocular information, reduces the visual field, and does not allow time for adaptation to the lack of binocularity. The study of subjects with reduced or absent stereoacuity (primarily due to strabismus) has demonstrated that some degree of adaptation does occur, as those with a long-term stereodeficits on average have better fine motor skill performance compared to monocularly occluded normal controls [64]. While this may suggest a linear relationship between stereoacuity and motor skill performance, in fact there are data to suggest that reduced stereoacuity results in slightly impaired in performance, whereas nil stereoacuity results in a large decline in fine motor skills [70].

Gait may also be affected by stereoacuity; reduced stereoacuity is associated with a more hesitant penultimate step and higher toe clearance when walking among obstacles, suggesting a more careful strategy for obstacle avoidance [71]. Additionally, there is evidence to suggest that monocular cues potentially are sufficient to localize ground level but stereoacuity is necessary to localize heights of steps and obstacles above ground level [72].

In addition to the improvements in functional skills, there is also the potential benefit of requiring less ophthalmological intervention, where the presence of stereoacuity results in better long-term stability of eye alignment, preventing the development of constant strabismus [37, 42]. While the rates of strabismus are high in the congenital cataract population, with multiple reports demonstrating rates of >50% [73–75], the presence of strabismus does not preclude the presence of ste-

Table 21.3 Stereoacuity and fine motor skills

	Outcome measure	Normal stereoacuity	Reduced stereoacuity	Nil stereoacuity	Monocular occlusion (short-term)
Threading beads [64] mean ± SD	Time to thread 30 large beads (s)	48.87 ± 4.93	52.45 ± 4.72	57.62 ± 7.14	64.83 ± 11.0
	Time to thread 22 small beads (s)	57.7 ± 8.49	61.36 ± 6.88	72.02 ± 9.51	79.4 ± 15.47
Buzz wire task [66, 67] mean ± SD	Time (s)	42.5 ± 12.4		61.7 ± 9.9	55.3 ± 11.1
	Errors (number)	6.75 ± 4.37	12.4 ± 13.9	40.8 ± 15.4	
Fine motor skills score [65] mean ± SD	Age-standardized scaled scores	40.32 ± 1.00	34.81 ± 1.39	35.82 ± 1.02	
Catching a ball [63] mean ± SD	% Successful catches at 14.6 m/s	83.3 ± 14.6	54.1 ± 28.7	45.1 ± 24.8	
Surgical task: EYESi simulator [69] Median (quartiles)	Pea-on-a-peg (number placed)	12.12 ± 1.64		9.09 ± 1.9 (LT)	9.9 ± 2.4
	Score out of 60 (higher = more accurate)	Task 1: 51.0 (33.0, 59.0) Task 3: 31.0 (8.0, 47.0)	Task 1: 6.0 (0.0, 33.0) Task 3: 0.0 (0.0, 0.0)		
Reach to grasp common household items [56]	Error rate (velocity & path)	0.43 ± 0.03	0.43 ± 0.03	0.80 ± 0.04	0.70 ± 0.04

reoacuity, as the strabismus may be intermittent or a sufficiently small angle to facilitate the development of some stereoacuity. Preserving stereoacuity, and in turn maintaining good eye alignment, therefore has the additional benefit of improved levels of health related quality of life. There is a wealth of evidence demonstrating that strabismus that is noticeable is associated with lower levels of health related quality of life [76, 77], impacting on many facets such as self- image, self-confidence, employment opportunities and satisfaction in interpersonal relationships.

In addition to the risk of developing strabismus, any interference with the development of stereopsis also may result in the onset of nystagmus [78–81]. Two recent longitudinal studies of children treated for congenital or infantile cataracts that included eye movement recording reported that 71 % developed nystagmus [78, 82]. Congenital or infantile onset cataracts and duration of visual deprivation that exceeded 6 weeks were significant risk factors for strabismus and nystagmus [78]. Monocular versus binocular visual deprivation was a significant risk factor only for asymmetric severity of nystagmus [78]. Thus, the development of stereopsis also plays a critical role in fixation stability and maintenance of accurate alignment of the visual axes.

21.5 Summary

Visual deprivation due to congenital cataracts significantly disrupts binocular cortical development during a critical period of maturation, typically resulting in reduced or nil stereoacuity. Early treatment and visual rehabilitation are crucial for the development of stereoacuity. Even the attainment of reduced rather than nil stereoacuity can afford a range of advantages, including better fine motor skills, more confident gait while walking, and reduced risk for strabismus and nystagmus.

References

1. Fox R, Aslin RN, Shea SL, Dumais ST. Stereopsis in human infants. Science. 1980;207(4428):323–4.
2. Held R, Birch E, Gwiazda J. Stereoacuity of human infants. Proc Natl Acad Sci U S A. 1980;77(9):5572–4.
3. Birch EE, Wang J. Stereoacuity outcomes after treatment of infantile and accommodative esotropia. Optom Vis Sci (Official Publication of the American Academy of Optometry). 2009;86(6):647–52.
4. Birch EE, Gwiazda J, Held R. Stereoacuity development for crossed and uncrossed disparities in human infants. Vision Res. 1982;22(5):507–13.
5. Granrud CE. Binocular vision and spatial perception in 4- and 5-month-old infants. J Exp Psychol Hum Percept Perform. 1986;12(1):36–49.
6. Birch E, Petrig B. FPL and VEP measures of fusion, stereopsis and stereoacuity in normal infants. Vision Res. 1996;36(9):1321–7.
7. Birch EE, Morale SE, Jeffrey BG, O'Connor AR, Fawcett SL. Measurement of stereoacuity outcomes at ages 1 to 24 months: Randot Stereocards. J AAPOS. 2005;9(1):31–6.
8. Birch EE, Salomao S. Infant random dot stereoacuity cards. J Pediatr Ophthalmol Strabismus. 1998;35(2):86–90.
9. Ciner EB, Ying GS, Kulp MT, et al. Stereoacuity of preschool children with and without vision disorders. Optom Vis Sci. 2014;91(3):351–8.
10. Ciner EB, Schanel-Klitsch E, Herzberg C. Stereoacuity development: 6 months to 5 years. A new tool for testing and screening. Optom Vis Sci. 1996;73(1):43–8.
11. Afsari S, Rose KA, Pai AS, et al. Diagnostic reliability and normative values of stereoacuity tests in preschool-aged children. Br J Ophthalmol. 2013;97(3):308–13.
12. Anketell PM, Saunders KJ, Little JA. Stereoacuity norms for school-age children using the Frisby stereotest. J AAPOS (The Official Publication of the American Association for Pediatric Ophthalmology and Strabismus/American Association for Pediatric Ophthalmology and Strabismus). 2013;17(6):582–7.
13. Birch E, Williams C, Drover J, et al. Randot Preschool Stereoacuity Test: normative data and validity. J AAPOS. 2008;12(1):23–6.
14. Saunders KJ, Woodhouse JM, Westall CA. The modified frisby stereotest. J Pediatr Ophthalmol Strabismus. 1996;33(6):323–7.
15. Simons K. A comparison of the Frisby, Random-Dot E, TNO, and Randot circles stereotests in screening and office use. Arch Ophthalmol. 1981;99(3):446–52.
16. Fawcett SL, Birch EE. Validity of the Titmus and Randot circles tasks in children with known binocular vision disorders. J AAPOS. 2003;7(5):333–8.
17. Leske DA, Holmes JM. Maximum angle of horizontal strabismus consistent with true stereopsis. J AAPOS. 2004;8(1):28–34.
18. van Doorn LL, Evans BJ, Edgar DF, Fortuin MF. Manufacturer changes lead to clinically important differences between two editions of the TNO stereotest. Ophthalmic Physiol Opt. 2014;34(2):243–9.
19. Read JC. Stereo vision and strabismus. Eye (Lond). 2015;29(2):214–24.

20. Mollenhauer KA, Haase W. Preliminary report: dynamic stereopsis in patients with impaired binocular function. Strabismus. 2000;8(4):275–81.
21. Tidbury LP, Black RH, O'Connor AR. Perceiving 3D in the absence of measurable stereo-acuity. Br Ir Orthopt J. 2014;11:34–8.
22. Hubel DH. Exploration of the primary visual cortex, 1955–78. Nature. 1982;299(5883):515–24.
23. Wiesel TN. Postnatal development of the visual cortex and the influence of environment. Nature. 1982;299(5884):583–91.
24. Horton JC, Hocking DR. An adult-like pattern of ocular dominance columns in striate cortex of newborn monkeys prior to visual experience. J Neurosci (The Official Journal of the Society for Neuroscience). 1996;16(5):1791–807.
25. Rakic P. Prenatal genesis of connections subserving ocular dominance in the rhesus monkey. Nature. 1976;261(5560):467–71.
26. Tao X, Zhang B, Shen G, et al. Early monocular defocus disrupts the normal development of receptive-field structure in V2 neurons of macaque monkeys. J Neurosci (The Official Journal of the Society for Neuroscience). 2014;34(41):13840–54.
27. Wang BS, Sarnaik R, Cang J. Critical period plasticity matches binocular orientation preference in the visual cortex. Neuron. 2010;65(2):246–56.
28. Hubel DH, Wiesel TN, LeVay S. Plasticity of ocular dominance columns in monkey striate cortex. Philos Trans R Soc Lond B Biol Sci. 1977;278(961): 377–409.
29. LeVay S, Wiesel TN, Hubel DH. The development of ocular dominance columns in normal and visually deprived monkeys. J Comp Neurol. 1980;191(1): 1–51.
30. Daw NW, Fox K, Sato H, Czepita D. Critical period for monocular deprivation in the cat visual cortex. J Neurophysiol. 1992;67(1):197–202.
31. Guire ES, Lickey ME, Gordon B. Critical period for the monocular deprivation effect in rats: assessment with sweep visually evoked potentials. J Neurophysiol. 1999;81(1):121–8.
32. Gilbert CD, Li W. Adult visual cortical plasticity. Neuron. 2012;75(2):250–64.
33. Espinosa JS, Stryker MP. Development and plasticity of the primary visual cortex. Neuron. 2012;75(2): 230–49.
34. Birch EE, O'Connor AR. Critical periods for visual development and the timing of congenital cataract surgery. In: Wilson ME, Trivedi RH, editors. Pediatric cataract surgery. Techniques, complications and management. 2nd ed. Philadelphia: Lippincott, Williams and Wilkins; 2014. p. 48–54.
35. Allen RJ, Speedwell L, Russell-Eggitt I. Long-term visual outcome after extraction of unilateral congenital cataracts. Eye (Lond). 2010;24(7):1263–7.
36. Birch EE, Swanson WH, Stager DR, Woody M, Everett M. Outcome after very early treatment of dense congenital unilateral cataract. Invest Ophthalmol Vis Sci. 1993;34(13):3687–99.
37. Brown SM, Archer S, Del Monte MA. Stereopsis and binocular vision after surgery for unilateral infantile cataract. J AAPOS. 1999;3(2):109–13.
38. Gregg FM, Parks MM. Stereopsis after congenital monocular cataract extraction. Am J Ophthalmol. 1992;114(3):314–7.
39. Hartmann EE, Stout AU, Lynn MJ, Yen KG, Kruger SJ, Lambert SR. Stereopsis results at 4.5 years of age in the infant aphakia treatment study. Am J Ophthalmol. 2015;159(1):64–70.e1–2.
40. Hosal BM, Biglan AW, Elhan AH. High levels of binocular function are achievable after removal of monocular cataracts in children before 8 years of age. Ophthalmology. 2000;107(9):1647–55.
41. Hussin HM, Markham R. Long-term visual function outcomes of congenital cataract surgery with intraocular lens implantation in children under 5 years of age. Eur J Ophthalmol. 2009;19(5):754–61.
42. Jeffrey BG, Birch EE, Stager Jr DR, Stager Sr DR, Weakley Jr DR. Early binocular visual experience may improve binocular sensory outcomes in children after surgery for congenital unilateral cataract. J AAPOS. 2001;5(4):209–16.
43. Lesueur L. Visual outcome after paediatric cataract surgery; is age a major factor? Br J Ophthalmol. 1998; 82:1022–5.
44. Merino P. Strabismus and congenital cataracts. Arch Soc Esp Oftalmol. 2007;82:623–8.
45. Wright KW, Matsumoto E, Edelman PM. Binocular fusion and stereopsis associated with early surgery for monocular congenital cataracts. Arch Ophthalmol. 1992;110(11):1607–9.
46. Zubcov AA, Stahl E, Rossillion B, et al. Stereopsis after primary in-the-bag posterior chamber implantation in children. J AAPOS. 1999;3(4):227–33.
47. Birch EE, Cheng C, Stager Jr DR, Felius J. Visual acuity development after the implantation of unilateral intraocular lenses in infants and young children. J AAPOS (The Official Publication of the American Association for Pediatric Ophthalmology and Strabismus/American Association for Pediatric Ophthalmology and Strabismus). 2005;9(6):527–32.
48. Ondráček O, Lokaj M. Visual outcome after congenital cataract surgery, long- term clinical results. Scripta Medica (BRNO). 2003;76(2):95–102.
49. Pratt-Johnson JA, Tillson G. Unilateral congenital cataract: binocular status after treatment. J Pediatr Ophthalmol Strabismus. 1989;26(2):72–5.
50. Kim DH, Kim JH, Kim SJ, Yu YS. Long-term results of bilateral congenital cataract treated with early cataract surgery, aphakic glasses and secondary IOL implantation. Acta Ophthalmol. 2012;90(3):231–6.
51. Bradford GM, Keech RV, Scott WE. Factors affecting visual outcome after surgery for bilateral congenital cataracts. Am J Ophthalmol. 1994;117(1):58–64.
52. Lundvall A, Kugelberg U. Outcome after treatment of congenital bilateral cataract. Acta Ophthalmol Scand. 2002;80(6):593–7.
53. Nishina S. Stereopsis after early surgery for bilateral congenital cataracts. Transactions of the XIth

International Strabismological Association; 2010, p. 282–6.
54. Ye HH, Deng DM, Qian YY, Lin Z, Chen WR. Long-term visual outcome of dense bilateral congenital cataract. Chin Med J (Engl). 2007;120(17):1494–7.
55. Gnanaseelan R, Gonzalez DA, Niechwiej-Szwedo E. Binocular advantage for prehension movements performed in visually enriched environments requiring visual search. Front Hum Neurosci. 2014;8:959.
56. Grant S, Suttle C, Melmoth DR, Conway ML, Sloper JJ. Age- and stereovision- dependent eye-hand coordination deficits in children with amblyopia and abnormal binocularity. Invest Ophthalmol Vis Sci. 2014;55(9):5687–57015.
57. Keefe BD, Watt SJ. The role of binocular vision in grasping: a small stimulus- set distorts results. Exp Brain Res. 2009;194(3):435–44.
58. Melmoth DR, Finlay AL, Morgan MJ, Grant S. Grasping deficits and adaptations in adults with stereo vision losses. Invest Ophthalmol Vis Sci. 2009;50(8):3711–20.
59. Melmoth DR, Grant S. Advantages of binocular vision for the control of reaching and grasping. Exp Brain Res. 2006;171(3):371–88.
60. Watt SJ, Bradshaw MF. Binocular cues are important in controlling the grasp but not the reach in natural prehension movements. Neuropsychologia. 2000;38(11):1473–81.
61. McIntire JP, Wright ST, Harrington LK, Havig PR, Watamaniuk SNJ, Hefta EL. Optometric measurements predict performance but not comfort on a virtual object placement task with a stereoscopic three-dimensional display. Opt Eng. 2014;53(6): 061711-061711-061718.
62. Drover JR, Stager Sr DR, Morale SE, Leffler JN, Birch EE. Improvement in motor development following surgery for infantile esotropia. J AAPOS. 2008;12(2):136–40.
63. Mazyn LI, Lenoir M, Montagne G, Savelsbergh GJ. The contribution of stereo vision to one-handed catching. Exp Brain Res. 2004;157(3):383–90.
64. O'Connor AR, Birch EE, Anderson S, Draper H. The functional significance of stereopsis. Invest Ophthalmol Vis Sci. 2010;51(4):2019–23.
65. Webber AL, Wood JM, Gole GA, Brown B. The effect of amblyopia on fine motor skills in children. Invest Ophthalmol Vis Sci. 2008;49(2):594–603.
66. Joy S, Davis H, Buckley D. Is stereopsis linked to hand-eye coordination? Br Orthopt J. 2001;58:38–41.
67. Murdoch JR, McGhee CN, Glvoer V. The relationship between stereopsis and fine manual dexterity: pilot study of a new instrument. Eye. 1991;5(5):642–3.
68. Read JC, Begum SF, McDonald A, Trowbridge J. The binocular advantage in visuomotor tasks involving tools. Iperception. 2013;4(2):101–10.
69. Sachdeva R, Traboulsi EI. Performance of patients with deficient stereoacuity on the EYESi microsurgical simulator. Am J Ophthalmol. 2011;151(3):427–33. e421.
70. Piano ME, O'Connor AR. The effect of degrading binocular single vision on fine visuomotor skill task performance. Invest Ophthalmol Vis Sci. 2013;54(13):8204–13.
71. Buckley JG, Panesar GK, MacLellan MJ, Pacey IE, Barrett BT. Changes to control of adaptive gait in individuals with long-standing reduced stereoacuity. Invest Ophthalmol Vis Sci. 2010;51(5):2487–95.
72. Ooi TL, He ZJ. Space perception of strabismic observers in the real world environment. Invest Ophthalmol Vis Sci. 2015;56(3):1761–8.
73. Demirkilinc Biler E, Bozbiyik DI, Uretmen O, Kose S. Strabismus in infants following congenital cataract surgery. Graefes Arch Clin Exp Ophthalmol. 2015; 253(10):1801–7.
74. Tartarella MB, Britez-Colombi GF, Milhomem S, Lopes MC, Fortes Filho JB. Pediatric cataracts: clinical aspects, frequency of strabismus and chronological, etiological, and morphological features. Arq Bras Oftalmol. 2014;77(3):143–7.
75. Lambert SR, Lynn M, Drews-Botsch C, et al. A comparison of grating visual acuity, strabismus, and reoperation outcomes among children with aphakia and pseudophakia after unilateral cataract surgery during the first six months of life. J AAPOS. 2001;5(2): 70–5.
76. McBain HB, Au CK, Hancox J, et al. The impact of strabismus on quality of life in adults with and without diplopia: a systematic review. Surv Ophthalmol. 2014;59(2):185–91.
77. Durnian JM, Noonan CP, Marsh IB. The psychosocial effects of adult strabismus: a review. Br J Ophthalmol. 2011;95(4):450–3.
78. Birch EE, Wang J, Felius J, Stager Jr DR, Hertle RW. Fixation control and eye alignment in children treated for dense congenital or developmental cataracts. J AAPOS. 2012;16(2):156–60.
79. Tusa RJ, Mustari MJ, Burrows AF, Fuchs AF. Gaze-stabilizing deficits and latent nystagmus in monkeys with brief, early-onset visual deprivation: eye movement recordings. J Neurophysiol. 2001;86(2):651–61.
80. Tychsen L, Richards M, Wong A, Foeller P, Bradley D, Burkhalter A. The neural mechanism for Latent (fusion maldevelopment) nystagmus. J Neuroophthalmol (The Official Journal of the North American Neuro-Ophthalmology Society). 2010;30(3):276–83.
81. Felius J, Busettini C, Lynn MJ, Hartmann EE, Lambert SR. Nystagmus and related fixation instabilities following extraction of unilateral infantile cataract in the Infant Aphakia Treatment Study (IATS). Invest Ophthalmol Vis Sci. 2014;55(8):5332–7.
82. Abadi RV, Forster JE, Lloyd IC. Ocular motor outcomes after bilateral and unilateral infantile cataracts. Vision Res. 2006;46(6–7):940–52.

MIX
Papier aus verantwortungsvollen Quellen
Paper from responsible sources
FSC® C105338

If you have any concerns about our products,
you can contact us on
ProductSafety@springernature.com

In case Publisher is established outside the EU,
the EU authorized representative is:
Springer Nature Customer Service Center GmbH
Europaplatz 3, 69115 Heidelberg, Germany

Printed by Libri Plureos GmbH
in Hamburg, Germany